AGELESS

*What Every Woman
Needs to Know
to Look Good
and Feel Great*

ALSO BY ELAINE BRUMBERG

Take Care of Your Skin
Save Your Money, Save Your Face

AGE*LESS*

*What Every Woman Needs
to Know to Look Good
and Feel Great*

ELAINE BRUMBERG

HarperCollins*Publishers*

DISCLAIMER

The information contained in this book represents the author's attempt to consolidate complex, detailed information into practical suggestions for consumers and represents the author's best-efforts research.

The author's opinions are expressed in an effort to provide helpful guidance to consumers. However, each individual has different needs concerning cosmetics, skin care, hair care, nutrition, exercise, and medical advice. Nothing in this book should be interpreted as a substitute for the care and guidance of a qualified medical professional.

The author has recommended products throughout this book based upon personal preference, independent product sampling, and the advice of relevant professionals. These recommendations were not based upon independent comparative research and represent the author's opinion only. The author assumes no responsibility or liability for products that do not perform as expected.

All price ranges given in this book are approximate and as manufacturers change formulations frequently to assure accurate information, consumers should contact the manufacturer directly. All products listed in this book, to the best of the author's knowledge, are trademarks.

HarperCollins books may be purchased for educational, business, or sales promotional use. For information, please write to: Special Markets Department, HarperCollins Publishers, Inc., 10 East 53rd Street, New York, New York 10022.

FIRST EDITION

Designed by Laura Lindgren

Library of Congress Cataloging-in-Publication Data
    Brumberg, Elaine.
    Ageless : what every woman needs to know to look good and feel great / Elaine
Brumberg. — 1st ed.
        Includes index.
        ISBN 0-06-270159-2
    1. Middle aged women—Health and hygiene. 2. Aged women—Health and hygiene. 3. Beauty, Personal. I. Title.
    RA778.B925 1997   96-52182
    613'.04244—dc21   CIP

97 98 99 00 ❖/RRD 10 9 8 7 6 5 4 3 2 1

This book is lovingly dedicated to my husband, Norman, who had to share his home and my time and attention with a mountain of cosmetics; and to our children, Harriet Brumberg & Robert Kramer, Bruce Brumberg & Karen Axelrod, Amy & Mark Seiden, and Scott Dimetrosky, as well as our five beautiful grandchildren, Ilyse Beth Kramer, Laurel Paige Kramer, Benjamin Ethan Seiden, Hilary Dana Brumberg, and Lindsay Hannah Seiden.

To the memory of my mother-in-law, Dorothy Brumberg, who loved me and treated me like her own.

CONTENTS

ACKNOWLEDGMENTS

Every book is the product of many months of hard work, most of which is not done alone. This book, in particular, because of the many and varied topics and products that are included, required the cooperation, skill, and patience of hundreds of people to whom I am indebted. Julia Coopersmith is truly this book's godmother. When I was insisting on writing a menopause book, Julia convinced me to expand the focus. I was instantly successful in finding a home for my idea with Linda Cunningham at HarperCollins, who had the foresight to see that this was a book mature women would want to read. Beth D'Addono has a talent for bringing people together. Some call it networking, she calls it connecting — and I am thankful to Beth for her connections. The most important person I want to thank is my friend Lauralee Dobbins. Her research, organization, talent, and hard work made this book possible.

Thanks also go to my agent, Diana Finch, from the Ellen Levine Literary Agency, and to the many people at HarperCollins, my editor Tricia Medved, Rose Carrano, Joana Jebson, Patty Leisure, who answered my relentless questions, and Joseph Montebello for his elegant book design.

Many, many professionals gave generously of their time and expertise, supporting my efforts well beyond the call of duty or even self-promotion. Chief among them have been Dr. Toby Shawe, Gary Grove, Ph.D. of the KGL Skin Study Center in Broomall, Pennsylvania, Barbara Greene of NeoStrata, Joyce Ayoub of the Skin Cancer Foundation, and my trainer Karen Lane.

Jack Shalita, Fred Cohen, and Jack Meehan from Beth Ayres Pharmacy answered more questions than any of us care to remember. Kathleen Ferguson of Barnes and Noble in Jenkintown, Pennsylvania, spent hours helping me sift through cookbooks. Thanks to you, too.

Dozens of physicians and other professionals around the country, after long days with patients and clients, spent their evenings giving interviews that made this book more complete. I want to thank: Rosario Acquista, Mari Aldin, Denise Austin, Dr. Wilma Bergfeld, Dr. Steven Bloch, Dr. Walter Bortz, Dr. Betty Broder, Bobbi Brown, Marlene Cahill, Dr. Alastair Carruthers, Dr. Gustave Colon, Dr. H. James Day, Dr. Dale DeVore, Dr. Zoe Draelos, Dr. Melvin Elson, Laura Geller, Dr. Ross Goldstein, Ellen Goodman, Dr. Charles Gudas, Matthew Gurrola, Dr. Teg Hager, Dr. Neal Handel, Ilana Harkavi, Linda Hellings, Dr. Steven Hernandez, Dr. Barnett Johnson, Phillip Kingsley, Dr. Henry Kowamoto, Helen Lee, Dr. Robert Leonard, Muggs Lerberg, Dr. Thomas Loeb, Jan Marini, Dr. James McGuire, Megan McLellan, Dr. Lorraine Meisner, Beth Minardi, Dr. Mark Mitchnick, Dr. Gary Monheit, Dr. Warwick Morison, Dr. Ferdinand Ofodile, Dianne Osborne, Janet Paolucci, Janice Pastorek, Dr. Nicholas Perricone, Dr. Doren Pinnell, Dr. Sheldon Pinnell, Francine Porter, Tina Potter, Dr. Thomas Rohrer, Dr. Thomas Romo III, Jill Ross, Dr. Larry Rotenberg, Betsy Rubenstone, Dr. Aaron Shapiro, Dr. John Skouge, Dr. Mark Solomon, Dr. Sheldon Solomon, Cheryl Stuart, Joyce Vedral, Marie Ward, Lynda Farrington Wilson.

It is the job of public relations professionals to provide people like me with products and information. Too often, those departments, agencies, and individuals go unthanked and unrecognized for the work they do to make projects like this possible. I'd love to name them all individually, but the list would be as long as the book — so thank you one and all for sending products, information, and most of all, well-wishes.

Countless women, many of whom I had never met before, volunteered to sample the products sent by the public relations people. I thank them for being brave enough to try something new and for caring enough about someone else's pet project to return their comments and questionnaires on time.

Thanks also to John Bailey of the FDA's Cosmetic Division, Dr. Ara Dermarderosian of the Philadelphia College of Pharmacy, and Norma Borne, the secretary to the late Erma Bombeck, who shared my interview request with a woman whose work I've always admired and respected. Erma Bombeck was warm, funny, and an inspiration to this writer who hopes that she, too, can contribute something meaningful to other women.

Thanks also to photographer Sigreid Estrada, who took the cover photos, and hairdresser and makeup artist Lori Klein, and to my regular team at La Papillon, manicurist Cheryl Mehaffey, stylist Joseph Langendorf, and colorist Toni Sanchez, who are the only ones who really know for sure.

And finally, a loving thank you to Norman and Mo who survived the invasion and to my fun, wise, wonderful friends Shelley, Frieda, Tessie, Jeanne, Ruth, Carol, Sylvia, Annalee, Bobbi, Cheryl, Lois, and Gladys, who are my inspiration and cheering section, as well as to the wives of Mubic for their insight. They, like the many other women whose stories are told in these pages, are truly Ageless in their own right and I am proud to know them and share their lives.

INTRODUCTION

My life started to fall apart when I turned fifty.

Until then I had enjoyed a successful career as a cosmetics consultant, written two books, one of which was a best-seller, made frequent television appearances, and lectured around the country. I had four great children, two grandchildren, a wonderful, loving husband, and to top it all off, people were genuinely surprised to find out I was a grandmother. Life was good.

Then menopause hit. And it hit me like a head-on collision.

It happened just two months after my big fiftieth birthday bash. For the first time in my life I felt old, not to mention bloated, unattractive, irritable, and hot—good lord, was I hot. (My husband says we could take a vacation in Paris with the money he saved on the heating bills while I was going through the change.)

After talking to countless women and trying all kinds of remedies, including trying to tough it out, I finally found the right hormones to get me back on track. Now, at fifty-seven, life is good again.

My experience with menopause got me thinking about writing another book. I discovered that there's a reason that they call it "the change." My libido took a nosedive and everything, yes, I mean everything, dried up. My hair changed, my skin changed, my coloring changed, and my weight changed. Everything changed when my periods stopped.

Even though I know a lot about cosmetics, skin care, and beauty in general, I was often at a loss about what to do about these changes. Products I had used and liked no longer worked. Colors suddenly looked funny on me and my once lustrous hair became dull and coarse almost overnight. I didn't know what to do and to top it all off, I was discovering at least a wrinkle a week and sitting *shiva* (complete with covered mirrors) for my dying looks. (When a Jewish person dies and the family gathers in one home to mourn the loss, that's known as sitting *shiva*. Tradition has it that during *shiva*, you cover the mirrors because you should not concern yourself with how you look while you are mourning.)

That's when it dawned on me. If I was unprepared to deal with the beauty challenges of menopause, certainly Mother Nature was torturing other women the same way.

So, I started working on a plan for a menopause beauty book — it sounded like a great idea, all my friends liked it, but I couldn't get a publisher to bite.

Finally, after the trauma of menopause had somewhat worn off, I started to look beyond the change and realized that my body wasn't the only thing that had changed in recent years. The cosmetics industry itself had changed tremendously since *Take Care of Your Skin*.

The aging baby boomers were beginning to have their way with the cosmetics industry and you'll read in Chapter 1, the lure of their collective pocketbook was spawning the development of all kinds of new ingredients and new products that really work. These women, many of whom had never paid much attention to cosmetics, in addition to my menopausal cohorts, were in need of some guidance because, let's face it, the cosmetics counter can be a pretty intimidating place.

What's more, Melanie Griffith was imploring us to defy aging and while that sounded like a great idea, who knew whether Melanie's cream was better than Elizabeth Hurley's?

I discovered that there is a lot we all need to know if we are going to be smart consumers. The over-forty set is the fastest growing segment of the population, which means that more and more products are being developed just for us. We've never had so much to choose from and so much to know about in order to make an informed choice.

So, I started to look at the audience for my book in broader terms and decided to share my wisdom (which is a side effect of turning fifty) with the legions of women who are about to cross that road.

Now that menopause is really behind me I can look ahead to the next thirty to forty years of my life with anticipation — mostly.

I'd be less than honest if I told you that there's nothing better than life after fifty. Some days when I look in the mirror, the only thing I see are my sagging jowls—more often though, I see a vibrant woman who looks great at fifty-seven. I'm faithful to my exercise routines, not because I love to sweat or ride a bike that's going nowhere, but because if I don't do it, my weight will certainly be heading down a path I'd rather not go. If I could get away with it, I'd pull the plug on my Life Cycle and eat dessert every night of the week.

Still, there's a lot to be said for being over fifty. Like many women my age, I have the time, energy, and good health to do just about anything I want. I am more confident than ever before and also more productive, because, with fewer demands on my time, I am more focused on attaining my goals. My children are grown now and giving me wonderful, beautiful grandchildren to spoil.

I now consider turning fifty a fork in the road, not the end of it.

I wrote this book to help other women navigate the often confusing world of beauty products, services, and challenges. We can all remember a time in our lives when looking great meant a good haircut and a tube of lip gloss. Now it takes a little more know-how, but it's not mission impossible. I wanted to write a book that would be an easy-to-use, hands-on shopping guide as well as an informative resource for growing older. When I think of this book, I think of the spaghetti sauce commercial that says, "it's in there." If there's anything you want to know about looking your best as you grow older, "it's in there."

The lion's share of the cosmetic industry's advances have been in skin-care products and there's a lot we need to know. By the time you're finished with Part 1, Face Facts, you'll know everything you need to know about taking care of your skin, protecting it from the sun, treating fine lines and wrinkles, and your cosmetic surgery options, should you decide to exercise them.

In Chapter 2, you'll find out what really happens to your skin as you age and how to check your skin type periodically to be on the alert for changes. You'll learn easy skin-care routines and find out how to adapt your skin-care regimens to changes in climate and season. I've made recommendations on the best cleansers, eye-makeup removers, toners, moisturizers, and eye creams. I've also listed some products that I feel are nice to have versus those you must have, so that you don't waste your money on products you don't really need.

Nothing promotes aging more than the sun and that's why I devoted all of Chapter 3 to sun-care products and sun-safe practices, along with a list of recommended products courtesy of the Skin Cancer Foundation. This is serious business that has come home to roost in women who baked in the sun slathered in iodine and baby oil. You know who you are.

Because so many of us worshipped the sun, wrinkle-fighting products have evolved even more quickly than traditional skin-care products. That's why I made a separate chapter for them. While companies once sold hope-in-a-jar, there are now a lot of products that really work. In Chapter 4, you'll find out everything you need to know about Retin-A, alpha hydroxy acids (AHAs), and the newest wrinkle-fighting ingredients—vitamins. I've recommended the best products in three categories: drug store/mass market brands, department-store brands, and products offered through doctors' offices and 800 numbers. You'll even get a bonus civics lesson when I tell you about the FDA and its regulation, or lack thereof, of the cosmetics industry.

Thanks to the demands placed on the cosmetics industry by the baby boomers, products are being developed and marketed faster than we can grow gray hairs. Many of them are terrific—I really can't believe how well they work. And, as always, some products are just not what you would expect.

In order to recommend products, I gathered as many name-brand products as I could possibly find and had them tested by women all over the country to see how they liked the products. I asked them how the products felt, smelled, applied, lasted, and if they felt the products worked. In the case of products that promised wrinkle-removing benefits, we took before and after pictures and compared them. I also took those same products to a well-known college of pharmacy and asked their chemists to tell me which products contained the ingredients to substantiate the label claims.

When I set out to write this book, I had hoped to be able to tell consumers how to read labels and know if a product would really work. I thought for sure there would be some guidelines I could share to help women know if the product really contained enough alpha hydroxy acid or vitamins to make a difference. What I found out was that the science of skin care has changed so dramatically that, without a masters degree in chemistry, you really can't learn enough about a product to make a good choice simply by reading the labels.

After all of this sampling and testing, I chose what I felt were the best products in each category and these are the ones that I am recommending to you. I may not be able to help you read a package label, but I've met with those who can and have provided some insider tips to help you get the most for your cosmetic dollar.

Men and women are lining up at doctors' offices to find out more about the latest and greatest wrinkle-removing options. Cosmetic surgeries and services are covered extensively in Chapter 5, where I've listed cost ranges and recovery times for almost every procedure you could ever think about having. I've talked to some of the top surgeons and dermatologists in the field to give you a realistic idea of what to expect. Magazines are full of articles about laser peels or the unusual service du jour, but this chapter provides a comprehensive look at all of your alternatives.

If you are physically unfit or in poor health, smooth, wrinkle-free skin and the perfect nose are relatively unimportant. That's why I devoted Chapters 6 and 7 in Part 2, More Than Just A Pretty Face, to the very basics of good looks—nutrition and exercise. I've also included low-fat dessert recipes from spas and restaurants around the country, recommendations for choosing walking tapes and exercise videos, and guidelines for buying the proper footwear and selecting a health club.

Also in this section, I'll tell you about caring for your feet, identifying and treating varicose veins, give you the scoop on miracle thigh creams, and even recommend some hand and nail products in Chapter 8.

Because it is a topic that every woman faces eventually, I've set aside Chapter 9 to look at menopause and the pros and cons of hormone replacement therapy. Even if you're not quite ready to think about these issues, if you read up on it now, you'll be better prepared when the time comes.

Skin care, cosmetic surgery, menopause, diet, and exercise can all be pretty involved subjects, which is why I saved the fun stuff for last. Part 3, Finishing Touches, talks about hair and makeup. I don't know too many women who don't enjoy getting a new haircut or finding a great tube of lipstick, but as we get older, even those simple pleasures can become a little more challenging.

I'll help you learn to alter your color selections as you age and offer some great tips for making up a more mature face in Chapter 10—About Face. Just because certain colors worked for you when you were thirty, doesn't mean they're still fabulous at forty or fifty. I've examined dozens of foundations, lipsticks, powders, eye shadows, and much more to select the best brands for your changing skin tones. When you're finished, you'll know how to keep your lipstick out of the lines around your lip, and how to select makeup that doesn't get trapped in your wrinkles.

We'll also look at hairstyles, coloring products, styling aids, shampoos, and conditioners, and help you buy the right products for your changing needs. If you've ever gone to the beauty supply store and tried to select hair color, you'll love Chapter 11 because I'm going to help you make the right choice every time.

In writing this book, I consulted with experts in every field— diet doctors, nutritionists, dermatologists, plastic surgeons, exercise specialists, chemists, analysts, cosmetic company researchers, the FDA, the Cosmetic Ingredient Review Board, makeup artists, hairstylists, and nail technicians—but because I'm new at this growing-older-gracefully stuff, I turned to my friends and their friends for the expert information on the final chapter. These women are the experts at growing older gracefully and I've set aside a full chapter for their advice and ideas. Many of their thoughts, tips, and words of wisdom (they too, are over fifty and are therefore wise) are included in these pages because I really believe that we can be tremendous resources to one another.

There has never been a better time to be growing older. Our opportunities are limited only by what our bodies and minds are willing to try. Consequently we are busier and more active than we ever dreamed we would be. Did you know that the over-fifty set represents 4 percent of college undergraduates? I suspect the baby boomers will make that number explode in the next few years.

We also want to look as great as we feel, but who has time to read beauty magazines every week to stay up to date on the latest and greatest skin-care products? That's where this book comes in.

With this one resource, you can learn what you need to know to make informed purchases and use them properly to look your best as you grow older. We all know there's no fountain of youth, but with your own little fountain of knowledge, you can look your best forever.

Throughout *Ageless* you'll meet some of my friends, interesting and inspiring women I've known for years and some I've just met. They'll talk about their first gray hairs, their first wrinkles, becoming grandmothers, enduring the changes that menopause brings, and a host of other topics that we can all relate to.

Bea claims to have thrown out her magnifying glass when it pointed out her first wrinkle and Erma Bombeck says she called her hairdresser at 911 when she spotted her first gray hair. Tessie says that the grayer she became, the blonder she turned. (Her hair looks like Loni Anderson's now.) We've all been there. I still check my makeup mirror for cracks because I'm certain that those accordion pleats on my upper lip can't be wrinkles.

Listening to and learning from other women is one of the fastest and most rewarding ways we can continue to grow. That's why I'm including these women in this book. They are, one at a time, redefining what it means to be growing older in this society and their experiences have enhanced their beauty and, more importantly, enriched their lives.

I hope that as you read *Ageless,* you'll think of someone else to share it with. Whether she's thirty-five and can use the information as a preventive guide, or eighty and in search of a new moisturizer, I think there's something in here for everyone. I urge you to continue the spirit of sharing in which this book was conceived and written and pick up a copy for your mother, your daughter, your granddaughter, sister, or best friend.

No one likes to think about growing old, so I suggest that we all discard that notion and start to think of ourselves as simply — Ageless.

Chapter 1

AGING IN THE NINETIES

"The really frightening thing about middle age is the knowledge that you'll grow out of it."

—DORIS DAY

"I have always thought that a woman has the right to treat the subject of her age with ambiguity until, perhaps, she passes into the realm of over 90. Then it is better she be candid with herself and with the world."

—HELENA RUBINSTEIN

Ask almost anyone, from an informal gathering of ordinary women to best-selling author and anthropologist Gail Sheehy, and they'll all tell you the same thing: Grandmothers, and older women in general, just ain't what they used to be.

In fact, thanks to longer lives, better health, and greater affluence in later years, most older Americans are living younger and better than ever before. Grandma has traded in her knitting needles for a pair of Nikes and is just as likely to be spending her afternoons surfing the Net as channel-surfing for soaps.

Take my friend Jeanne, for example. She's seventy and has a full and active life that includes a regular exercise class, bridge parties, and charity work. Bea is eighty, still drives a car, has lunch with her friends, plays cards, and goes shopping. Both of these women consider old age to be a state of mind, not a number. Bea says, "A person stops being young when their energy and sense of humor leave them. There's no such thing as being old, unless you are very sick."

In her book *New Passages,* Gail Sheehy described for the first time what people everywhere have been noticing and feeling for years, that fifty is what forty used to be, forty is what thirty used to be, and so on.

Some, like Dr. Ross Goldstein, founder of Generations Insights, a market research firm in San Francisco, call this phenomenon "the downaging of America." While many factors have contributed to it, the undeniable truth is that both men and women can reasonably expect to live active, vital lives well into what was once considered the "golden years."

At the turn of the century, the average life expectancy was forty-seven years, which meant that forty was old. By contrast, a girl born in 1995 can expect to live to be eighty-one. In an article published by the National Institutes of Health, Dr. James Vaupel of Odense University Medical School in Denmark maintains that forthcoming advances in treating coronary disease and cancer could push life expectancy to ninety or one hundred years in the foreseeable future. But you don't need government statistics to prove just how meaningless chronological age can be, as eighty year olds run marathons and men in their seventies run for president of the United States.

"Vitality is not age-related, it's health-related," says Dr. Larry Rotenberg, chief of psychiatry at Reading Hospital in Reading, Pennsylvania, and a clinical psychiatry professor at Temple University. "Preventive health, as well as a revolution in medical care, has made it possible to maintain youthful activities far into what was once considered old age," said Rotenberg. "Jogging, walking, and working out were never part of the equation for older people. Now, we don't think anything of people doing aerobics at seventy."

The downaging phenomenon also manifests itself in younger Americans. Just look at the number of women having their first child in their late-thirties and forties. At a time in life when I was helping my daughter shop for a prom dress, these women are arranging day care and going to Mommy and Me classes.

According to Dr. Goldstein, "The numbers don't mean what they used to—it's part of a larger trend of age irrelevance. Mick Jagger is fifty and still singing rock 'n' roll; Lauren Hutton is over fifty and still modeling. People are defining ages for themselves and saying 'this is what it's like to be fifty.' "

Sophia Loren is a great example of someone for whom age has become irrelevant. She had her children in her late thirties and, even though her career keeps her busy, she's still very much a full-time mom to her college student sons. Although her birth certificate will tell her she's past her sixtieth birthday, the idea still comes as somewhat of a surprise to her.

Age is also irrelevant for my friend Tessie, who at seventy-eight is a superb role model for "growing older gracefully." She takes an aerobics class three times a week and does a two-mile walk whenever the weather permits. She fights the loneliness of being a widow by staying involved with friends and art. Getting older doesn't bother her in the least.

"We grow older whether we want to or not," she says. "As long as you can maintain good health and a clear mind, growing older is acceptable. If you are physically well and still mentally alert, then growing older is not threatening and can be a positive experience. You can see your grandchildren grow into adulthood."

"You can't avoid getting older," said centenarian George Burns, puffing on a cigar, "but you don't have to get old."

SAFETY IN NUMBERS

"The number of people over sixty-five will continue to grow over the next twenty to twenty-five years," says Rotenberg. "We're seeing a trend now of older people continuing to do various jobs. Look at Barbara Walters. She's in her sixties and still doing a great job. Twenty years ago she would have been canned."

Rotenberg is right. In case you missed this bit of demographic trivia, here it is again. One person will turn fifty every 7.5 seconds through the year 2006, and by 2030 there will be about seventy million people age sixty-five or over. Millions of healthy and fit people with years of experience will not be dismissed as "past their prime" or no longer useful, especially when they are the majority and there are fewer people in the age groups behind them to fill their shoes.

TOUR GUIDES FOR THE GROWING-OLD-GRACEFULLY ROAD TRIP

"The secret to staying young is to live honestly, eat slowly, and lie about your age," Lucille Ball once said. Until fairly recently, women tried to hide their age and admitted to nothing over twenty-nine. Today women are infinitely more comfortable with acknowledging their age, particularly if they think they look good.

Perhaps women like Jane Fonda, Linda Evans, Joan Collins, and the like, who turned forty and fifty and began boasting about how great they looked, should get some of the credit for helping drive the "downaging of America." They helped many of us to realize that turning forty or fifty isn't the end of the world, but can actually mean the start of a new life.

But it wasn't just the "beauties" whose names came up when I asked women to name their "growing old gracefully" role models. Almost unanimously, they identified women of substance and accomplishment who look good, but aren't trying to look "young." Women like Barbara Walters, Barbara Bush, Jessica Tandy, Lena Horne, and Katharine Hepburn were the names I heard most often.

In a study conducted by the Yankelovich Partners for Clinique, called the Truth/Beauty survey, respondents listed many of the same names and added a few others, including Jacqueline Kennedy Onassis, Tina Turner, Hillary Clinton, Audrey Hepburn, Helen Hayes, Georgia O'Keeffe, Elizabeth Taylor, Joan Rivers, Sophia Loren, and Raquel Welch. Katharine Hepburn received the most responses with 37 percent of the vote.

When I asked the late Erma Bombeck about her aging gracefully role model, she too surprised me with her answer. "Don't hang up on me," she said. "Mother Teresa is my role model. She has the most interesting face and it reflects what she is: humility, beauty, kindness. Even if I didn't know what she did, her face tells a lot about her. I would know what she does. It comes from being productive and being interested and being interesting. The other role model is my mother. She's not Mother Teresa, but has a great sense of pride and independence. She keeps very busy and it shows in her face. We watch our mothers all of our lives and I see the same light in her eyes now as when she was younger."

Time and again, everyone I spoke to identified women of intelligence and accomplishment who are known for what they have done rather than their looks. Looking *good* was important, but looking *young* was not.

"Women today are looking at beauty as something more than just physical appearance," said Jann Leeming, president and editor-in-chief of *About Marketing to Women* magazine. "It's about confidence, intelligence, sense of humor, accomplishments — much more than just how a person looks."

At fifty-seven, Ruth is one of the busiest women I know. She's a wife, mother, and grandmother who also works as a cooking teacher and writer. She plays tennis and golf, is well read, and gets involved in charitable efforts. Like everyone, she wants to look her best, but she's not obsessed with looking younger. "I want to look better," Ruth says. "I want my body to stay healthy, but I'm not fixated with looking younger."

The Clinique Truth/Beauty study illustrates Ruth's feelings in a statistically valid study. In it, 74 percent of the women surveyed said they accepted aging as a natural part of life and were not concerned with looking *young,* but 97 percent said they wanted to look the best they can *for their age*.

A study of women's attitudes done by *Self* magazine found that:

> women seem to be following a path of increased self-acceptance when it comes to aging, acknowledging that they don't look as attractive as they did, but stressing other assets that appreciate as they age and keeping the focus on physical and mental health. Aging is still an issue for women, but there's more to the process than losing one's looks. Achievements and involvement in other areas of their lives help to soften the impact of the inevitable changes in physical attractiveness.

CREDIT THE BOOMERS

Just as the baby boomers defined the youth movement, they continue to impact our culture in enormous ways. Dr. Goldstein observed that this group, who once didn't trust anyone over thirty, now lives in a world where everyone is over thirty and another twelve thousand of them turn forty every day.

These baby boomers continue to flex their considerable economic muscle and manufacturers rush to bring them appealing products. Lady Clairol has downaged into Miss Clairol, and roomy Oldsmobiles have a sporty look now so that they won't be confused with "your father's Oldsmobile."

"As the baby boom generation gets older, we're demanding that age be okay," said syndicated columnist Ellen Goodman. "Just as we changed attitudes about childbirth and work, we have a strong desire to make the experience of aging different."

Dr. Goldstein describes this different aging experience as remaining "attitudinally young." According to him, it's all about staying in touch. "One of the most important factors is maintaining an openness to new stimulation, a willingness to be flexible. When I was growing up, my parents' attitude toward my dress, music, and style was really negative; that was called the generation gap. Now, being willing to reach across generations and understanding that your generation isn't the only generation and realizing that your generation doesn't have the inside road on truth—that keeps people attitudinally young," says Goldstein.

CASHING IN AT THE COSMETICS COUNTER

Perhaps more than any business, other than medicine, the cosmetics industry has and will continue to benefit from these blooming boomers who want their appearance to match their youthful attitudes.

According to Packaged Facts, in 1994 the cosmetics industry took in $3.4 billion for skin-care products in the United States alone. By the year 2000, experts predict that Americans will spend $4.6 billion for skin care, while the rest of the world antes up another $27 billion— and that doesn't include the billions spent on hair care, makeup, or nail care. In fact, the introduction of mass-market alpha hydroxy acid products in 1992 created a skin-care category that had not existed previously, but in 1995 accounted for $630 million in U.S. sales.

According to Dianne Osborne, vice president of skin-care marketing for Estee Lauder—whose customers range in age from eighteen to eighty, with an emphasis on the over-thirty-five set—the target market has not changed much over the years, but their objectives in purchasing skin-care products have.

"I don't think the basic profile has changed much, but what I am seeing is the customer is getting into serious skin care at an earlier age," said Osborne. "There is a change in emphasis from correction to prevention. I hear that in all of the focus groups—greater concern at an earlier age for protection."

While Barbara Bush, with her wrinkle-hiding pearls, has led the way for women to be comfortable with years of good living showing on their faces, don't expect the boomers to "let it all hang out" as they once did. They're gobbling up skin-care products at an amazing rate, allowing cosmetics companies to post double-digit sales increases year after year.

Ninety-six percent of the respondents in the Clinique Truth/Beauty survey said that you don't have to look young to be beautiful, but seven in ten plan to do everything they can to stay young-looking. Our minds seem to be comfortable with being part of the aging crowd, but our egos want us to be the fairest of them all.

This explains the dichotomy between our apparent comfort with aging and the stampede at the cosmetics counter. "Aging is less threatening, but it's not *un*threatening at all," says Dr. Goldstein. "People still want to look good and enhance their beauty. But there's been a large shift in approach. There's been a dissolution of the illusion that you can stop aging, toward the idea of *controlling* aging. It may sound like semantics but it's an important difference. If you look at ads for Oil of Olay, they're talking about controlling aging, not stopping it. Consumers know that aging happens and they don't expect to be able to stop it, but they are finding products that help them to control it."

Goldstein added that "remarkable advances in cosmetics and anti-aging agents make it possible to actually control aging. The research done on free radicals and antioxidants are good examples. We've just scratched the surface of understanding the aging process and the research will be propelled in the coming years by the marketplace."

The economic imperative of appearing youthful for the job market is perhaps the most powerful incentive. With companies constantly downsizing, many fifty-year-old employees find themselves on the street at a time when they expected to be comfortable in their careers. Add to that the likelihood of retirement being pushed back to age seventy and you'll understand why men are also beginning to fill up plastic surgeons' schedules.

"Looking fifty is great," says comedian Joan Rivers, "if you're sixty."

BETTER LIVING THROUGH CHEMISTRY

The application of science to the cosmetics business has been the best thing that's ever happened to the industry. "Years ago, the industry in skin care had a reputation of being hope-in-a-jar — creamy, fluffy hope-in-a-jar — and that's changed dramatically," said Lauder's Osborne. "In 1982, Estee Lauder led the way with Night Repair. That was the first time any skin-care product came straight from scientific research. I remember the product reviews saying that with Night Repair, Estee Lauder sent all of its competitors into their laboratories. That was the start of scientific research in skin care."

"Without the economic driver of seventy-six million baby boomers, I think the developments would be slower coming along," said Goldstein. "Take male-pattern hair loss, for example. It's been around as long as there have been male patterns, but no one's done much about it except for toupees and some tonics that didn't work. The good research is just getting started. I expect there will be really good products in the next five to ten years. There have been powerful innovations driven by the fact that every year for the next ten years, another two million males will turn forty."

According to TGE Demographics of Ithaca, New York, as cited in the Official Guide to American Incomes, 72 percent of households headed by someone age forty-five to fifty-four had discretionary income averaging $4,500 per person. While slightly fewer households headed by fifty-five to sixty-four year olds had discretionary income (71 percent), those who did had close to $5,500. It's those discretionary dollars buying wrinkle creams, thigh thinners, and hair tonics that will push cosmetics companies' sales figures over the $4 billion mark next year.

The forces of the marketplace have created a near revolution in the skin-care business. Ten years ago, companies were just beginning to dabble in alpha hydroxy acids (AHAs) and antioxidants had yet to arrive on the scene. I used to advise women to apply sunscreen in addition to foundation and moisturizer. Now, almost every moisturizer and foundation has some sunscreen in it and it's hard to find a skin-care product without some kind of exfoliating acid. In fact, in 1994 cosmetics companies introduced fifty new products containing AHAs. Millions of people living longer, healthier, more productive lives are demanding multipurpose products that actually do what they promise and the skin-care industry is developing them faster than any of us can keep up.

In 1995, Ortho Pharmaceuticals announced that they had finally received approval from the Food and Drug Administration (FDA) for Renova, a Retin-A based product, that has been proven to reduce fine lines, wrinkles, and age spots. (For a full discussion of Retin-A and Renova, see Chapter 4.) The approval of Renova as a prescription wrinkle formulation is a significant milestone in the application of science to cosmetics. For the first time ever, the FDA is attesting to the fact that a product actually reduces wrinkles. That Ortho had Renova on pharmacist's shelves only six weeks after receiving FDA approval is a testament to the product's vast appeal.

You can bet the ranch that, with someone turning fifty every 7.5 seconds through the year 2006, additional approvals won't be far behind and they'll soon make skin-care products that not only repair your skin, but teach you to tango, too.

While it's true that the application of science to skin care has raised the bar considerably, it's important to remember the very nature of the cosmetics customer. Hope does spring eternal. Who among us hasn't bought something that seemed too good to be true only to find out that it was? By the same token, none of us will buy something a second time if it didn't work the first time and companies know that.

That's why we are bombarded with newspaper, television, and magazine ads selling every kind of age-defying, youth-enhancing, wrinkle-smoothing, gray-covering, tired-muscle soothing, corn-removing product imaginable. We are living longer, healthier, more productive lives and Madison Avenue is ready to show you ten new things that will help you do it more comfortably and beautifully.

That's also why *Ageless* was written. With so much advertising attention focused on aging women, it's nearly impossible to sort through all of the information so that you can avail yourself of the best products without making it your life's work to make an informed selection. After all, Granny's got to get in a workout before heading to computer class, that's over just in time to pick up the grandchildren from school. . . .

Part 1

FACE FACTS

Chapter 2

THE SKINNY ON SKIN CARE

*A Common Sense Approach
to Saving Face*

"My dream is to save women from nature."

—CHRISTIAN DIOR

It's true that beauty is only skin deep. That also means that the key to looking great at any age is taking good care of your skin. If your heart is like a car's engine that drives your body, then your skin is the steel and fiberglass body that keeps what's inside safe and dry. Unfortunately, your skin isn't as tough as steel or fiberglass, but it still has to stand up to the damaging effects of pollution, weather, and sunlight. Before I take this automotive analogy too far, remember this: Your skin is your body's largest organ, weighing approximately six pounds and covering twenty-five square feet, and just as you take healthful precautions to keep your other organs functioning properly, you should also take good care of your skin.

Since your skin is 90 percent water, keeping the skin well hydrated both internally and externally is an important step on the road to great skin. But other factors, particularly diet, exercise, smoking, exposure to sunlight, and overall good health play key roles in how your skin looks. The good news is that we can control all of those things fairly well.

Now for the bad news. Even if you lived in a biosphere, ate a well-balanced diet, exercised regularly, did not smoke, and drank alcohol only in moderation, as you grew older, your skin would still eventually begin to dry up, wrinkle, and sag. It's just nature.

Since there is no fountain of youth and you cannot stop the clock, should you just turn in your beauty bar, party all night long, and go to bed with your makeup on? Absolutely not. There are no miracles, but there is a whole lot you can do to make your skin look its best.

HOW AGE AFFECTS YOUR SKIN

As we age, the skin naturally becomes thinner and less elastic. As body functions slow down, so too does the skin's ability to replace old cells with new ones. On top of all that, gravity also takes its toll. Hence the lines start to show, the jowls start to sag, and skin tone goes limp.

Essentially, the skin is comprised of two layers, the epidermis, or top layer, and the dermis, the supporting structure. The epidermis is the body's first line of defense against the environment, disease, and ultraviolet light. The top layer is comprised of dead cells that serve as the body's barrier to ultraviolet rays, pollution, etc., and it is called the stratum corneum. New cells are produced every day at the base of the epidermis and over a period of a few weeks, the cells your body builds today will make their way to the surface of your skin. When they reach the surface, they die and are sloughed off to make room for new cells. That's called turnover and when you hear ads for cosmetics that promote turnover or cell renewal, that's what they're talking about.

In a twenty-year-old woman, turnover takes approximately thirty days; by the time a woman is sixty, the process takes 50 percent longer and, in addition to having a hard time holding in moisture, the cells look dull and flaky.

The dermis, made mostly of collagen and elastin, supports the epidermis, stores water, and protects your body from injury. Think of an orange: it has a top layer, the zest, that is orange in color and has certain characteristics that further identify the fruit as an orange (not a grapefruit or a lemon); underneath the zest is the rind, which supports the zest and protects the juicy fruit within. As an orange sits around for a while, it begins to dry out, lose its firmness, and eventually wrinkles, much like your skin.

The dermis is the home of blood vessels, sweat glands, nerve endings, and hair follicles. The collagen and elastin in the dermis give skin its strength and elasticity, but over time the sun damages these tender fibers, causing them to lose their bounce, just as a stretched-out waistband refuses to snap back into shape. These sun-damaged fibers manifest themselves as wrinkles. To demonstrate this, pinch the skin on the back of your hand and notice how slowly it flattens out again. Try that on someone who is ten or twenty years younger than you and notice the difference. What you are seeing on your own hand is a loss of elasticity.

Although skin-care products often claim to penetrate the skin, making it sound as if beneficial ingredients could actually reach this important layer of skin, most molecules, including water, are too large to reach the dermis.

Menopause and the Skin

Despite the lack of published research on the topic, dermatologists do know that declining estrogen levels are associated with the breakdown of collagen. Physicians like Arthur Balin, who works at the Center for the Rejuvenation of Aging Skin in suburban Philadelphia and is also a microbiologist, observe that declining estrogen levels coincide with a decrease in oil production. That's why many menopausal women experience dullness, dryness, thinning, and a seemingly overnight loss of elasticity.

Women who take estrogen replacement therapy, however, report big gains in skin quality, such as better hydration and plumpness, as well as more youthful hair and nails, according to Dr. Wilma Bergfeld, head of clinical research at the Cleveland Clinic's department of dermatology.

If you've already been through menopause, probably none of this is a revelation, but if you're one of the millions of women yet to arrive at that crossroads, you can be on the lookout for these additional symptoms and factor them into your decision to use or not use Hormone Replacement Therapy (HRT). (This is discussed in Chapter 9.)

Time Marches On

As I said earlier, over time, no matter how well you care for your skin, you're going to start seeing the telltale signs of aging. At first it's just a fine laugh line, then it's a furrow in the brow and a few age spots. If you're in your fifties or sixties, you know how these things creep up on you. However, so that you know what to expect in the future and can figure out if you're beating the odds, here's a decade-by-decade list of what you can expect.

THIRTIES
- **Prime time for adult acne. According to studies done by Ortho Pharmaceuticals, two-thirds of Americans with acne are age twenty-five to forty-nine.**
- **Cell renewal and circulation begin to slow.**

- First expression lines appear.
- Eyelid-bagging can begin.

FORTIES
- Lines and wrinkles become more apparent.
- Elasticity slackens.
- Blotching and forehead furrows appear.
- Ears and neck begin to become crepe-like.
- Chin may start to droop.

FIFTIES
- Menopause and its changing hormones takes its toll on skin with slacking jawline and the furthering of crepiness.
- Existing wrinkles deepen, frown lines appear, turkey neck starts.
- Wrinkles around nose, earlobes, and chin become more apparent.
- Skin color may begin to fade.
- Age spots begin to appear.

SIXTIES
- Overall dryness and lack of toning exacerbate wrinkles, which begin to appear on cheeks.
- Skin can take on a chapped look.
- Bones can shrink, increasing slackness of skin.
- Skin thins, which allows capillaries and redness to show through.

SEVENTIES
- Skin loses elasticity and overlapping wrinkles can give face a road-map look.

SKIN TYPES

Many of us had oily skin as teenagers, but by the time most women reach their forties, their skin, like everything else, has changed. Most mature women have either dry or combination skin—a mix of dry or normal and oily skin. Typically the cheeks are one skin type and the T-zone (the forehead, nose, and chin) are slightly oily.

Because our bodies change so much as we age, it's a good idea to check your skin type every few years just to be sure you are using the right products. Many of us find a skin-care regimen that we like and we stick with it, which is fine. But in our quest for simplicity we sometimes fail to notice that products are not working as well as they once did. That could be because our skin type has changed and we didn't notice.

When I was looking for women to try the products that are recommended in these pages, I was shocked to learn that 90 percent of the women who volunteered to sample products didn't know their skin type. Before they could sample the products, I told them how to determine their skin type with this simple test.

Elaine's Exclusive

EASY SKIN TYPE TEST

1. Wash your face with lukewarm water and a mild soap such as Dove or any other mild cleanser.
2. Rinse your face by splashing it fifteen times with lukewarm water and pat dry. Do not moisturize or apply a toner.
3. Wait for three hours.
4. Number four one-inch pieces of facial blotting paper, onion skin, or cigarette paper for each of four areas of your face: forehead, cheeks, nose, chin.
5. One at a time, hold the appropriate piece of paper to the corresponding area of your face for a slow count of ten.
6. Take the papers into a good light and look at them.
   - *If the papers have a very faint oil residue, then your skin is normal.*
   - *If the papers have a slight, but definitely discernible oil residue, then your skin is oily.*
   - *If the papers have an obvious oil residue, then that area of your skin is very oily.*
   - *With truly dry skin, all of the papers will be dry.*
   - *If you have combination skin, the forehead, nose, and chin papers will come up oily and the cheek paper will be dry.*

Dry Skin

Hydration is the key for women who have dry skin and that's the vast majority of Caucasian women over forty. Dry skin is one of nature's nasty little tricks that is exacerbated by hormonal changes, pollutants, and a lifetime of exposure to the sun. The best thing you can do for your skin is to keep it well hydrated inside and out, and protect it from the sun. Drinking plenty of water is important for overall good health, and it's especially helpful in maintaining healthy skin. Be particularly diligent about applying moisturizer and sunscreen.

Combination Skin

Balancing the needs of dry or normal skin with some normal or oily areas is the most important thing you can do for combination skin. Each section needs to be treated a little differently. Your main goal is to keep the T-zone free from oil and clogged pores without drying out the rest of your face.

Normal Skin

Maintenance is the key if you are one of the few women blessed with normal skin. Remember that the best thing you can do for your skin is to maintain the balance. Keep it simple and use as few products as possible on your face (mild cleanser and sunscreen). The more you apply to your skin, the more likely you are to experience an adverse reaction.

Oily Skin

Oil-free is what you want to be. By the time most Caucasian women reach their thirties, oily skin is a thing of the past. But some women, particularly Black, Hispanic, and Asian women, and some Caucasians with darker complexions, still struggle with shiny faces even into old age. Your goal is to sop up unwanted oil and tame any breakouts that occur. If you think you have oily skin, or have always had oily skin, be sure to do the skin type test periodically and be on the lookout for changes.

Sensitive Skin

There's no true definition of sensitive skin, but 70 percent of all women say they have it. Sensitive can mean that skin often reacts to cosmetics, is prone to blemishes, burns easily in the sun, or many other things.

Dermatologists report that they see more and more people complaining of sensitivity that is probably due to all of the products people are using on their skin. Everything contains some kind of preservative and lots of chemicals that have the potential to cause reactions. Furthermore, alpha hydroxy acids (AHAs) are included in products to slough off the top layer of dead skin cells. Those cells do serve a protective purpose and for some people, too much sloughing can enable other chemicals to penetrate the skin farther than they should.

If you're having sensitivity problems, start eliminating skin-care products, starting with cleansers, which can be harsh and cause redness or irritation. If you're having problems with pimples, eliminate your moisturizer first—it could be too heavy. Continue eliminating products a week at a time, until you can identify which product is causing the problem. The shorter route to identifying the irritant is to pack up all of your products and head straight to a dermatologist, who may be able to identify the offending ingredient just by reading the product labels.

It's true that AHA products are likely to sting and that skin will become desensitized to that sting over a short period of time. Redness, blotchiness, itching, and breakouts, however, should not be tolerated. So stop using any product that gives you that kind of reaction.

NeoStrata, the company that pioneered the research on alpha hydroxy acids, and the use of AHAs in skin care, recently introduced a line of department store products, called Exuviance. Exuviance's sensitive-skin products contain a patented ingredient called gluconolactone, which works like glycolic acid but is less irritating. The products are wonderful and according to NeoStrata's marketing director, Lynda Farrington Wilson, this is the only truly sensitive formula in the prestige line of cosmetics. Many other sensitive-skin formulas are merely less potent versions of the original product.

Dark Skin

Whether you're Black, Hispanic, Asian, or Mediterranean, if you have dark skin, you are fortunate to have more melanin to protect your skin from the sun's withering rays than fair-skinned people. Despite the fact that dark skin tends to be thicker, it can run the gamut of skin types and can be sensitive as well. Treat your skin gently by cleansing, moisturizing, protecting, and exfoliating based upon the needs of your skin type.

Dark-skinned women are more likely to be plagued with acne longer and often struggle with the drying effects of the acne products. According to Dr. Loretta Pratt of the Center for the Rejuvenation of Aging Skin in Media, Pennsylvania, Black women in particular should be sure not to overmoisturize in response to dry, ashy patches.

"The best moisturizer is water," says Dr. Barnett Johnson, a Philadelphia dermatologist. "To prevent ashiness, hydrate with splashes of water and then seal it in with something that retards evaporation." Oil-free products are good for women with acne problems, but others will find petrolatum-based products do the job well.

In addition, Black women want to be sure to keep hair dressings off the skin. Dr. Pratt tells her clients who wear heavy hair dressings to change pillowcases daily or cover their hair when sleeping. The oil from the hair dressings can aggravate acne and cause brown spotting.

Benzoyl peroxide, a common ingredient in acne medicines, can discolor the skin. Instead, choose salicylic acid-based acne products.

Dark-skinned women should be careful not to take their genetic sun protection for granted. While you are naturally resistant to the sun's drying rays, you are not impervious and should still apply sunscreen and wear a hat and sunglasses.

FOUR BASICS OF SKIN CARE

Caring for your skin is not difficult, or complicated, nor does it have to be expensive or involve a medicine cabinet full of products, but it is something you should do faithfully for best results over a lifetime. Despite the fact that there are thousands of different skin-care products, there are really only three things you *need* to do for your skin and a fourth practice that is a good idea.

CLEANSING
Removing oils, pollutants, makeup, dirt, and dead cells.

MOISTURIZING
Sealing in the skin's own moisture and enhancing it will keep it looking fresh and supple.

PROTECTING
Protecting your skin from the sun's harmful rays is the single most effective thing you can do to preserve your skin.

EXFOLIATING
Sloughing off dead cells so that fresher, younger cells are visible on the skin's surface helps eliminate fine lines and pigmentary problems.

COMPLETE PRODUCT LINES

Some consumers hesitate to mix and match products from several different lines, preferring instead to buy everything from one company. While this kind of synergy is not necessary and does not really give the consumer superior results, the companies themselves are thankful for the brand loyalty, and it does simplify things for the consumer.

Some companies make a few, several, or many good products and a select few make everything well. I've listed those product lines here to eliminate a lot of repetition in the individual product recommendations. Whether you mix and match products or are brand-loyal, you can't go wrong with anything you buy in these lines.

Product samplers who tested these products unanimously agreed that the products worked well, were aesthetically pleasing, and are exceptionally good values. Each product line offers a complete line of products for every skin type, including antiagers and specialty items such as sunscreens and skin lighteners.

The product lines that are listed in bold are my top recommendations because they are quality products that are attractively priced. Other product lines produce quality products, but are more expensive. For product lines that are only available from professionals, use the 800 numbers shown here to find a dispensing physician near you.

Skin Type Key: N normal; D dry; VD very dry; C combination; S sensitive; R Renova, Retin-A
Price Key: $ under $10; $$ $11–$21; $$$ $21–$30; $$$$ $31–$40; $$$$$ $41–$50; $$$$$$ over $50
(unless otherwise specified)

PRODUCT	WHERE AVAILABLE	PRICE	PHONE
Alpha Hydrox	Drugstore	$	800-55-ALPHA
Aqua Glycolic	Drugstore/800 #	$$	800-253-9499
BioMedic	Physicians	$$–$$$$$$	800-736-5155
Exuviance	Department stores	$$–$$$	800-225-9911
Glyderm	Physicians	$–$$$$$	800-321-4576
Hymed/Hylunia	Physicians/estheticians	$$$–$$$$$$	800-547-1232
Jan Marini	Physicians/estheticians	$$$–$$$$$$	800-347-2223
Kiehls	Select salons & department stores nationwide	$–$$$$$$	800-KIEHLS-1
M.D. Formulations	Physicians/estheticians	$$–$$$$$$	800-253-9499
M.D. Forte	Physicians	$$–$$$$$	800-253-9499
Murad	Physicians/ estheticians/800 #	$–$$$$$	800-33-MURAD
NeoStrata	Physicians/800 #	$$–$$$	800-865-8667

CLEANSING

The purpose of cleansing is to remove oils, pollutants, dirt, makeup, and dead skin cells. Regardless of your skin type, you should select the mildest product that will do the job well and rinse off completely with water.

"Cleansing without dehydrating is the first step to good skin care," said Dr. Mary Lupo, a New Orleans dermatologist and assistant clinical professor of dermatology at Tulane Medical School in Louisiana. "Select a water rinsable cleanser that does not require a toner, balancer, normalizer, or other extraneous products. If you're using a cleanser that requires toner to complete the process or correct something the cleanser is doing—get another cleanser."

Many skin-care regimens include toners or toning lotions that, in my opinion, are extraneous, wasteful unless your skin is oily, and can be drying to mature skin.

If you have dry skin, it's easy to overcleanse the face and exacerbate the dryness. A thorough cleansing in the evening to remove makeup, pollution, etc., and a few gentle splashes of water in the morning are sufficient. Unless you had a really wild night, your skin doesn't pick up dirt and pollution while you're sleeping, so there's no need to go through the cleansing ritual in the morning unless you have oily skin.

There also is no need to purchase an expensive dry-skin cleanser, although many women like the AHA cleansers sold with the physician-dispensed regimens. Choose a gentle bar or milky cleanser with an emollient. Dove and Neutrogena are good, gentle bar cleansers and Cetaphil or Aquanil are good, inexpensive liquid cleansers that were recommended by every dermatologist I interviewed. Others recommended Ponds products, too.

Tissue-off cream cleansers were once useful for removing the heavier, oil-based makeup that was made for dry skin. Today, however, makeup for dry skin is much lighter, and a heavy cream cleanser is no longer needed to remove it. If you are still wearing a heavy foundation that needs a cream cleanser, treat yourself to a new foundation. (I've recommended plenty of products for you to try in Chapter 7.)

Women with oily skin can use common soaps like Neutrogena for oily skin, Aveeno or Phisoderm, which help tame the bacteria, or specially formulated oily-skin cleansers. And, because oil can build up overnight, you may wish to recleanse in the morning. Also, use a toner or astringent after cleansing to help keep the oil under control.

Treat your combination skin to a cleanser that addresses the normal or dry parts of your skin, like Ponds or Alpha Hydrox Foaming Face Wash, and take care of the oily spots by swiping a little toner across the area to whisk away the excess oil.

Normal skin is best cared for with a gentle nondrying cleanser like Dove, Ponds, or Neutrogena.

If your skin tends to be sensitive, choose the mildest product available for your skin type. My dermatologist, Dr. Toby Shawe, recommends Aquanil, physician-dispensed NeoStrata, or Hymed for the most sensitive skin.

Finally, a clean face should feel fresh and supple. If it feels extremely tight, dry, or greasy after cleansing, choose another product. Listen to your skin. If it feels good and looks good, stick with whatever you are using.

Cleansing for Retin-A and Renova Users
If you use Retin-A or Renova, ask your doctor for specific cleanser recommendations because those products work best when applied to skin that is properly prepared with an acid pH cleanser. Retin-A tends to be extremely drying, so alkaline products only exacerbate the problem. Renova and AHAs are formulated to be nondrying, but

they still benefit from properly cleansed skin that is ready to soak up the wrinkle-fighting ingredients. (See the next section in this chapter, The Dope on Soap, for more information about the pH of cleansing products.)

Neutrogena makes a line of products for sensitive skin that are compatible with Renova use. The Non-Drying Cleanser, Moisture SPF 15, Light Night Cream, and Sensitive Skin Sunblock SPF 17 are all pre-existing Neutrogena products that were tested for Renova compatibility and have recently been marketed that way. The Renova Compatible Skin Care Kit—2 ounces of cleanser and 2 ounces of sunscreen packaged in a nice box for $9.95—is a good way to sample the products without spending extra money for the full-size bottles. However, the full-size products are not very expensive and you will probably like them, so you could go ahead and skip the trial package. Mary Kay has also introduced a line of Renova-compatible products.

The Dope on Soap

A soap by any other name would still clean as well. With apologies to William Shakespeare, the fact of the matter is that we tend to lump a whole lot of cleansing products under the category of simple soap. But these days soap takes on so many forms it's hard to know what to buy. Again, if you're using something that works for you and is at a price you're willing to pay—by all means, stick with it.

To select a good cleanser, you need to know a few things about your skin's pH—the measure of alkalinity or acidity. Normal balanced pH is 7.0. Anything below 7.0 is considered acidic and anything above is considered alkaline. Healthy skin is normally between 4.5 and 6.5, which means that skin is naturally acidic. When we use products like alkaline soaps or acidic toners, we temporarily upset the balance of the skin's pH. Most of the time that's okay, because healthy skin will quickly (within minutes) restore its own balance. As skin matures, however, getting back in balance may take longer.

Since skin has an acid pH, if you have normal or dry skin, it is best to choose a product that is similar in pH to the composition of your skin. Soap, by definition, has an alkaline pH. So if your skin is already dry, it is wise to steer clear of anything labeled "soap" because its alkaline pH will exacerbate the problem. Conversely, if you have oily skin, you *should* choose a soap to cleanse your face because it will help dry up some of the excess oil.

A product that is truly *soap* is made by combining an alkali (mineral salts) with a fat, usually vegetable oil, and water. Products like good old Ivory soap fall into this category, and sodium bicarbonate, listed on the ingredients, is a tip-off that a product will have an alkaline pH.

Detergent soaps are often called "soapless" soaps because they don't contain the mineral salts used in soap. Most people would probably cringe at the idea of using a detergent on their face, because they associate detergent with cleaning clothes and dishes, not their skin. Although detergents can be harsh, manufacturers can easily balance the pH of detergent soaps and add in some emollients to create mild products like Dove.

Most moisturizing beauty bars and liquid cleansers fall into the category of detergent soaps, and many of these market themselves as non-alkaline, which really means that they are pH-balanced and therefore, theoretically, less irritating. Two common detergent ingredients are sodium laurel sulfate and laureth 4. If you see those ingredients listed on a product's label, you'll know you're getting a product that is not likely to be too alkaline, although sodium laurel sulfate can be drying.

Many product lines now offer alpha hydroxy acid (AHA) *cleansers* to be used with the entire skin-care regimen. Most of the doctors I spoke with, however, say they are a waste of money because the acid is not on the skin long enough to exfoliate. A few doctors disagree, saying that even the minute or two of deep cleaning with an AHA product can be beneficial in loosening up dead cells.

Despite what the doctors say, I have used an AHA cleanser that I truly believe helped to exfoliate my skin. I really saw a difference.

RECOMMENDED CLEANSERS

Skin Type Key: N normal; D dry; VD very dry; C combination; S sensitive; R Renova, Retin-A; AR Acne Rosacea
Price Key: $ less than $5; $$ $5–$10; $$$ over $10

DRUGSTORE BRANDS

PRODUCT	SKIN TYPE	SIZE/FORM	PRICE
Alpha Hydrox Foaming Face Wash	all	6 oz	$$
Aqua Glycolic Facial Cleanser (12% AHA)	N/D	8 oz	$$$
Aquanil Cleanser	S/AR	8 or 16 oz	$$
Aveeno Cleansing Bar	O	bar	$

PRODUCT	SKIN TYPE	SIZE/FORM	PRICE
Basis Vitamin Bar	N/D/VD	bar	$
Basis Sensitive Skin	S/AR	bar	$
Basis Comforting Clean Face Wash	N/D	6 oz	$$
Cetaphil Cleanser	N/D/S	8 oz	$$
Cetaphil Gentle Cleansing Bar	N/D/S	4.5 oz	$
Dove Beauty Bar	N/C/S	bar	$
Ethocyn Skin Treatment Gel Cleanser	all	6.7 oz	$$$
Flori Roberts My Everything Treatment Foaming Gel Cleanser	N/D	6 oz	$
L'Oréal Plenitude Clarify A3 Facial Gel Foaming Cleanser	N/D	4 oz	$$
Lowila	N/C/S	bar	$
Lubriderm Body Bar	N/C/S	bar	$
Neutrogena	N/C/S	bar	$
Neutrogena Non-Drying Cleansing Lotion	D/S/R	5.5 oz	$
Neutrogena	D/S/O	4 oz	$
pHisoderm	O	4 oz	$
Pond's Cleansing Lotion & Moisturizer	N/D	7 oz	$$
Pond's Fresh Start Daily Wash	N/D	5 oz	$
Pond's Self-Foaming Facial Cleanser	all	4 oz	$$
Pond's Foaming Cleanser & Toner	all	7 oz	$$
Purpose	N/C/S	bar	$

DEPARTMENT STORE BRANDS

PRODUCT	SKIN TYPE	SIZE/FORM	PRICE
Borghese Gentle Makeup Remover	N/D	8.4 oz	$$$
M.A.C. Foaming Cleanser	N/VD	4 oz	$$$
Lancôme Ablutia Fraicheur Purifying Foaming Cleanser	N/D	6.8 oz	$$$
Shiseido Benefiance Creamy Cleansing Emulsion	D/VD	6.7 oz	$$$

SPECIALTY/SALON BRANDS

PRODUCT	SKIN TYPE	SIZE/FORM	PRICE
Hymed Liquid Soap*	S/AR	8 oz	$$$
Nova Skin Facial Cleanser*	all	8 oz	$$
Paul Mitchell White Oak Facial Cleanser	N/D	8 oz	$$
Redken One 2 One Oil Free Cleansing Gel	O	5 oz	$$
Sebastian Trucco Skin Basix—The Cleanser	N/D	5.7 oz	$$

*Only dispensed by physicians

TONERS

While most mature women would steer clear of something called an astringent—assigning it, rightfully, to oily-skinned teenagers—many women still use toners for that wonderful, tingly feeling or because the salesperson at the cosmetics counter sold it as part of the total package. The skin-care business is full of people who still subscribe to the very old notion that two products are needed to thoroughly clean the face. I understand salespeople wanting to sell more product and believing what their company training manuals tell them, but there are also plenty of others who should know better and still try to convince dry-skinned consumers that they need a toner. Not too long ago, an esthetician performing a facial on a colleague of mine insisted that toners were absolutely necessary for all skin types to restore the pH balance.

The fact of the matter is that toners are astringents and their job is to take oils and dirt off of your skin. And there's a place for that. If you have oily skin, by all means, use a toner to sweep away excess oil.

The problem is that almost every department store skin-care regimen will include a toner regardless of skin type. A toner will only tighten your skin by drying it and it absolutely will not shrink oil glands or decrease oil production. Despite what the esthetician had to say, it's just not necessary for most mature women.

In the last few years, cosmetics companies have changed their product lines to include toning *lotions*, alcohol-free preparations for dry or combination skin types. As the name lotion implies, these products are not as drying as their predecessors, but if you rinse your face thoroughly (fifteen splashes), there's no real need for this additional step in your routine or the added expense of another product.

That having been said, if you insist on using a toner, keep these things in mind:

- Most toners contain coal tar dyes that are not approved for use around the eyes because they can be comedogenic (acne inducing) and irritating. If you're using toner because your skin is oily, you should be steering clear of comedogenic ingredients anyway.
- Many toners contain camphor, menthol, sodium borate, and other ingredients that are irritating, very drying, and have no proven effect on acne breakouts. Some toners contain anti-acne ingredients and should be avoided if you're using a benzoyl peroxide medication.

- Retin-A users, especially, should avoid toners.
- Black women should avoid toners with resorcinol because it can leave a brownish scale to the skin.
- If you have dry skin, be sure to choose an alcohol-free toner.
- The least expensive, best, nonirritating, noncomedogenic toner you can use is plain old-fashioned witch hazel. But, even witch hazel is 17 percent alcohol, so I recommend cutting it with 50 percent rose water. If it makes you feel more pampered, pour it into an old bottle of the department store stuff.

TONERS/FRESHENERS

Skin Type Key: N normal; D dry; VD very dry; C combination; S sensitive
Price Key: $ under $10; $$ $11–$21; $$$ $21–$30; $$$$ $31–$40; $$$$$ over $40

PRODUCT	SKIN TYPE	ALCOHOL	SIZE (OZ)	PRICE
Lancôme Tonique Controle	O	yes	6.8	$$
Lancôme Tonique Respectee	N/C	no	6.8	$$
L'Oréal Plenitude Clarigy A-3	O	yes	8	$
M.A.C. Purifying Toner	N/C	no	4	$$
Physicians Formula Captyane Purifying Facial Toner	N/C	no	6	$
Physicians Formula Oil Control Conditioning Skin Toner	O	yes	8	$
The Body Shop Hydrating Freshener	N/D	no	6.7	$
The Body Shop Exfoliating Lotion	all	no	6.7	$
Nova Skin Oily Skin Toner* (12% glycolic acid)	O	yes	4	$$

*Only dispensed by physicians

EYE MAKEUP REMOVER

Your regular soap or cleanser is designed to remove makeup, but if you wear heavy eye makeup or waterproof mascara, it's a good idea to use an eye makeup remover before cleansing. What's more, if you use a facial cleansing product with an AHA, you should be careful to avoid the eye area when washing with that product. Be sure to read your cleanser's label, or, if you're using physician-dispensed products, ask your doctor if the cleanser will irritate your eyes.

If you use waterproof mascara or an AHA cleanser, you should consider eye makeup remover a beauty essential. Unfortunately many of these products sting the eyes, which is why many women avoid them. The products I've recommended here do not sting. They remove waterproof mascara very well without pulling out delicate eyelashes, and they actually leave lashes feeling soft. I know, because I tried them all personally.

EYE MAKEUP REMOVERS

Price Key: $ less than $5; $$ $5–$10; $$$ over $10

DEPARTMENT STORE BRANDS

PRODUCT	SIZE (OZ)	PRICE
Christian Dior Clear Eye Makeup Remover	2.5	$$
Clarins Gentle Eye Makeup Remover Lotion	4.4	$$
Clarins Gentle Eye Makeup Remover Cream Gel	2.7	$$
Clinique Extremely Gentle Eye Makeup Remover	2	$
Elizabeth Arden Conditioning Eye Makeup Remover	4	$$
Lancôme Bifacil Eye Makeup Remover	4	$$
M.A.C. Eye Makeup Remover	4	$$
Shiseido Absolute Eye Makeup Remover	1.7	$$

DRUGSTORE BRANDS

Almay Eye Makeup Remover Pads	60 pads	$
Maybelline Moisturizing Mascara Remover	2.3	$
Revlon 30-Second Eye Makeup Remover	2.0	$

MOISTURIZING

Next to sunscreen, moisturizer is probably the single most important product you can apply to your skin, and of course many of today's products include a sunscreen in their formulation. As with everything else, you needn't spend a fortune to buy a good moisturizer unless it is a product that you particularly like, that makes you feel good, or contains an AHA. Some of the simplest, least expensive ingredients like petrolatum, mineral oil, lanolin, glycerin, and urea are the basis for the best moisturizers.

The main function of moisturizer is to add moisture to the skin and keep it from evaporating. You can improve the quality of your skin by as much as 16 percent simply by moisturizing it. Many people mistakenly believe that the purpose of moisturizing is to add oil to the skin. Mineral oil and petrolatum are included in moisturizers to prevent evaporation of the skin's own moisture; other ingredients in the formulation are intended to add to the skin's moisture.

Today, moisturizers include any number of ingredients that supposedly nourish the skin, fight free radicals, and leap tall buildings at a single bound. Unfortunately, most of the ingredients' molecules are far too large to ever penetrate the skin and reach the dermis—the most any of them do is plump up the stratum corneum.

Even water can't penetrate the skin. If it could, we'd be like giant sponges in the bathtub. Keep that in mind when you're buying skin-care products. The skin is your body's natural barrier; it's not supposed to let anything in. So don't be fooled into buying some fancy collagen complex thinking that it will increase the collagen in your skin. Collagen is a good moisturizer, but it can't penetrate the epidermis to join its fellow collagen molecules in the dermis.

Moisturizers used to be the biggest thing in skin care, but now that alpha hydroxy acids have entered the scene in such a big way, it's difficult to separate the moisturizers from the wrinkle creams. In addition to exfoliating the skin, these acids are also excellent moisturizers and have been proven to help correct surface roughness, fine lines, and pigmentation problems. That's why I strongly recommend AHA products to everyone and if you use one that also includes a sunscreen, so much the better.

Even though I recommend AHA products to everyone, there are still plenty of women who have such sensitive skin that they can't tolerate even the mildest AHA products and others who don't want or feel they need them. In addition, AHA products should be used only as directed, which usually means one daily application before going to bed. Consequently a non-AHA cream or lotion is needed for daytime use. That skin-care strategy is exactly what Ponds had in mind with its two-in-one packaging of a day-and-night cream. The top part of the jar is a moisturizer/sunscreen cream and the bottom part of the jar is an AHA moisturizer. They're good products at a good value. (There's more on them in Chapter 4.)

Specific Moisturizing Needs

If you have dry skin, always, always, always use a moisturizer and apply it to damp skin. Most lotions work well, but in cold months, for example, and if your skin is extraordinarily dry, a cream may be better for you. Select a moisturizer with petrolatum or lanolin as these ingredients help reduce evaporation of the skin's own fluids. Also look for products with hyaluronic acid, which binds one thousand times its weight in water to the skin, and liposomes, which do penetrate the skin and help deliver moisture to the driest parts.

Oil-free moisturizers are made with silicone derivatives, and they're good, but not quite as good as simple mineral oil or petrolatum and should be saved for normal to oily skin.

If you have normal or combination skin, choose a light oil-free moisturizer that will seal in your own moisture without adding any unnecessary oils to your face. If your combination skin means you have an oily T-zone, don't apply moisturizer there. Again, look for hyaluronic acid, NaPCA, glycerin, and urea, all of which bind water to the skin.

If you have oily skin, skip the moisturizer.

Some women who are undergoing treatment for acne may experience dryness as a result of the medication, even though they have oily skin. If that's the case, try a little oil-free moisturizing lotion on those areas only and a little moisturizing eye cream if necessary.

Lotion or Cream?
Moisturizing lotions generally have more water than creams, and that's about the only difference. In fact, within a product line, the cream and lotions may contain identical ingredients, only the percentage of water makes them different. Especially in the summer months or in hot and sunny climates, lotion is often a better choice, even for mature skin. Creams are best reserved for the driest, most mature skin and for the coldest, driest seasons and climates. If you alternate between cream and lotion, depending on the season, you may want to buy only the cream and apply a small amount of it to a very wet face, so it feels more like lotion.

Whether you choose a cream or a lotion, always remember to moisturize your throat, neck, and chest since those areas are exposed to the elements almost as much as your face.

For the sake of simplicity, I've listed what I think are the best non-AHA moisturizers in this chapter and have listed the AHA products in Chapter 4.

MOISTURIZERS

Skin Type Key: N normal; D dry; VD very dry; C combination; S sensitive; R Renova, Retin-A

Price Key: $ under $10; $$ $11–$21; $$$ $21–$30; $$$$ $31–$40; $$$$$ over $40

DRUGSTORE BRANDS

PRODUCT	SKIN TYPE	SPF	SIZE (OZ)	PRICE
Almay Time-Off Age Smoothing Moisture Lotion	N/D	15	4	$
Alpha Hydrox Oil-Free Lotion	O		4	$
Alpha Hydrox Moisturizing Daily Lotion	N/D	15	4	$
Alpha Hydrox Night Replenishing Creme	N/D		2	$
Basis All Night Face Cream	N/D		4	$
Basis Face the Day Lotion	N/O		4	$
Eucerin Daily Facial Moisturizing Lotion	D/VD	25	4	$
L'Oréal Plenitude Excell-A3 Skin Revealing Lotion	N/D		2	$$
L'Oréal Plenitude Active Daily Moisture Lotion	N/D/O	15	4	$
Neutrogena Healthy Skin Face Lotion	N/D	15	2.5	$$
Neutrogena Healthy Skin Face Lotion without SPF	N/D		2.5	$$
Neutrogena Moisture Facial Moisturizer	S/R	15	4	$$
Neutrogena Light Night Cream	S/R		2.25	$$
Nivea Visage Optimale Cumulative Care Creme	D	6	1.7	$$
Oil of Olay Daily UV Protectant Beauty Fluid	N/D	15	5.35	$
Physicians Formula Vital Defense Moisture Concentrate	VD	15	2	$$
Revlon Results with alpha recap Rest & Renewal Night Cream Concentrate	N/D		2	$$
Revlon Results with alpha recap Daily Requirement Moisture Cream	N/D	8	2	$$
Revlon Results with alpha recap Day Light Replenisher Moisture Lotion	N/D	8	2	$$
St. Ives Collagen-Elastin Essential Moisturizer	D/VD		1.4	$
Sudden Change Liposome Action Facial Moisturizer	N/D		2	$

DEPARTMENT STORE BRANDS

PRODUCT	SKIN TYPE	SPF	SIZE (OZ)	PRICE
Bobbi Brown Essentials Face Cream	N/D		2.2	$$$$
Chanel Day Lift Plus Multi-Hydroxy Refining Lotion	N/D	8	1	$$$$$
Christian Dior Capture Rides Multi-Action Wrinkle Creme	N/D	8	1	$$$
Clarins Double Serum Total Skin Supplement	VD		.5	$$$$$
Clarins Multi-Active Night Lotion	D		1.7	$$$$
Estee Lauder 100% Time Release Moisturizer	N/D		1.7	$$$$
Flori Roberts My Everything Treatment Revitalized Protection Moisturizer	N/D		4	$$
Iman All Day Moisture Complex	N/D		3	$$
Iman Night Time Complex Oil-Free Moisturizer	O		1.8	$$
Iman PM Renewal Cream	N/D		1.8	$$
Iman Oil Free Advanced Moisture Complex	O		3	$$
Lancôme Bienfait Total Well-Being Day Creme Hydration Radiance	N/D	15	1.7	$$$$
Lancôme Bienfait Total Well-Being Day Fluide Hydration Radiance	N/D/O	15	1.7	$$$
M.A.C. EP-2 Day Emulsion	N		2	$$$
M.A.C. CR-2 Night Emulsion	N/O		2	$$$$
Monteil Skin Reform Fluid Energizer	O		6.7	$$$
Prescriptives All You Need for Oily Skin	O		1.7	$$$$
Princess Marcella Borghese Cura Forte Moisture Intensifier	D/VD		1	$$$$
Shiseido Benefiance Revitalizing Emulsion	VD		2.5	$$$$

HOME SALES/SALON BRANDS

PRODUCT	SKIN TYPE	SPF	SIZE (OZ)	PRICE
Mary Kay Nighttime Recovery System	VD		2.8	$$$
Matrix Age Recovery Alpha Renewal Lotion	C/O	8	1	$$$$
Matrix Hydrating Lotion	O		2	$$$
Matrix Regenerating Skin Supplement	all	8	1	$$$$
NuSkin MHA Revitalizing Lotion with SPF	N/D	15	1	$$
NuSkin MHA Revitalizing Lotion	N/D		1	$$
Paul Mitchell Night Moisturizer	D		1	$$
Sebastian Trucco Skin Basix—The Moisturizer	N/D/O		2.1	$$

PROTECTION

Protecting the skin from the sun will help keep the years from showing on your face and if you don't believe me, compare the skin on your derriere with the skin on your face or forearms. There's a reason why your posterior is smoother, more supple, and more evenly pigmented. Unless you've been sunbathing in the nude, this area of your body doesn't often see the light of day.

Even though Caucasians are twenty times more likely to develop skin cancer than Blacks, that doesn't mean that black or darkly pigmented women can sunbathe freely. The sun still dries up dark skin, causing it to look weathered, so you should protect it with sunscreen to keep yourself from becoming a victim of skin cancer.

TWO FOR THE PRICE OF ONE: MOISTURIZERS WITH SUNSCREEN

Many moisturizers today have sunscreen in them and the SPF is usually clearly listed on the front of the package. Sometimes a product will claim to prevent the signs of aging—that's also an indication that the product has sunscreen in it.

Because sunscreen is so important to good skin care, I strongly recommend buying a moisturizer with a sunscreen in it, particularly if you live in Florida, Arizona, Southern California, or other hot, sunny locations. These products save time and money and you don't have to remember to apply a separate sunscreen because it's already there. Unfortunately, many of the moisturizers with sunscreen only have an SPF of 8, so you may want to supplement the sun protection.

Certainly you don't need a sunscreen at bedtime, but if you don't want to spend the extra money for a separate night cream, using a moisturizer with sunscreen won't hurt. (Please see Chapter 3 for more information on sunscreens and sun protection.)

EXFOLIATION

Mechanical or chemical, exfoliation is the removal of dead cells from the surface of the skin. Without the benefit of a loofah sponge, buff puff, or exfoliating acid, dead cells build up on the skin's surface, leaving it looking dull and lifeless.

Many older women have relied on any number of scrub products to give skin that bright, polished look, but today, alpha hydroxy acids have taken over as more effective exfoliators that actually help to thicken the skin by increasing collagen in a way that scrubbing never will.

In addition, many women scrub their faces like they're scrubbing pots and pans and they leave behind reddened skin and broken capillaries. That's why I recommend that older women stick with the alpha hydroxy acid products that are discussed at length in the next chapter.

If you really like the feel of an occasional scrub and you promise to be gentle, go for it, but no more than once a week and don't use your acid product for at least twenty-four hours after the scrub. Rinse well and apply a nonacid moisturizer afterwards.

Women with acne should avoid scrubs on their sensitive skin.

OTHER TREATMENTS
Masks
There are a variety of masks marketed today that promise to "remove impurities," or provide "deep cleansing," exfoliating, or hydrating effects. While masks are nice for enforced relaxation—you can't run errands with egg white or green clay on your face—they are certainly not a necessity. If you like the relaxation of a mask, keep these things in mind.

Elaine's Exclusive

DRY SKIN MASK FOR PENNIES

- *Beat 1 egg yolk with 1 tablespoon cod liver oil and 1 tablespoon honey.*
- *Using a small clean pastry brush, apply to clean skin, avoiding eye area.*
- *Leave on for 15 minutes.*
- *Rinse with tepid water.*
- *Moisturize over damp skin.*

For the most part, clay masks are great for oily skin because they really do help unclog pores and pull excess oil out of the skin. Most older women, however, should stay away from clay masks for just that reason—they pull oil out of the skin. If you have combination skin, use the clay mask only on the oily areas. Since clay is clay no matter where it comes from, don't bother spending big bucks for "Cassius" clay or whatever else the cosmetics companies dream up to separate you from your money.

Hydrating masks are another story because they can provide a nice boost to the skin. There is, however a certain amount of pulling and stretching associated with any mask that just isn't necessary for mature skin. All of that action on your face can cause capillaries to break. There are plenty of other ways to exfoliate or moisturize your skin, so why take unnecessary risks with your face?

If you have dry skin, choose a hydrating or moisturizing mask containing glycerin, amino acids, and oils. Some of the newer masks also contain clay (listed in the ingredients as kaolin), herbs, and AHAs for exfoliation. St. Ives makes the best mask I've ever used and it is the least expensive product on the market. Avoid clay masks with alcohol or witch hazel—those products are only for oily skin.

Regardless of your skin type, don't use a mask more than once a week and certainly not after or before a scrub.

HYDRATING MASKS

Skin Type Key: N normal; D dry; VD very dry; C combination; S sensitive; R Renova, Retin-A
Price Key: $ under $10; $$ $11–$21; $$$ $21–$30; $$$$ $31–$40; $$$$$ over $40

PRODUCT	SKIN TYPE	SIZE (OZ)	PRICE
Alpha Hydrox Purifying Clay Masque	N/D	4	$
M.A.C. VM-2 Hydrating Mask	N/D	2	$
The Body Shop Intense Moisture Mask	N/D	3.38	$
St. Ives Firming Masque	N/D	5	$

Eye Cream and Eye Gel

Because your skin is thinnest around your eyes, there are some special skin-care challenges that occur in that area, including dryness, puffiness, dark circles, bags, and crow's-feet. Before shopping for an eye cream or gel, you need to identify your problem because all dark circles and bags are not created equal.

Dr. Draelos explains, "dark circles are usually pigmentation. If your circles are brown, they are caused by pigmentation, which is heredi-tary and that means your best bet is a good concealer. Laser work is not particularly helpful and hydroquinone fade creams tend to work only if the circles are caused by sun damage."

If your circles are purple, however, they're probably from broken blood vessels. Essentially they are a bruise and may be helped by a vit-amin product like the one developed by Dr. Melvin Elson, medical director of the Dermatology Center in Nashville. His eye cream con-tains vitamin K, which helps strengthen the blood vessels, and vita-min C, which helps stimulate collagen production.

Still other circles are shadows caused by the architecture of the face. Those are the dark rings normally seen around deep-set eyes. In that case, again, makeup is the best solution.

Circles are also caused by fat deposits in the eyelids and your skin's natural melanin. It's important to note that stress can have an impact on melanin production, which may explain why dark circles can be more apparent during stressful times in your life.

Because the skin is thinnest around the eyes, sometimes the dark-ness you see is actually your facial muscles, says Dr. Elson. "As skin gets more sun damaged, it gets thinner, and as we get older gravity starts pulling that tender skin toward the cheek. Often what you're actually seeing is muscle through the skin." In this case, a product that con-tains an AHA or vitamin C, which will help build collagen, may be your best bet for crepiness and dark circles.

Other eye products are designed to reduce puffiness through the use of plant extracts like comfrey, marigold, and chamomile, which have dehydrating effects on the skin. Other products have moisturiz-ers to soften the skin and reduce the appearance of crow's-feet and tiny wrinkles. Clearly, it would not do you any good to buy a cream that's formulated to reduce puffiness if your eye area is too dry, so read the label.

NeoStrata's Exuviance eye cream is the first to include an acid, gluconolactone, which is a poly hydroxy acid, not an alpha hydroxy acid. It acts like an AHA, but is not irritating.

Before you spend extra money on an eye cream or eye gel, be sure to identify your problem correctly.

EYE CREAMS AND GELS

Price Key: $ under $10; $$ $11–$21; $$$ $21–$30; $$$$ $31–$40; $$$$$ over $40

DRUGSTORE BRANDS

PRODUCT	SIZE (OZ)	PRICE
Alpha Hydrox Hydrating Eye Gel	.5	$
Ethocyn Skin Treatment Eye Cream	.5	$$$
L'Oréal Plenitude Eye Defense Gel Cream with liposomes	.5	$$
Neutrogena Intensified Eye Moisture	.5	$
Nivea Visage Optimale Eye Cream (SPF 6)	.5	$
Oil of Olay Revitalizing Eye Gel	.5	$$
Revlon Results with Alpha Recap Brighten-Up Eye Cream	.75	$$

DEPARTMENT STORE BRANDS

PRODUCT	SIZE (OZ)	PRICE
Chanel Creme-Gel Firming Eye Cream	.5	$$$$$
Christian Dior Capture for Eyes	.5	$$$
Estee Lauder Resilience Eye Creme	.5	$$$$$
Lancôme Renergie Specific Anti-Wrinkle and Firming Eye Creme	.5	$$$
M.A.C. EZR Day/Night Emulsion Eye Zone Remoisturizer	1	$$$$
Monteil Activance Energy Concentrate for Eyes	.5	$$$
Prescriptives Px Eye Specialist	.5	$$$$

HOME SALES/SALONS/SPECIALTY ITEMS

PRODUCT	SIZE (OZ)	PRICE
Aveda Botanical Kinetics Pure Vital Moisture Eye Creme	.5	$$$
Avon Lighten Up Eye Cream	.5	$$
Avon Anew Perfect Eye Care Cream (SPF15)	.5	$$
Matrix Nourissa Age-Defying Eye Creme	.5	$$
Mary Kay Triple-Action Eye Enhancer	.5	$$
Nova Skin Smoothing Eye Cream*	.5	$$
Sebastian Trucco Skin Basix The Eye Cream	.5	$$

*Only dispensed by physicians

Elaine's Exclusive

7 SIMPLE STEPS FOR SUPER SKIN

1. Use a mild cleanser that can be rinsed off with water.
2. Splash your face fifteen to twenty times with *tepid* water to remove all cleanser residue. (Hot water can dry the skin.)
3. Only use a toner on oily areas.
4. Use an alpha hydroxy acid moisturizer instead of a scrub.
5. Apply sunscreen, unless it is included in your moisturizer.
6. Use products that are appropriate for the climate and season. (Creams in cold/winter, lotions in hot/summer.)
7. Choose products formulated for special needs. Allergic? Avoid fragrance and lanolin. Using Retin-A or Renova? Sunscreen is a must.

ENVIRONMENT AND LIFESTYLE

Environment and lifestyle play a big part in skin care. Whether you spend most of your time indoors or out, how much stress you endure, whether or not you smoke or drink alcohol, if you maintain a consistent and appropriate weight, how much exercise you get, and much more determine, in great part, how good your skin looks.

"If skin is healthy it will look good," says Dr. Lupo. "Healthfulness is key. Just as you can't be in shape by simply dieting, you can't expect to have good skin just by using the right products. It's more important avoiding things that are bad for you and doing things that are good for your skin."

First and foremost, she encourages patients to avoid the sun and use proper protection when the sun can't be avoided. Quitting smoking is second on her list, followed by sleeping on your back.

"Don't sleep on your face because it impedes circulation and that's when your skin has a chance to breathe—your pores aren't clogged, there's no makeup, and your body is recovering from the day. Try sleeping on two or three pillows, and put pillows under each arm. Plant yourself into the bed so you can't flip over. Sleeping on your face is one of the most physical, bad things you can do for your skin."

If you avoid the sun, don't smoke, and sleep on your back, she believes you'll look ten years younger than your contemporaries who sunbathe, smoke, and sleep on their faces.

The Sun
There's so much to say about the damaging effects of the sun on your skin and yet, many of us still love nothing more than lazing by the pool or at the beach. There's so much you should know about protecting yourself from the sun and its harmful rays, that Chapter 3 focuses exclusively on the sun and its effects. Nothing damages the skin more over a lifetime than exposure to the sun. It's that simple. And the more you do to protect your skin from the sun's drying rays, the smoother and less wrinkled you are likely to be as you grow older.

Pollution
While researching this book, I went for an acid peel to see what it was like. I was advised to cleanse in the morning, but not to apply any moisturizer or makeup. When I got to the doctor's office, and she cleansed my face again, I was amazed by how dirty the cotton balls became. I had only been outside between my house and the car, and the car to the doctor's office — and I don't even live in a city! Just imagine how much pollution accumulates on your skin over the course of a day.

But, since no one is likely to relocate for the sake of their skin, I'd simply caution you to be particularly diligent about cleansing your skin no matter where you live, but especially if you live in a city or other highly polluted area.

Smoking
Tobacco companies still try to glamorize smoking as something chic or sexy, but there's nothing less attractive than a cigarette dangling out of someone's mouth. Aesthetics aside, if the threat of lung cancer and heart disease aren't enough to get you to quit smoking, add the promise of extra wrinkles to the list of good reasons to kick the habit. Smoking harms your skin in several ways.

- *First*, nicotine depletes the amount of oxygen flowing through your blood and to your skin.

- *Second,* because of the puffing and squinting involved in smoking, smokers tend to develop more laugh lines and an accordion-pleated upper lip.
- *Third,* collagen, which is the main component of the dermis, requires vitamin C to synthesize. Smoking depletes vitamin C to such an extent that smokers need 50 percent more vitamin C than nonsmokers, just to stay even.
- *Fourth,* smoking decreases estrogen levels, which also damages collagen.
- *Fifth,* smoke in the air accumulates in your hair and on your skin, which dulls the shine and smells bad.

Diet

Dramatic weight gain or loss causes the skin to stretch out of proportion and can cause stretch marks. Furthermore, your skin needs proper fluids, vitamins, and minerals to rebuild itself and stay moist. While it is a myth that chocolate and fatty foods *cause* pimples, these things can *aggravate* acne in some people. Eat a well-balanced, low-fat diet, but make sure it's *low* fat, not no fat. A healthy complexion needs some essential fatty acids (EFAs) to prevent parching, cracking, and scaling. Some research has linked a low-fat diet to a lessened likelihood of age spots. Older people, in particular, tend to run the risk of skin problems because of spartan, low-fat diets. See further in this chapter for more on xerosis and other skin conditions.

Climate

Seasons and geography should be factored in to your skin-care plans because temperature, elevation, and humidity all affect your skin.

Cold climates and winter months: These rob your skin of its own natural moisture, so it's wise to take extra precautions. Use a cream moisturizer that contains lanolin or petrolatum to help prevent evaporation. Regardless of your skin type, try working a little moisturizer into your foundation for some extra protection.

Shield your face from the skin-chapping wind by wearing a silk, not a woolen scarf. (Silk is less abrasive on your skin and holds in your own warmth.)

Hot climates and summer months: Sunscreen and a wide-brimmed hat should be the most important part of your skin-care ritual during the summer or if you live in places like Florida, Southern California, or Arizona. Like the American Express commercial says—don't leave home without them.

Switch to a moisturizing lotion in the summer or apply a small amount of cream to a very damp face to get the same results.

Because even the driest skin can become a little moist in the heat and humidity of summer, try blending a little bit of translucent powder into your foundation. It will make the foundation a little lighter, and the powder is absorbent.

Also, be sure to drink plenty of water. It's important for your overall health and your skin needs to constantly replace the moisture that is naturally evaporated from your skin.

Rainy climates and cloudy days: Whether you live in jolly old England or the Pacific Northwest, don't let the endless dreary days fool you into thinking you can skimp on the sunscreen. Harmful rays sneak through the clouds and can still do cumulative damage to your skin.

The moistness in the air can be great for your skin, enabling women with dry skin to use a lotion instead of cream, and allowing normal skin to remain normal without the benefit of moisturizer. But, if you spend most of your time indoors with the heat on, it's best to stick to the usual routine.

High altitudes: The air "up there" can be especially drying to your skin. From Denver to the desert, women who live in high altitudes often complain that their skin feels taut or parched. That's the same sensation many people experience after being on an airplane. Misting can help relieve the feeling temporarily and keeping a humidifier going in the home and office is also helpful.

COMMON SKIN CONDITIONS

Aging skin isn't the only thing mature women have to contend with. I've listed below some of the more common skin problems that adult women sometimes face.

Elaine's Exclusive

SKIN CARE TO-DO LIST

- *Do cleanse thoroughly every night. In the morning, a few splashes with tepid water are all that is needed.*
- *Do use as few products as possible in your skin-care regimen.*
- *Do choose a moisturizer with a sunscreen and some kind of AHA.*
- *Do wait twenty-four hours after using a facial scrub before applying an AHA.*
- *Do select products that are vitamin-enriched.*
- *Do be gentle with your skin.*
- *Do keep your hands off your face.*
- *Do avoid pinched or frowning expressions.*
- *Do drink plenty of water.*
- *Do quit smoking.*
- *Do exercise.*
- *Do enjoy a glass of wine, if you drink alcohol, but avoid overindulging.*
- *Do take warm showers and wash your face with tepid water. Cooler temperatures clean just as well as hot water without the drying effects.*
- *Do be realistic about what you expect from skin-care products.*

Rosacea

Rosacea is often called "adult acne." It is very common among individuals in their thirties and forties and is sometimes mistaken as simple skin sensitivity. Typically, rosacea is characterized by dilated blood vessels on the nose, cheeks, and chin, causing a harsh but "rosy" look to the face, and little red and white bumps that look like cysts, which is why some people think of it as acne. Stress, hormones, physical exertion, alcohol, caffeine, hot and cold beverages, blasts of heat, and infections can cause rosacea to flare up, but no one knows for sure what causes it, although it is most common in fair-skinned people of Celtic origin.

A dermatologist can prescribe any number of remedies, including

Hymed products, formulated especially for sensitive or problem skin, and oral medications, to soothe the symptoms of rosacea. Lasers are also being used to treat the dilated blood vessels. For mild cases, cool milk or chamomile tea compresses may provide some comfort. Typically the condition will gradually fade away, but it often takes five to ten years to do so.

If you have chronic red spots that seem like a simple irritation, first, be careful not to irritate the area further, and, second, see a dermatologist for a proper diagnosis. If it turns out that you have rosacea, be careful not to irritate your skin by overcleansing, scrubbing, or having a salon facial that involves pinching and squeezing pores.

Acne

While many of us assumed that one of the benefits of growing older would be growing out of acne, the sad truth is that's not always the case. Hormones as well as stress contribute to two of the more common forms of systemic acne and just as our teen years were full of raging hormones, menopause and postpartum hormonal fluctuations can cause skin to erupt all over again. Although acne at any age can be disturbing, keep in mind that you are particularly sensitive to it and it usually appears worse to you than to anyone else.

Most simply, acne is a hair follicle or pore that has become clogged with sebum (oil from beneath the dermis), dead skin cells, and bacteria. Most lesions fall into the whitehead or blackhead categories and, contrary to what many people think, blackheads are not black because of dirt, but due to melanin in your skin.

For your reference, here are the kinds of acne you may still encounter even as an adult.

COMMON ACNE This is the adolescent type of acne that can still flare up in your thirties and forties even if you never had an outbreak as a teenager. For an occasional, mild breakout, try an over-the-counter benzoyl peroxide preparation. For regularly occurring, more severe acne, a dermatologist can prescribe topical (Retin-A) or oral (tetracycline or Accutane) medications.

If you choose to treat acne yourself, be sure to wait at least thirty minutes after cleansing your face to apply a benzoyl peroxide pimple cream. Also, if you are using benzoyl peroxide products, check your other skin-care products and avoid anything with salicylic acid or resorcinol. The combination can be very irritating.

COSMETIC ACNE As its name suggests, cosmetic acne (acne cosmetica) describes breakouts caused by cosmetics and skin-care products. Whenever possible, select products that are labeled noncomedogenic or non-acnegenic. Even a woman with dry skin can experience acne cosmetica if she's using heavy, creamy cleansers or heavy moisturizers.

Sometimes the most troublesome thing about acne cosmetica is isolating the offending product, which is why it's a good idea to introduce only one new product at a time to your skin-care and makeup routines. When all else fails, pack up all of your cosmetics and take them to your dermatologist. He or she may be able to identify the culprit by reading the ingredients.

DRUG ACNE Also known as chemical acne, these flare-ups can be caused by any number of chemicals, including steroids like cortisone and medications like danazol, lithium carbonate, phenobarbitol, and dilantin. Even marijuana has been implicated in causing drug acne. Iodine is a well-known culprit, so be aware of foods that are high in iodine, including salty foods, shellfish, and beef liver. The normal use of table salt should not put enough iodine in your diet to cause a flare-up, but be sure to check your multivitamin for extra iodine.

OTHER ACNES Tropical acne is acne triggered by tropical climates, just as sun-related acne can crop up due to exposure to the sun. Industrial acne can be caused by exposure to industrial compounds like insoluble cutting oils and coal tar derivatives. Acne mechanica is a kind of acne caused by repeated rubbing against the skin. Belts, straps, even eyeglasses, can cause acne mechanica.

RETIN-A THERAPY FOR ACNE While most older women know Retin-A as a wrinkle remover, its initial and approved purpose is to fight acne. Although your doctor will tell you, as will your prescription package inserts, it bears repeating: Always wear a noncomedogenic sunscreen with at least SPF 15 when using Retin-A. Better yet, stay out of the sun altogether.

DOS AND DON'TS FOR ACNE-PRONE SKIN
- **Don't overcleanse. This can further irritate your skin.**
- **Don't use a scrub unless prescribed by your doctor. They'll do little to unclog acne-clogged pores and may cause additional irritation.**

- Do use a toner, but watch out for salicylic acid if you're using a benzoyl peroxide medication.
- Don't pick at blackheads or whiteheads.
- Do use an oil-free moisturizer if the benzoyl peroxide dries you up too much, but only apply it to dry areas.
- Do be especially careful about self-treating acne if you are Black. Benzoyl peroxide can darken skin and Retin-A, a commonly prescribed acne treatment, can lighten skin— so don't use a friend's prescription. Try a 2.5 percent benzoyl peroxide solution first. Don't jump right in with a 5 or 10 percent preparation.

Xerosis

Older men and women experience xerosis, or extremely dehydrated skin that is characterized by flaking, scaling, itchiness, and redness. Older people who eat very little because they lack an appetite, and who try to stick to a low-fat diet because of heart conditions, often turn up with this skin problem, especially on their arms and legs. Adding fat to the diet and taking quick, tepid showers instead of hot showers or baths can help tremendously. Lactic acid-based moisturizers like Lac-Hydrin or Lacticare and Cetaphil cleanser will also help, while a mild cortisone ointment can help with the itchiness.

Seborrheic Dermatitis

A red, scaly, itchy rash on the neck, back, chest, scalp, or in the smile area between the eyes is a characteristic of this usually hereditary condition. Those who had oily skin as teenagers are most likely to turn up with this problem, which is worsened by stress and often associated with parkinsonism. The condition is easily treated with topical ointments, but cannot be cured.

Keratosis

Keratosis is a skin growth that is normally seen in elderly people and is usually caused by the overproduction of keratin, a main skin protein.

ACTINIC KERATOSES These red, scaly growths are seen only on sun-exposed areas and are usually precancerous. Don't fool around with this kind of a lesion. Seek medical advice immediately.

SEBORRHEIC KERATOSES Although unsightly, these seborrheic warts are completely harmless. They tend to be flat, dark brown, and sometimes covered with a greasy, removable crust. They normally develop on the body. These "warts" can be removed through cryosurgery, chemical treatment, or laser treatment.

SOLAR KERATOSES Small, red, or flesh-colored wartlike bumps appear on sun-exposed areas (arms and head) as a result of cumulative sun exposure. They occasionally develop into a squamous cell carcinoma, so they should be removed, usually through cryosurgery.

Skin Tags

For reasons no one seems to know, tiny, but sometimes unsightly, pouches of flesh-tone or slightly pigmented skin sometimes sprout out on the face and body, usually on areas that are exposed to the sun, but also under the arms and breasts, too. Although unsightly, skin tags are usually harmless, but they can interfere with routine grooming like underarm shaving. Skin tags are common among pregnant and postmenopausal women and those with diabetes.

Skin tags can be zapped with an electrical current, or frozen off. Some people have been known to tie a thread around them and cut off their circulation, although I wouldn't recommend that particular method. A dermatologist can also snip them off. While the electrodessication will hurt a little, cryosurgery tends to leave behind a tiny white mark which, depending on your skin color, could be worse than the skin tag.

Age Spots

After years of sun exposure, brown spots, sometimes called liver spots or more properly known as solar lentigines, tend to appear, particularly on the head, face, and hands. While they are harmless, they are part of the reason that the hands give away the secrets of even the most ageless women.

If the spots pop up from nowhere, change shape, become raised, or bleed, be sure to have a physician check that they are not an early form of skin cancer. If they are not cancerous, count your blessings, because you now have any number of remedies to get those telltale spots to fade from sight.

Lasers are the latest weapon against age spots, but you may first want to try a fade cream with hydroquinone, Retin-A, or Renova since any of these remedies will be less expensive than a laser treatment. Doctors can also freeze the spots off or use trichloroacetic acid (TCA) to treat them. Freezing and TCA can, however, leave white spots in their place.

SKIN CARE FOR CANCER PATIENTS

When the doctor confirms that you have cancer, skin care may not be the foremost among your concerns, but once the chemotherapy and radiation begin, and your hair falls out and your skin dries up, it quickly moves higher on the list of priorities.

Chemotherapy is poison designed to kill cancer cells, but it also affects the rest of your body, including sweat glands and hair follicles, causing skin dryness and hair loss.

A good moisturizer will help ease the dryness, flaking, and itchiness associated with cancer treatment and you can safely use your usual skin-care products so there is no medical reason to buy any special skin-care products. If your therapy leaves you especially dry, you may want to ask your doctor to prescribe Lac-Hydrin, which is a well-formulated, 12-percent lactic acid moisturizer used for patients with the driest skin, or treat yourself to something special, just for the pampering.

SKIN-CARE INGREDIENTS

Just as you read food labels to compare products and find out how much fat, salt, and fiber are in a particular product, so too should you read the labels of your skin-care products. Whether you're checking out the advertising claims on the front of the package or the ingredient list on the back, you almost need a scientific encyclopedia to sift through the unpronounceable ingredients listed on any given product.

Alpha Hydroxy Acids

This is the generic term for lactic, malic, and glycolic acids. These acids are compounds derived from natural ingredients like grapes, mangoes, apples, sour milk, sugar, and citrus fruits. They are used in skin-care products for three reasons: They are natural exfoliants, they are good moisturizers, and they help thicken the skin. Products that claim to reduce fine lines, or restore youthful skin, usually contain some concentration of alpha hydroxy acid.

Amino Acids

Amino acids are the primary components of protein and are used in cosmetics in an effort to nourish the skin. Although topically applied amino acids probably don't help rebuild the skin's substructure because they cannot penetrate the skin, they do help the surface cells retain moisture and give them a nice, plumped-up look.

Collagen

Collagen is the basis of the dermis and is an excellent topical moisturizer, but that's all. Applied as a cream or lotion, collagen cannot penetrate the skin because the molecule is too large. It has no long-term effect on your skin's structure, and certainly cannot diminish the look of wrinkles unless it is injected.

Elastin

Like collagen, elastin is a protein found in the body. It is a good moisturizer but, also like collagen, it cannot penetrate the skin to provide any significant benefit to the dermis.

Enzymes

Different enzymes do different things including exfoliate, protect against sun damage, metabolize fat, build collagen and elastin, break down collagen and elastin, and lots more. Chemists are busy adding enzymes to products and trying to keep them stable and active so that they actually work. Look for a big burst of products with enzymes in the near future.

Esters

There are more than a dozen esters used in skin-care products. These ingredients often sound like forms of alcohol, which they are — esters are formed when an organic acid combines with alcohol. They are often included in skin-care products because they aid the skin in absorbing creams and lotions. Some commonly used esters are isopropyl myristate, spermaceti, octyl palmitate, isodecyl neopentanoate, butyl stearate, and isopropyl isostearate.

Lipids

Lipids are oils, including cholesterol, glycolipids, phospholipids, and free fatty acids that occur naturally on the epidermis. Many

skin-care products include lipids because they are excellent moisturizers.

Liposomes/Niosomes

Liposomes and niosomes are technically not ingredients at all—they're
a delivery system—tiny, hollow lipid spheres, to be precise, although
you'd be hard-pressed to know that by reading a product label. Liposomes and niosomes are capsules, like the tubes at the bank's drive-
thru window, that deliver moisturizing ingredients to the skin.

Mucopolysaccharides

Certain compounds that are found in the dermis are called
mucopolysaccharides. The most common is hyaluronic acid, which
binds a thousand times its weight in water to the skin. Many skin-care
products, from the outrageously expensive prestige lines to the least
expensive drugstore brands, include hyaluronic acid or chondroitin
sulfates because they are good moisturizers.

Hyaluronic acid is beginning to get media attention because it is
such a beneficial ingredient, and I suspect that we will soon see companies promoting the inclusion of this compound in their products'
formulations. Mucopolysaccharides are considered natural moisturizing factors (NMF) because they occur naturally in the skin.

Silicones: Dimethicone and Cyclomethicone

As in car wax, silicones in skin-care products provide a seal on the
skin to keep moisture in and pollutants out. When a moisturizer, for
example, claims to be oil-free, it usually contains one of these ingredients. The substances are slick, and trap moisture in the skin like mineral oil and petrolatum do, but they are not oils and are therefore
better for oily or sensitive skin that might react to lanolin, mineral oil,
or petrolatum.

Thymus Extracts

According to cosmetics companies, the thymus glands of some animals can stimulate cell renewal and may have some benefit to the
skin. Although independent studies have not confirmed this, it's hard
to imagine a company seeking out animal glands for skin-care products unless they were pretty convinced that it worked.

Water

Although it may seem silly to mention, water is usually the number one ingredient in skin-care products, because replacing moisture is one of the main goals in skin care.

Emollients

Emollients are ingredients that trap moisture in the skin and are included in any skin-care products made for normal to dry skin.

LANOLIN Derived from sheep's wool, lanolin is chemically very close to sebum, the skin's natural oil, and is very effective at preventing moisture loss—that's why it's included in so many products. Unfortunately, lanolin can be comedogenic and irritating to some women. If you're not sure and you have sensitive or acne-prone skin, you may want to avoid products containing lanolin of any kind. Otherwise, it's a great ingredient.

MINERAL OIL Simple mineral oil is less sensitizing than lanolin and hardly comedogenic. It's pretty good as an occlusive agent as well, although not as good as petrolatum or lanolin. Because it's inexpensive, not as sticky as petrolatum, and not as sensitizing as lanolin, many of the skin-care products made still include some mineral oil.

PETROLATUM Probably the most effective, least irritating product in skin care is good old petrolatum—petroleum jelly, also known by it's brand name, Vaseline. Petrolatum is the best occlusive agent, which means it prevents evaporation of the skin's own moisture and it helps to moisturize as well. Although it's normally associated with the thick stickiness of pure petroleum jelly and reserved for chapped lips in wintertime, a great many quality products contain petrolatum and there's nothing sticky about them.

SQUALANE This is a common emollient.

Humectants

Humectants are compounds that attract moisture to the skin. They are also included in most products for normal to dry skin because of their ability to pull moisture from the atmosphere to the skin. If you're in an unusually dry atmosphere—desert, high altitude, airplane, etc.—you may want to avoid products with a lot of humectants because they will begin drawing moisture from your skin when there is none in the atmosphere.

GLYCERIN The most common humectant, glycerin is found in almost every moisturizer.

NAPCA *Sodium pyrrolidone carboxylate* is a giant name for another NMF that is found in many products.

PROPYLENE GLYCOL Another commonly included humectant, propylene glycol has been cited as an allergen by some women. Most often, the women who experience irritation live in very dry areas where the propylene glycol begins to steal moisture from the skin. At low levels, propylene glycol is not likely to be irritating and since it helps facilitate the penetration of other ingredients, it's often found at the end of the ingredient list even for sensitive skin products.

UREA Many products include urea because it is not only an effective humectant, but it also softens the skin and is nongreasy. It is considered an NMF because it is found naturally in the body. Yes, urea is found in human urine, but cosmetics companies have a more hygienic way of obtaining it.

Moisturizing Agents

ALLANTOIN Allantoin is a nonirritating skin softener, used in many products for sensitive skin because it seems to weaken the effects of some ingredients that are skin sensitizers. It was originally used for wound treatment because of its healing and soothing properties.

ALOE The aloe vera plant secretes two different substances, but the one used in skin-care products is a clear, gelatinous substance that is loaded with mucopolysaccharides, enzymes, minerals, and amino acids. While there are numerous claims made about the beneficial properties of aloe, one thing is for sure: It's a good moisturizer. It may also soothe burns and inflammation, and undiluted may be helpful in treating liver spots. Used continuously, it may also increase the level of soluble collagen in the skin. All of these benefits aside, aloe is a common allergen, so if you have sensitive skin, read your labels.

FATTY ALCOHOLS By definition, these ingredients do not have the drying properties of other alcohols found in oily-skin formulations. They include stearyl, cetyl, and myristyl alcohol.

JOJOBA OIL Jojoba is another plant extract with excellent moisturizing properties, and it is not comedogenic, making it even more valuable to skin-care manufacturers. Companies are still working with jojoba (pronounced *ho ho ba*) to see if it has any function in oily-skin products.

TRIGLYCERIDES This is the catchall name for a number of oils commonly used in skin-care products. Some of the oils that are considered to be triglycerides are: apricot kernel oil, avocado oil, castor oil, cocoa butter, coconut oil, corn oil, grape seed oil, soybean oil, mink oil, olive oil, sesame oil, sea butter, sweet almond oil, wheat germ oil, and peach kernel oil.

VITAMINS

Every time you turn around there's another magazine or newspaper article about vitamins, especially antioxidants. While the research is just starting to deliver meaningful results, I think that it's going to be a long time before we stop hearing news about vitamins as cancer-fighters, life-extenders, and wrinkle-removers. If you've been bombarded with the lingo, but haven't taken the time to figure out what all of the fuss is about, read on. The science of skin care is really fascinating.

When your car gets old and the protective paint and wax chip away, oxygen begins to oxidize the metal. It's known as rusting. When your body is exposed to unstable molecules caused by smoke, pollution, and a number of other environmental factors, it reacts much the same way — cells become damaged, even diseased. These free-spirited molecules are called free radicals and they attack otherwise healthy cells, causing them to break down, altering their DNA, and ultimately causing the cell to age and become vulnerable to disease.

Antioxidants are the body's own can of Rustoleum — they stabilize free radicals and prevent them from wreaking havoc on your cells. If your body is stockpiled with sufficient amounts of antioxidants (vitamins A, C, D, E, and beta-carotene), the free radicals will have less power to destroy fat and protein molecules and damage the collagen support system of the dermis.

Dr. Nicholas Perricone, a clinical professor of dermatology at Yale Medical School and a well-known antiaging researcher, has learned that after forty-five minutes in the sun, 80 percent of the body's vitamin C reserve is used up, and even when study participants ingested megadoses of vitamin C, the sun still depleted the supply in under an hour. After that, free radicals that are caused by exposure to the sun are left to run amok virtually unchecked.

Because free radicals beat up on healthy cells, antioxidants are now being added to moisturizers, sunscreens, lip balms, and eye gels to help minimize their effects on the skin. But most products use vitamin C in its ascorbic acid form, which can sting, is difficult to stabilize, and is only soluble in water, which means it cannot penetrate the epidermis.

Dr. Perricone's studies have shown that topically applied ascorbal palmitate, a combination of ascorbic acid (vitamin C) and a fatty alcohol, can actually reach beyond the stratum corneum. Because it remains stable and penetrates the stratum corneum, he says that the ascorbal palmitate is forty times more effective at protecting against future cell damage and stimulating collagen production to repair existing damage than ascorbic acid.

Vitamin E (alpha tocopherol) has been added to skin-care products for years, but Dr. Perricone has discovered that tocotrienol, another derivative of vitamin E, works better as a topically applied free-radical fighter. Because vitamin E is fat-soluble, it doesn't have the same trouble getting below the skin's surface as vitamin C. Tocotrienol is hard to come by, however, and Dr. Perricone predicts that it will be another year before it is available in sufficient quantity to be included in cosmetics.

Coenzyme Q10, which you may have read about in relation to exercise, is another antioxidant that Dr. Perricone believes will be making a big splash in the skin-care market in the coming years. Researchers agree that Q10 helps vitamin E to protect cells from free-radical damage much the way vitamin C does.

Research continues to mount up in support of the theory that topically applied vitamins can repair previously damaged cells and prevent future cell damage. Scientists are working feverishly to apply their growing knowledge of vitamins to skin-care products, so don't expect the deluge of information and new and improved products to end any time soon.

Over the next few years, I believe that the biggest breakthroughs in skin care will come from antioxidant research and the formulation of products that include several different antioxidants, since they all attack free radicals differently. Just as doctors and researchers found a way to make vitamin A work on the skin, by developing Retin-A, I am convinced that safe and powerful vitamin-enriched products are right on the horizon.

Until then, what's sold in the store today won't make your wrinkles disappear overnight, and most don't have the exfoliating properties of an alpha hydroxy acid, but these vitamin-enriched products can't hurt and just might help, so why not give them a try? In Chapter 4, I'll tell you more about a few wrinkle-fighting products whose magic ingredient is vitamin C.

LIPOSOMES' GIANT LEAP FORWARD

For years now, companies have proudly announced the presence of liposomes and niosomes in their moisturizers. But, since most people don't know a liposome from a Flintstone, that little detail passes without much interest. Liposomes are microscopic, spherical envelopes, if you will, that were first engineered by scientists at Harvard to exactly mimic a human cell, says Dr. Ted Hager, chairman of IGI, Inc., of Buena, New Jersey. The purpose behind creating a liposome was to make a delivery vehicle that would encase ingredients, particularly moisturizers, and escort them beyond the outermost layers of the skin where they could actually provide some benefit.

The good news is that liposomes do just that. The bad news is that human cells turn over constantly and because liposomes mimic cells exactly, they also turn over quickly. Consequently liposomes tend to be unstable. They fall apart quickly, and they are expensive to make.

A few years ago, Dr. Hager teamed up with Dr. Donald Wallach, the Harvard scientist who first created liposomes, and together they built the proverbial better mousetrap. The new technology is called a novasome, which essentially does the same thing that a liposome does without falling apart. Novasomes can also be made inexpensively, so companies can afford to put more of them into their formulations. According to Dr. Hager, when companies make products with liposomes, they may put an eyedropperful into a vat of product. As a result, the amount in any given jar is minuscule.

Today, companies like Estee Lauder are using this new novasome technology in thirty or forty products, including their 100 Percent Moisturizer, Prescriptives All You Need Moisturizer, and Virtual Skin makeup. Almay's Time Off and Revlon Results also include novasomes. Dr. Hager has also developed his own line of skin-care products, called NovaSkin, that include novasomes. NovaSkin products are available only from dermatologists, plastic surgeons, or estheticians.

It's impossible to read an ingredients label to find liposomes or novasomes because they are made from different ingredients, depending on the application, but if you see package labeling that proclaims aquaspheres or novaspheres, that means that the novasomes are in there.

In addition to cosmetics, novasome technology is being used in fat-free treats like Girl Scout cookies, Richard Simmons low-fat cookies, as well as low-fat Hydrox and Vienna Fingers. The novasomes allow bakers to substitute calorie-free novasome-encapsulated material for fat.

Novasomes are a particularly exciting advance because, according to Dr. Hager, the tiny spheres can be engineered to deliver material to any layer of the skin and even beyond. Among the obvious possibilities are using novasomes to deliver vaccinations and other medications that are normally injected. He also anticipates applying novasome technology to the work being done by the "gene jockeys." Using novasomes, scientists could deliver material to the genes to stimulate a desired response or block an undesired action. An improved version of minoxidil that uses novasomes to deliver six times as much medication to the hair shaft is currently under development, and some day novasomes could be used to cure everything from psoriasis to cancer.

MARKETING SKIN-CARE PRODUCTS: YOUR CHOICE

There is no right or wrong way to buy cosmetics. Some people feel ripped off when they realize that a certain drugstore brand has ingredients that are equivalent to a much more expensive department store brand. Other women don't care much about price and enjoy the experience of shopping for and sampling department store cosmetics. Still others swear by a certain line of products and wouldn't switch brands if you gave them a lifetime supply of something else for free. Whether you enjoy the pretty jars on your vanity, or choose products based solely on results, only you can decide how much you're willing to pay for cosmetics. Even if your reasoning seems frivolous to someone else, who cares? It's your skin. Pamper it with products that make you feel good inside and out.

Despite all of the beauty experts telling consumers that skin care need not be expensive, millions of women still purchase expensive,

department store goods because they think the products do something extra for their skin—and some of them do. Over the past ten or
fifteen years, cosmetics companies have poured billions into research
that has yielded great products that do indeed improve the look of
the skin.

On the whole, skin care based on science instead of marketing is
good for consumers. It does, however, make things awfully confusing.
Not too long ago, we approached skin-care products with a healthy
degree of skepticism, realizing that we were buying hope-in-a-jar.
Today, that jar is starting to look more like a magic lamp that just
might release an ageless genie to do our bidding.

Even though science has upped the ante in the skin-care business, it's still not necessary to spend a fortune on quality skin-care
products if you don't want to. At the end of this chapter, I've listed
modestly priced products that will give good results.

If you do choose to splurge on skin care, or makeup for that matter, consider a few of the factors that contribute to their price.

In a department store, you can sample products, have a makeover,
and take home samples. But those free samples really aren't free, they're
just factored in to the price you pay for the product. That's part of the
reason many drugstore cosmetics, which are just as good as department store products, can be offered at considerable savings. The down-
side is that if you pick up a tube of moisturizer at your local drugstore
or supermarket and it's too thick for you, you probably won't bother to
return it. By the same token, if you've already sampled a department
store product, you probably won't need to return it.

Prestige skin-care products and cosmetics also tend to be over-
loaded with packaging. Bottles, jars, and tubes come in attractive
boxes, but these are entirely unnecessary, and can add to the cost of
the product—sometimes the jars, tubes, and pump dispensers can
cost more than the product that's in them.

Cosmetics companies spend obscene amounts of money to sell
their products to you through magazine ads and television commercials. Consider that a one-page ad in a magazine like *Good House-
keeping* will cost more than $50,000, and that companies buy several
pages in several magazines every month in addition to TV commercials, newspaper ads, etc., and you see that the advertising dollars are
staggering.

THE HAVES AND THE HAVE-NOTS

With so many products on the market, it's easy to find yourself buying things you really don't need. The advertising is compelling and the prospect of better-looking skin causes many of us to end up with a vanity table full of stuff we never use. Here's a quick reference to help you sort through the maze. There are some things you must have to maintain clean, healthy skin, others are nice luxuries, and still others, in my opinion, are a waste of hard-earned money.

HAVE TO HAVE	NICE TO HAVE	WASTE OF MONEY
Gentle cleanser	Eye-makeup	Toner (except for
Moisturizer	remover	oily skin)
Sunscreen	Eye gel or cream	Throat cream
AHA or scrub	Hydrating spritz	Separate day & night
product	Hydrating masks	cream
Hand & body		
moisturizer		

ALTERNATIVE OUTLETS

Television shopping, dermatologists, and 800 numbers are popular vehicles for marketing cosmetics. If you've found products you like, you may wish to comparison shop among these outlets because the prices can vary wildly.

Many of the skin-care products sold by doctors are available directly from the manufacturer by calling their 800 number. Before buying from your doctor, check prices with the manufacturer. If the doctor's markup is minimal, the convenience may be worth the extra dollar or two, but if the markup is significant, you may wish to order directly from the company.

If it were not for the unconditional money-back guarantees offered by electronic retailers like QVC and Home Shopping Network, I would not recommend buying skin-care products or color cosmetics via television. But, because the prices are good and they do honor the guarantees without question, it's a good option—and millions of women are taking advantage of the choice. A survey of five hundred women done by *Allure* magazine showed that women buy more skin-care products at home then they do in department and specialty stores combined. That statistic also includes home sales companies like Avon and Mary Kay.

At Home Shopping Network (HSN) cosmetics accounted for 10 percent of the company's 1995 sales with more than $100 million worth of skin creams and makeup shipped nationwide. Adrien Arpel sold a record $4.5 million worth of her skin-care products in just nineteen hours. Beauty Tech, HSN's own brand of makeup, which was created to compete with brands like M.A.C. and Bobbi Brown, sold at an astonishing $2,000-per-minute clip when it was first introduced.

Betty Broder, QVC's director of Cosmetics and Health and Beauty Aids says that her company assures quality products by staying up on the latest news and technology of the industry and then putting any product line they are considering through rigorous legal and quality-assurance review. QVC will only sell products that can substantiate any claims they make.

One of the many things I like about television shopping is that manufacturers, endorsers, or inventors are featured on the beauty shows demonstrating the products and offering application tips. On QVC, a model removes her makeup to reveal a large strawberry mark on her face that was totally unnoticeable when she was wearing Dermablend. This kind of "before your very eyes" demonstration makes it easy for you to see how products might actually work for you.

Electronic retailers often sell products at significant savings because the manufacturers don't have to pay sales commissions or develop in-store marketing materials, so they pass the savings on to QVC and HSN, who in turn pass the savings on to consumers. Additionally, the networks receive volume discounts for buying so much product.

When it comes to makeup, however, you can go through a lot of trial and error via return mail if you're trying to buy a new foundation, and Broder admits that QVC is still working on the best way to sell color cosmetics so that customers are getting products that work for them. Having to return products, after all, is not convenient—which is what the C stands for in QVC. Aside from foundation and lipstick, which are extremely dependent upon your own coloring, buying makeup from television retailers is simple, cost-effective, and informative—there's always a makeup artist demonstrating application techniques.

SHOPPING STRATEGIES TO PREVENT
OVERSPENDING FOR COSMETICS

It's easy enough to do. You're having a bad hair day and you had an argument with your husband. Or, your last child just went away to college. Or, new wrinkles appeared overnight along with ten new gray hairs right in front. You're feeling old, tired, and not very attractive. You hit the department store looking for a lift and here comes one of those cosmetics salespeople with the lab coats. You figure, oh well, let's see what they've got. The next thing you know this lab-coated glamour-puss is promising to revitalize your looks, give your skin a lift, and make you look ten years younger in a week. But she doesn't have any samples of the miracle cream, so you say, what the heck, I deserve this, and plunk down your $50.

It's easy to be wooed into buying cosmetics especially these days when they really can improve the look of your skin. But not every product works equally well for every person. Sometimes choosing cosmetics is a lot like dating. You have to try out a few before you find the right one.

SIMPLE SKIN-CARE SHOPPING SECRETS

1. **Plan your skin-care shopping trip in advance and go without any makeup. That way the salesperson can get a good look at your skin and make appropriate recommendations.**

2. **Whenever you buy cosmetics, be sure to use a credit card instead of cash to pay for your purchase. And, by all means, save the receipt. If the product doesn't do what you were promised, take it back. You may get a hard time from the salesperson, but stand firm. They'd rather have the chance to steer you toward another product that might suit you better than lose you altogether. If you can't get satisfaction from the salesperson, ask to see the department manager or the store manager. If worse comes to worst, you can always instruct the credit card company not to pay the charge. Most credit cards offer some kind of buyer protection service.**

3. **When shopping for cosmetics, you'll have much better luck if you look like someone who is likely to spend money on themselves. If you turn up at the counter in old sweatpants and a T-shirt, with your hair disheveled, don't be surprised if the salespeople don't spend much time with you and don't offer to give you samples. I know you can't judge a book by its cover, but commission salespeo-**

ple will always spend more time and energy on customers who look like real prospects.

4. When you've had a consultation, ask for samples of the product before spending $50 for a jar of cream. You can also bring your own small jars so that you can take home a dab from the tester bottle if the salesperson is out of samples. Be sure to ask for the salesperson's card and their schedule. After all, they do work on commission and if you like the products they've shown you, it's only fair to buy from them. If you're buying a product without trying a sample first, be sure to buy the smallest portion possible. You won't be saving anything if you only use half of the econo-size jar before switching brands.

5. Home-shopping clubs like QVC are especially good about returned products. They offer a money-back guarantee and they mean it. If you find it hard to stand your ground with salespeople, you may find it less stressful to buy products through one of these outlets, where you'll never have to confront anyone in person. Be sure to keep your receipt.

6. Listen carefully. Don't be taken in by sales pitches that promise unrealistic results. If a salesperson tells you a product contains some magic ingredient, ask what it is and what the long-term effects may be.

7. Nothing lasts forever. Unless your product has an expiration date stamped on it, date your skin-care products when you buy them. If a product separates, changes color, or has a funny odor, throw it away. Additionally, if a product has a new price tag stuck over an old one, leave it on the shelf. Prices typically change every six months and that particular jar or bottle may be a leftover from a prior shipment.

8. Keep your skin-care products in a cool, dry place. If you live in a warm climate, you may want to refrigerate them.

9. If you're thoroughly confused, or just don't want to bother shopping, you can see a dermatologist and buy products the doctor recommends or sells.

10. Check your mail for circulars and newspaper ads for specials at drugstores, supermarkets, and beauty outlets. Never buy at your local flea market. Those vendors often buy closeouts that may be out of date.

Chapter 3

SUN SMARTS

"It's a drag having to wear socks during matches, because the tan, like, stops at the ankles. I can never get my skin, like, color-coordinated."

—MONICA SELES

It doesn't matter how grown-up you are—you can still buckle under the weight of peer pressure. Take tanning, for example. Even though you're a grown woman, do you secretly hope that your friends will nod approvingly when you come back from vacation with a "great tan"? On the other hand, do you shudder when your longtime cohorts look at you in the middle of summer and exclaim, "Oh my gosh—you're so pale!" There's still plenty of pressure to get a tan and a good portion of the public continues to equate a tan with beauty.

Just the other day, I spotted a young woman lying on the slanted roof of her house, sunning herself. My first thought was, don't roll over, dear, or you might slide off. My second thought was, she probably has a big date or a wedding to attend, and thinks she has to get some color before the grand event. Some old habits die hard.

No matter what the latest trends dictate, here's some very simple advice if you want to retain your good looks as you grow older: Avoid overexposure to the sun. Although the aftereffects of sunlight may take up to twenty-five years to appear, you'll have to pay for them sooner or later. Forget what your friends say—after all, you're not supposed to follow the crowd at this stage in life anyway—and remember this simple, irrefutable fact: Sun exposure accelerates the aging process.

Think about it. If a tan is so great, why don't you see movie stars with tanned faces anymore? When a gorgeous woman appears on the big screen (or on any soap opera, for that matter), she has creamy, smooth skin. Do you think she got that from lying in the sun? Not a chance. Remember the beginning of *Gone With the Wind*? Scarlett

O'Hara brought a parasol to a picnic to protect her face from the sun. It certainly did the trick: Scarlett, played by Vivien Leigh, had flawless skin. In those days, pale skin was prized as a trophy of the upper class.

Now, you don't have to turn into Scarlett O'Hara, but you should pay attention to some basic facts: Prolonged sun exposure not only dries and wrinkles your skin, it also puts you at high risk for skin cancer.

In this chapter, you'll learn smart, practical tips about how to shelter yourself from the sun's harmful rays and preserve your skin for a lifetime.

Elaine's Exclusives

NO REPLY

When tan people mention how pale you are, smile sweetly and refrain from commenting about how wrinkled they are!

ALL BURNED UP

If someone you love ends up with a sunburn, resist the urge to say I told you so. Advise them to treat mild sunburns with cool baths, bland moisturizers, or over-the-counter hydrocortisone cream. Aspirin may also help. More serious sunburns require medical attention if accompanied by headache, chills, or fever.

SUNSCREENS AND SUNBLOCKS

Sunscreens are just what their name implies: products that screen your skin from the sun. Even though most of us still crave the "healthy glow" of a tan, the fact that the sun causes wrinkles and skin cancer seems finally to have sunk in. Americans spent close to $400 million on sunscreens and sunblocks in 1993 and, according to New York-based Packaged Facts, total sales are predicted to soar to nearly $800 million by 1997.

When the sun's ultraviolet rays penetrate your skin's inner layer, your skin produces more melanin—the substance that gives your skin color—to protect it from further damage. That's a tan, your body's survival gear kicking into action. Repeated exposure to the sun's rays causes changes in skin texture, which leads to wrinkling, loss of elasticity, and age spots.

Elaine's Exclusive

DETECTIVE WORK

If you are at risk for skin cancer because of exposure to the sun, there is a method of detection called dermatoscopy that can help uncover malignant melanoma at a very early stage. Using a handheld microscope, dermatologists can detect skin lesions not noticeable to the naked eye. While a complete physical examination of the skin is the first line of defense in detecting melanoma, dermatoscopy can help determine whether or not a biopsy is needed.

The ultraviolet light in sunlight includes: ultraviolet A (UVA), ultraviolet B (UVB), and ultraviolet C (UVC). Presently UVC doesn't reach the earth because it is blocked by the ozone layer, but it may become a factor in the future if the ozone layer continues to be depleted.

The original ingredient in sunscreens that protected the skin from the sun was PABA (para-aminobenzoic acid), but it tended to stain clothes and was replaced with newer, more refined ingredients called PABA esters, which rarely stain clothing. Some people with particularly sensitive skin may have an allergic reaction to PABA and its esters, or even to the fragrance in a sunscreen. The allergy may make your skin red and itchy about twenty-four hours after applying the sunscreen. If you are in this category, try sunscreen products containing other chemicals such as benzophenones, cinnamates, and salicylates. It may take a bit of trial and error to find a sunscreen product that does not irritate your skin. If you suspect you are highly allergic to PABA or its derivatives, ask your dermatologist to confirm it with a patch test.

You're bound to find a sunscreen that you like, because manufacturers are keenly aware of the value of customer satisfaction and have created sun-protection products that are more refined and user-friendly than in the past. You'll notice, for example, that sunscreens are absorbed into the skin much more easily than before.

When choosing a product, remember that there are different sunscreens for different skin types. Here's how dermatologists classify skin, so see where you fit in:

Type 1   Always burns and never tans

Type 2   Always burns and tans minimally

Type 3   Burns moderately and tans gradually and uniformly

Type 4   Burns minimally and always tans well

Type 5   Rarely burns

Type 6   Never burns

There are two types of sunscreens: physical and chemical. Physical sunscreens, or sunblocks, reflect sunlight, causing it to bounce off your skin. These include zinc oxide or titanium dioxide. Over the years, these ingredients have been improved so that they don't appear on the skin. Z-cote, made by SunSmart, is micronized zinc oxide, which is the broadest spectrum sunblock available and the active ingredient in 99 percent of the products that list zinc oxide as an ingredient. Zinc oxide is nontoxic and nonallergenic, which means that anyone can use it.

In fact, says SunSmart medical director Mark Mitchnick, the micronized zinc oxide works better than its nonmicronized sister, which appears white and pasty on the noses of lifeguards everywhere. The micronized particles are smaller, which is why you can't see them, but they spread over the skin better than the large particles that you can see. Dr. Mitchnick explains it this way: If you put a one-pound basketball on your head, you can't cover your feet. You could cover much more of your body with one pound of ping pong balls.

OH NO! THE OZONE

Research shows that the incidence of skin cancer may rise significantly in the future because depletion of the ozone layer is allowing more and more UV radiation to reach earth. In fact, over the last fifteen years, the average amount of UVB reaching North America increased by 4 percent, but in Argentina and Chile, the average amount increased by almost 10 percent.

Chemical sunscreens absorb the UVA or UVB energy using PABA, or its ester derivatives, cinnamates, benzophenones, and anthranilates. You should always choose a sunscreen that is labeled "broad spectrum" and includes a combination of ingredients because PABA and the cinnamates only absorb UVB rays and the benzophenones only scoop up UVAs. The anthranilates absorb both types of rays.

Use a sunscreen year-round, whenever you are in the sun—*not* just when you spend a day at the beach or by a pool. People tend to stock up on sunscreen during vacation, but seasonal use is not wise, say dermatologists. You need a sunscreen during any outing—walking at lunchtime, playing a quick game of tennis, or driving around in your convertible. UV rays even come through your car's windshield. Don't omit sunscreen on cloudy days, either. Eighty percent of the sun's ultraviolet rays pass through the clouds and onto your skin.

Also don't assume that a sunscreen works like a suit of armor and totally shields you from the sun's rays. Even with a sunscreen, the sun can be harmful, so don't think you have free rein to bake in the sun just because you applied sunscreen. Use the sunscreen as part of a conscious, well-rounded approach to sun-avoidance. For example, apply sunscreen, and then stay under an umbrella when you're sitting in the backyard reading a book.

Some experts warn that not all sunscreens protect you from UVA rays. Because the SPF rating system only measures protection from UVB rays, look for a sunscreen that also protects against UVA rays, the rays that penetrate deeper into your skin and add to skin wrinkling, burning, and cancer.

To make sure that sunscreens stay on your skin, look for a water-proof product, especially if you swim or sweat a lot. Also, if you take medications, suffer from a disease, or have a personal or family history of skin cancer, talk with your doctor about sunlight exposure because UV rays may affect you more strongly.

Why should you use sunscreen? Just hold up your palms and look at the softer side of your arm—notice how smooth and unwrinkled it is? That's how the rest of your skin could look if it were not exposed to the sun, says Manhattan dermatologist Barney J. Kenet.

BE ON THE LOOKOUT
If you have exposed your skin to an overdose of sun during your lifetime, be on the lookout for signs of cancer. Skin cancer may first appear as a dry, scaly patch, a persistent pimple, an inflamed area with a crusting center, or as a pearly, waxy nodule that can ulcerate or bleed.

I think I bought the very first bottle of sunscreen ever sold and smeared it on my children. When all of the other girls were oiling up for a day on the beach, my daughter Amy dutifully slathered on her sunscreen. She may have felt out of it at the time, but she thanks me now because even at thirty-four, her skin is much smoother than other women her age. Just imagine the difference there will be in twenty years.

There's no question that prevention is the best treatment for sun damage. But, even if you've already overexposed your skin to the sun, it's never too late to protect yourself. Every single time you bake or burn in the sun, you add more damage to your skin. By avoiding additional sun exposure, you minimize further damage.

Of course, in addition to keeping your skin softer and more youthful, sunscreens also protect you from cancer. The skin is the body's largest organ and skin cancer is the most common cancer— and also the most preventable. There is no doubt that skin cancer is linked to the damaging ultraviolet radiation from the sun and that skin cancer is reaching epidemic proportions in America with eight-hundred-thousand to one million new cases each year.

There are several types of skin cancer, including malignant melanoma. If not detected and treated early, it can be fatal. Other skin cancers, including basal cell carcinoma and squamous cell carcinoma, are less serious but can be disfiguring, especially on the face, neck, and hands. Because fair-skinned people do not have enough melanin to protect their skin, the rate of skin cancer and premature aging is higher among Caucasians.

But, even though people of color have a low incidence of skin cancer, the need for sun protection depends on the shade of your skin and whether or not you burn. Remember, people with dark skin are less likely to get melanoma, but no one is immune from it.

In a nutshell, repeated suntanning is an open invitation to wrinkling and skin cancer. You wouldn't knowingly expose yourself to radiation from a nuclear plant or an atomic bomb, would you? Then cover up with adequate sunscreen and other protection when you're out in the sun.

You don't need to go to the other extreme and become a hermit. After all, life on earth would not exist without the sun. Just make it a point to be smart and take precautionary measures when you're outdoors so you can truly enjoy the sun's warmth and maintain youthful, healthy skin.

KNOW YOUR ABCs

Skin cancer is one of the few cancers that you can see with the naked eye. You can help detect it early by taking note of moles or growths on your body. To detect changes, perform monthly skin self-exams in front of a mirror while holding a smaller mirror for a back view. A simple ABCD rule shows what to look for when you examine your skin:

***A* is for Asymmetry: One half of a mole or skin growth does not match the other half.**

***B* is for Border Irregularity: The edges of the mole are ragged, notched, or blurred.**

***C* is for Color: The pigmentation of the growth is not uniform.**

***D* is for Diameter: Greater than 6 millimeters (about the size of a pencil eraser). Be alert to any sudden or progressive increase in the size of a mole.**

THE SIMPLE SECRET OF SPF

You know that sunscreens have an SPF number, but do you know what SPF means? SPF stands for sun protection factor. SPF sunscreens protect you from UVB rays, the primary cause of sunburns and skin cancer. The SPF listed on a sunscreen's label is regulated and controlled by the FDA.

SPF numbers range from 2 to as high as 50. The numbers represent the sunscreen's ability to block out the sun's burning rays. The SPF is determined by comparing the amount of time needed to produce a sunburn on protected skin to the amount of time needed to cause a sunburn on unprotected skin. For example, if a fair-skinned person who normally turns red after ten minutes of exposure to the sun, uses a 2 SPF, multiply the ten-minute burn time by 2 and estimate that it will take about twenty minutes of exposure for the skin to turn red. Likewise, if the same person used a 15 SPF, it would take one hundred fifty minutes of exposure for her to burn.

But, while you're selecting an SPF number, keep this tidbit in mind: SPF protection does not increase proportionally with SPF numbers. For example, an SPF of 2 absorbs only 50 percent of the sun's rays. An SPF of 15 absorbs 93 percent and an SPF of 34 absorbs 97 percent. (Notice that there's only a four percentage point difference between a 15 and a 34.)

That means that you should forget about the bottles of SPF of less than 15 that are stashed away in your medicine chest because they *do not protect your skin.* If you have them, throw them away and replace them with SPFs of 15 or higher.

Of course, this information leads to the burning (pardon the expression) question: Do you *need* an SPF higher than 15? Dermatologists say that if you spend a lot of time outdoors, you may benefit from a higher SPF. Studies have shown that outdoor workers such as fishermen have a higher incidence of certain types of skin cancers and skin-aging than indoor workers. You might not be a fisherman, but if you spend a lot of time outdoors playing golf or tennis, or gardening, you may want to select an SPF that's higher than 15.

Also, if you tend to skimp on sunscreen application, a layer of a higher SPF may offer some added protection. (See the next section for information on applying sunscreen.)

If all of this seems a tad confusing, when you go to the store to select a sunscreen, remember this: The American Academy of Dermatology, the Skin Cancer Foundation, and the American Cancer Society *all* recommend an SPF of *at least* 15 to protect all skin types from the sun.

Elaine's Exclusives

PROOF POSITIVE

According to the Skin Cancer Foundation, an Australian study of patients over age forty showed that daily use (not just during recreation) of sunscreen with an SPF of 17 led to a significant decrease in the number of new precancerous solar keratoses over a seven-month period, as well as an increase in the number of remissions from existing lesions.

IT'S A DATE

Do you know that just like a carton of milk, some newer sunscreens have an expiration date? If you've been hoarding a bottle or tube of sunscreen for a while, check the date to make sure it is still effective. Open bottles may degrade and become less effective over time.

TYPECASTING: THE BEST SUNSCREEN FOR YOUR SKIN TYPE

Take a peek at the sunscreen section of your local drugstore or super-market and you'll find that there are plenty of products, including oils, lotions, creams, gels, and sprays, to choose from.

Experts are reluctant to say that one is better than the other because they feel sunscreen selection is mostly a personal choice (except, of course, for choosing one with an SPF of at least 15). So, much like your perfume or moisturizer, the sunscreen that's best for you depends on your taste.

Remember, however:

- Most sunscreens with oil *do not* contain enough sunscreen to protect you. They usually have an SPF 2 or 4. If you have dry skin, use a sunscreen with an SPF of 15 or higher that contains a moisturizer.
- You can sweat off or wash off gel sunscreens more easily than lotions, but they may be preferable if you have a history of acne. Be sure to reapply gels frequently.
- While sunscreens containing alcohol tend to dry your skin, creams tend to be more moisturizing.

Which type of sunscreen you use really depends on your own preference, activity level, and skin type. Keep in mind that sunscreens are over-the-counter drugs, and therefore, they all provide the same level of protection within a given SPF. A department store SPF 15 product will protect you just as well as the drugstore brand.

Elaine's Exclusive

THE SENSITIVE TYPE

If you are taking medications or suffer from a chronic illness, you may be particularly sensitive to ultraviolet radiation from the sun. Drugs, including some antihistamines, antibiotics, diuretics, and antidepressants, may cause photosensitivity (an excessive or acute skin reaction to sun exposure or artificial light). Ask your doctor if you are at risk for photosensitivity.

HOW TO PROPERLY APPLY SUNSCREEN

The experts may have differing opinions about which sunscreen is best for you, but they certainly agree on this fact: When applying sunscreen, most people don't use nearly the amount needed to protect them.

To remedy this, remember this credo: Don't be stingy!

Warwick Morison, M.D., professor of dermatology at Johns Hopkins in Baltimore, describes our sunscreen application habits this way: "When a patient asks me if they can use a sunscreen from last summer, I know they're not using enough!"

Here's a good rule of thumb, says Dr. Morison: An ounce of sunscreen covers an average adult wearing a bathing suit. Therefore, if your bottle of sunscreen contains eight ounces, figure on using it about eight times for full-body coverage.

Here's where the higher SPF numbers come in handy. If you have a tendency to be frugal with the sunscreen, a 30 SPF might give you a bit more protection, although remember, it won't be twice as much protection.

And don't wait until you're out in the sun to apply sunscreen. Do that about thirty minutes or more beforehand to give it a chance to bind to your skin. Besides, you're much more likely to cover those "hard to reach" spots in the privacy of your own home than on a beach or at a public pool.

Also, after about two hours in the sun, be sure to reapply sunscreen. Dermatologists say this is a practice that a lot of people neglect. Repeated applications won't give you another full period of protection against the sun's rays, but it will reinforce any areas where the product has washed or rubbed off.

Watch the men in your life when they apply sunscreen. They tend to treat it like aftershave, rubbing it into their hands and then applying it to their face and body, and ultimately getting more on their hands than anywhere else. While wrinkles on men are considered "distinguished" (talk about an aggravating double standard), tell him you don't want him drying up before his time.

Always remember the "forgotten" areas of you body that tend to get sunburned, including your head, neck (especially the back of the neck), ears, lips, face, hands, and feet. About 95 percent of metastatic basal cell cancers start on the head and neck, which receive the most sun exposure.

SUNSCREENS IN MOISTURIZER AND MAKEUP

Chronic exposure to the sun can cause your skin, and especially your face, to become thick, wrinkled, and leathery. Shielding your skin from the sun is *the* single most important step you can take to keep your face looking youthful.

To protect your face, some moisturizers on the market contain an extra ingredient: sunscreen. For many people, these moisturizers are fine for days when just a few minutes are spent in the sun walking from the car to the office.

But, says Dr. Morison, why not go another route (actually a vice-versa route) and use a sunscreen with a moisturizer every day to provide maximum protection for your face? Using a moisturizer with a sunscreen factor when you spend the day outdoors won't do the trick because it's thin and you're not likely to reapply it every two hours for adequate protection. For instance, if you're golfing, wear a sunscreen that contains moisturizer, not just your everyday moisturizer with an SPF.

By the way, applying a plain moisturizer *before* sunbathing actually increases the effects of ultraviolet light. So only moisturize using an SPF product before going in the sun.

The same goes for makeup with an SPF. It won't act as a complete sunscreen if you're planning to spend the day gardening, but it's fine for a normal day of minimal sun exposure. If you plan to spend more than twenty minutes outside, wear sunscreen under your makeup.

You can still find some products that claim on their labels to have sunscreen in them, but do not specify an SPF. That kind of worthless information will soon be a thing of the past because the FDA has said that companies cannot imply protection without specifying how much. That means that companies will have to remove the "with sunscreen" note on the product's label or replace it with an SPF number, which is good news for consumers.

Photo-aging, the premature wrinkling of the skin, is *not* an inevitable part of aging. Protecting your face from ultraviolet radiation can substantially minimize aging. So, use makeup and moisturizers with an SPF for daily minimal coverage; for better coverage when you are outdoors for extended periods, use a sunscreen with moisturizer.

Elaine's Exclusive

KISS THIS

Don't forget to cover your lips when you're protecting your skin from the sun. Use a lip balm containing sunscreen with an SPF of 15 to prevent your lips from burning.

CLOTHING WITH SUNSCREEN

Does clothing protect you from the sun's rays? T-shirts and shorts certainly won't. For instance, a white T-shirt offers as much protection as a 5 SPF (which means not much).

But some other clothes in your closet offer protection from the sun. Research shows that clothes made with unbleached cotton act as UV absorbers. High-luster polyesters and thin, satiny silk can also be highly protective because they reflect radiation away from your body.

Fibers such as polyester crepe, bleached cotton, and viscose, on the other hand, are quite transparent to UV rays and should be avoided in the sun.

Weave may be even more important when it comes to sun protection. In general, the tighter the weave or knit, the higher the SPF. To decide whether a fabric offers enough protection from the sun, hold it up to a window or a lamp and see how much light gets through. Dark clothes usually have a higher SPF.

For people who are sensitive to the sun or who spend a lot of time outdoors (pay attention, golfers, joggers, walkers, gardeners, and boaters!), UV-protective clothing is also available. Containing colorless compounds, fluorescent brighteners, or specially treated resins that absorb UV, these clothes may provide an SPF of 30 or more.

Ultraviolet Protection Factor (UPF), a new rating system for fabrics, is becoming the standard for sun-protective clothing in Australia (the country with the world's highest rate of skin cancer). If you are extremely sensitive to the sun, these garments may be the ticket for your sun-protection regimen.

One company, Sun Precautions, Inc., of Seattle, created a line called Solubra 30+ Ultra Sun Protective Clothing. The company's founder, Shaun Hughes, is an outdoor-lover who was diagnosed with malignant melanoma at age twenty-six. After he was treated and recovered, he was strongly advised to avoid sun exposure to prevent recurrence of the deadly skin disease. So working with dermatologists and cancer experts, he fashioned clothing that provides sun-sensitive people with light-weight, comfortable clothing so they can lead an active life in the great outdoors! The clothing line includes wide-brimmed hats, long-sleeved shirts, and long pants that provide 30+ SPF and block the entire UV radi-ation spectrum, even when damp or wet. If you are interested in sun-protective clothing, call Sun Precaution at 1-800-882-7860 for a catalog.

One important note: Most garments lose about a third of their ability to protect you from the sun when wet. Also, unless you are covered with a parachute, no clothing can completely protect you head to toe! Complement your protective clothing with sunglasses, a hat, and an SPF 15 (at least) sunscreen on all exposed areas for a com-plete sun-safe ensemble.

PROTECTING YOUR EYES FROM THE SUN

The sun is bad for your skin, but did you realize that it can also harm your eyes? Research shows that ultraviolet rays, including those that reflect on snow or water, increase the likelihood of certain cataracts. In fact, sun damage is responsible for a sizable portion of the more than one million cataracts operated on yearly in the United States. And, because the depletion of the ozone layer allows more and more radiation to reach the earth, sun damage to eyes may increase.

Cataracts are the loss of transparency in the eye's lens, which results in clouded vision. Surgery may correct cataract damage but if left untreated, cataracts can rob you of your vision.

Other eye problems caused by ultraviolet rays are eyelid cancers, conjunctival growths, corneal burns, and possible senile macular degeneration, a major cause of reduced vision for people over age fifty-five. The risk of getting any of these eye problems is reduced with proper eye protection that shields you from harmful UV rays.

When buying sunglasses, check the label for lenses that provide 99 to 100 percent UVA and UVB protection. This is an easy, compara-tively inexpensive and practical way to shield your eyes. Wraparound frames that closely fit your forehead area are best for maximum eye and eyelid protection. Also, look for sunglasses that are durable and impact-resistant, and lenses that allow you to have good color recognition. The most popular colors for sunglass lenses, neutral gray and amber brown, both generally provide good color rendition.

When selecting sunglasses, choose a pair that complement your face and shield your eyes—the windows to your soul—from the sun. Look for the Skin Cancer Foundation's Seal of Recommendation for sunglasses as a guide when shopping for protective eyewear.

In addition to wearing your sunglasses whenever you are in the sun (not just at the beach or when you're skiing in the mountains), use umbrellas and other shade devices to keep your eyes safe.

Elaine's Exclusives

NOW HAIR THIS

The sun not only damages your skin, it dries out your hair, too. So wearing a wide-brim hat to protect your face does double-duty by protecting your hair at the same time.

THE TRUTH ABOUT TANNING SALONS

OK, you want to sum up the benefits of tanning beds? In a word, none. (Except, of course, for the dermatologists who are paid to treat people suffering from the aftereffects.)

Forget what the advertisements say about "safe" tanning—artificial radiation in tanning salons carries all the risks of the sun's rays. About thirty minutes in a tanning salon equals about six to eight hours of nonstop sunning at the beach.

Here's what you'll get for paying to achieve a tanning-parlor tan: cataracts, sunburns, skin cancer, and premature wrinkling of the skin.

Many salon owners claim that the UVA radiation from tanning booths is safe. But that's not true. UVA radiation can pose long- and short-term risks to your skin. Unfortunately, dermatologists have noticed more young women with heavily damaged skin and skin cancers as the result of tanning salons.

A high rate of people who frequent tanning salons are also developing eye disorders such as cataracts, corneal burns, and retinal damage, apparently due to the failure of the salons to provide every patron with UV-protective goggles.

Most tanning salons are unregulated, so you enter at your own risk. Experts say that tanning booths can also damage your immune system and cause a reaction to certain fragrances, lotions, moisturizers, and medications.

Despite these facts, the indoor tanning industry brings in more than a billion dollars a year and the use of tanning parlors keeps growing.

Don't get suckered in—you and your skin will regret it.

> **WINTER SENSE FROM THE SKIN CANCER FOUNDATION**
> **The sun doesn't take a break just because it's chilly outside. Here are some recommendations from the Skin Cancer Foundation to keep your skin safe in the winter:**
> - **Half an hour before you go outside, generously apply a sunscreen with an SPF of 15 or higher over all exposed areas. Remember the underside of your chin and front of your neck, which are especially vulnerable to reflected UV rays.**
> - **Cumulative heat from sun exposure adds to skin damage, so take a break indoors at some point during the hottest hours of the day, reapply sunscreen, and go back out after an hour or so.**
> - **Wear wraparound sunglasses that block at least 99 percent of both UVA and UVB.**
> - **Wear your winter hat low to protect your ears from UV. If you don't have a hat on, and particularly if your hair is thin, use a sunscreen spray on your hair.**
> - **Don't visit a tanning parlor in an effort to increase melanin. UV from tanning machines has been shown to multiply the risks of skin cancer.**

NEW LIGHT ON SELF-TANNING

If life as you know it simply will not be the same without a tan, the safest way to accomplish your goal is with sunless tanning or self-tanning products. Why? Because dermatologists say that sunless tanning products are safe.

Elaine's Exclusive

NO JOKE

Some people kid around about the need to get a great tan, but the damage caused by the sun's ultraviolet rays is hardly laughable. In 1996, more than thirty-eight thousand people were diagnosed with malignant melanoma. Since 1973, the incidence rate of melanoma has increased about 4 percent a year. Researchers have found that many years can pass between the initial sun damage and the development of cancer. You are at risk if you had ultraviolet radiation exposure, especially in childhood and during your teenage years, or at infrequent intervals, even in adulthood.

Self-tanning products, whether they come in cream, lotion, or spray form, contain DHA, a compound that occurs naturally in the skin. When you apply the sunless product, DHA interacts with the amino acids in your skin's dead surface cells and a tan appears on your uppermost skin layer.

Although they produced orange-ish tans when they first appeared on the market (remember QT?), in recent years many of the new sunless products provide a more aesthetically pleasing light brown or golden shade. The products work so well now that health-conscious consumers snatched up close to $90 million worth of the products in 1993 and, according to Packaged Facts, sales for 1997 are projected to hit $137 million.

A WORD OF WARNING

Sunless tanning items do not offer protection from ultraviolet rays, even if the label says they contain sunscreen. If you use the sunless product and go out in the sun, you must also use a sunscreen to protect your skin, even if it appears tan.

Be sure to select a tanless product that indicates the exact color you will turn after using it. For example, the product's label may indicate that it will turn your skin a "deep golden bronze." If you are very fair-skinned, however, a "deep golden bronze" may appear very unnatural and you may want to select a product that is closer to your natural shade. You need not spend extra money for department store products unless you find a line that you particularly like. Essentially, it doesn't matter whether you buy Neutrogena, Bain de Soleil, or Estee Lauder. They all work the same way.

Application

To avoid streaking, it's best to shower and shave your legs before applying sunless tanning products. Apply in thin, even coats. Be sure to apply lightly around the elbows, ankles, and knees because too much in those areas may cause dark blotches. Wash your hands with soap and water immediately after application, paying particular attention to your knuckles, cuticles, and under your nails. Make sure your skin is completely dry before putting on clothes.

Some sunless products recommend several applications within one day. Reapply every three to six days if you want to deepen or maintain the color. If you use an AHA, you may have to reapply more frequently because the acid's job is to slough away the dead cells that the self-tanner colors. Also, to get maximum benefit from a self-tanner, do not apply moisturizer immediately before or after applying a self-tanner. It may dilute the effectiveness of the tanner.

Because everyone's skin is different, you may have to experiment with the amount and number of applications that are right for you, so don't use a sunless tanning product for the first time the night before your daughter's wedding.

OBEY THE TAN COMMANDMENTS
- **Stay out of the sun between 10 A.M. and 4 P.M., when the sun's rays are the strongest.**
- **Apply a broad-spectrum sunscreen with an SPF of at least 15.**
- **Reapply sunscreen every two hours when outdoors, even on cloudy days.**
- **Wear protective, tightly woven clothes, including long-sleeved shirts.**
- **Wear a four-inch wide broad-brimmed hat and sunglasses, even when walking short distances.**
- **Stay in the shade whenever possible.**
- **Avoid reflective surfaces because they can reflect up to 85 percent of the sun's damaging rays.**

Tanning Pills

Tanning pills and sunless tanning products are *not* in the same category. Tanning pills, with an active ingredient called canthaxanthin, a cousin of beta carotene, are illegal in the United States. While something derived from a form of beta carotene may sound healthy enough, it may actually cause nausea, diarrhea, severe itching, skin eruptions, night blindness, and hepatitis.

Forget about tanning pills—they are dangerous. If you simply must have a tan, stick to the sunless tanning products.

RECOMMENDED SUNSCREENS AND MOISTURIZERS

The Skin Cancer Foundation has given its Seal of Recommendation to the following products as "aids in the prevention of sun-induced damage to the skin." This list is updated each year.

PRODUCT	SPF
Amway Corporation	
Sunpacer Sunless Tanning Lotion	15
Sunpacer Ultra Sunscreen Lotion	15
Sunpacer Ultra Sunblock Creme	30
Sunpacer Ultra Sunblock Stick	15
Avon Products, Inc.	
Anew Perfect Moisturizer	15
Daily Revival Moisture Shield Creme	15
Daily Revival Moisture Shield Lotion	15
Daily Revival Tinted Moisture Shield Cream	15
Sun Seekers Children's Sunblock (pediatrician-tested, fragrance-free)	15
Sun Seekers Children's Ultra Sunblock (pediatrician-tested, fragrance-free)	30
Sun Seekers Face Ultra Sunblock Creme	30
Sun Seekers Sport Sunblock	30
Sun Seekers Sunblock Lotion	15
Sun Seekers Tote Pack Sunblock Lotion	15
Sun Seekers Ultra Sunblock Lotion	30

PRODUCT	SPF
Beirsdorf, Inc.	
Eucerin Daily Facial Lotion	20
Eucerin Facial Moisturizing Lotion	25
Blistex, Inc.	
Blistex OCT	20
Blistex Ultra Protection Facescreen	30
Chanel, Inc.	
Chanel Daily Protective Complex	15
Chanel Natureblock Cream	15
Chanel Oil-Free Sun Shelter Lotion	23
Chanel Spot Protector	30
Chanel Sun Shelter Cream	15
Chanel Sun Shelter Face Block	15
Chanel Total Protection Cream	15
Chanel Total Protection Matte Lotion	15
Clarins, U.S.A., Inc.	
Hydration Plus Moisture Lotion	15
Clarins Sunblock Ultra Protection	25
Self-Tanning Face Cream	15
Sun Care Cream Very High Protection	15
Sun Care Mist Very High Protection	19
Clinique Laboratories, Inc.	
City Block Oil Free Daily Face Protector	15
Full Service SunBlock	15
Full Service SunBlock	20
Oil-Free SunBlock	15
Special Defense SunBlock	25
Total Cover SunBlock	30
Elizabeth Arden, Co.	
Daily Moisture	15

Estee Lauder

Advanced Suncare SunBlock for Body	15
Advanced Suncare SunBlock for Face	15
Advanced Suncare SunBlock for Face	25
Advanced Suncare SunBlock Lotion for Children	25
Advanced Suncare SunBlock Lotion Spray	15
Oil-Free Sun Spray	15
Sunblock for Lips & Eyes	15
Waterworld Sport Sunblock	15

Fischer Pharmaceuticals, Ltd.

Babysol Cream	16
Babysol Lotion	16
Body Guard Lotion	15
Body Guard Cream	15
Ti Baby Natural Lotion	16
Ti Screen	15
Ti Screen Lotion	30
Ti Screen Natural Cream	16
Ti Screen Natural Lotion	16
Ultrasol Cream	15
Ultrasol Cream	16
Ultrasol Cream	34
Ultrasol Eye Cream	16
Ultrasol for Children Lotion	15
Ultrasol for Children Cream	15
Ultrasol Lotion	15
Ultrasol Lotion	16
Ultrasol Lotion	34

Mary Kay, Inc.

Intense Protection Sunblock	28
Sensible Protection Sunblock	15
Sun Essentials Lip Protector Sunblock	15
Ultimate Protection Sunblock	30

PRODUCT	SPF
Matrix Essentials, Inc.	
Biolage Sun A Day in the Sun	30
Biolage Sun Face The Sun	30
Biolage Sun Some Sun	15
Pfizer Consumer Health Care	
Bain de Soleil All Day For Kids Waterproof SunBlock Lotion	15
Bain de Soleil All Day Gentle Block Waterproof SunBlock Lotion	30
Bain de Soleil All Day Waterproof SunBlock Lotion	15
Bain de Soleil All Day Waterproof SunBlock Lotion	30
Procter & Gamble Co.	
Oil of Olay Daily UV Protectant Beauty Fluid	15
Oil of Olay Daily UV Protectant Fragrance Free Beauty Fluid	15
Oil of Olay Daily UV Protectant Fragrance Free Replenishing Cream	15
Oil of Olay Daily UV Protectant Replenishing Cream	15
Schering Plough Healthcare Products, Inc.	
Coppertone Sport Dry Lotion	15
Coppertone Sport Dry Lotion	30
Coppertone Sunblock Lotion	15
Coppertone Sunblock Lotion	30
Coppertone Sunblock Lotion	45
New Coppertone Oil Free Sunblock Lotion	15
New Coppertone Oil Free Sunblock Lotion	30
New Coppertone Skin Selects for Dry Skin	15
New Coppertone Skin Selects for Oily Skin	15
New Coppertone Skin Selects for Sensitive Skin	15
Shade UVA Guard Lotion	15
Shade UVA/UVB Sunblock Lotion	45
Shade UVA/UVB Sunblock Oil-Free Gel	30
Shade UVA/UVB Sunblock Stick	30
Water Babies Sunblock Lotion	15
Water Babies Sunblock Lotion	30
Water Babies Sunblock Lotion	45

Sun Pharmaceuticals

Banana Boat Active Kids Sunblock	30+
Banana Boat Active Kids Sunblock	50
Banana Boat Active Kids Sunblock Lotion	30+
Banana Boat Active Kids Sunblock Lotion	50
Banana Boat Aloe Vera Lip Balm	21
Banana Boat Baby Kote	30+
Banana Boat Baby Sunblock Lotion	29
Banana Boat Baby Sunblock Lotion	50
Banana Boat Broad Spectrum	50
Banana Boat Faces Plus for Normal to Dry Skin	31
Banana Boat Faces Plus for Normal to Oily Skin	15
Banana Boat Faces Plus for Normal/Combination Skin	23
Banana Boat Faces Sunblock	23
Banana Boat Maximum Sunblock	50
Banana Boat PABA-Free Broad Spectrum Sunblock	25
Banana Boat Sport Sunblock Lotion	30
Banana Boat Sport Sunblock Lotion	30+
Banana Boat Sport Sunblock Lotion	50
Banana Boat Sunblock Lotion	15
Banana Boat Ultra Sunblock	30
Banana Boat Ultra 30+ Super Sunblock	30
BioSun Maximum Sunblock Lotion	45

BioSun

BioSun Children's Ultra Sunblock Lotion	30
BioSun Faces	25
BioSun Moderate Sunblock Lotion	15
BioSun Ultra Sunblock Lotion	30

Tanning Research Laboratories, Inc.

Hawaiian Tropic Baby Faces	35
Hawaiian Tropic Baby Faces	50
Hawaiian Tropic Baby Faces and Tender Places	25
Hawaiian Tropic Baby Faces Natural Sunblock Lifeguard	15

PRODUCT	SPF
Hawaiian Tropic Baby Faces Sunblock Lotion	25
Hawaiian Tropic Bioshield Facial Sunblock for Normal Skin	15
Hawaiian Tropic Bioshield Facial Sunblock for Sensitive Skin	15
Hawaiian Tropic Just for Kids	30
Hawaiian Tropic Just for Kids	45
Hawaiian Tropic Land Sport Sunblock	20
Hawaiian Tropic Sport	15
Hawaiian Tropic Sport	45
Hawaiian Tropic Sunblock	15+
Hawaiian Tropic Sunblock	30+
Hawaiian Tropic Sunblock	45+
Hawaiian Tropic Sunblock Lip Balm	45

Westwood-Squibb Pharmaceuticals

PRESUN Active Sunscreen Gel	15
PRESUN Active Sunscreen Gel	30
PRESUN Block	21
PRESUN Creamy Sunscreen	46
PRESUN for Kids	29
PRESUN for Kids Spray Mist Sunscreen	23
PRESUN Sensitive Skin Sunscreen	15
PRESUN Sensitive Skin Sunscreen	29
PRESUN Spray Mist Sunscreen	23

Yves Saint Laurent

Yves St. Laurent Hydra-Fluid	15

Please note that these products are the recommendation of the Skin Cancer Foundation. However, there are plenty of quality sunscreens on the market that are not listed here. Remember, every product labeled SPF 15 will provide the same level of protection.

Chapter 4

IRONING OUT THE WRINKLES

"Lower the lights and change all of the bulbs to 25 watts."
—ERMA BOMBECK, ADVICE TO
THIRTY-FIVE-YEAR-OLD WOMEN ON GROWING OLDER

"This treatment, when made use of according to directions, gives an appearance of graceful plumpness to the form and a pearly blooming purity to the complexion, which is ever the admiration of the opposite sex. It will also remove freckles and wrinkles: in fact, it makes the beautiful still more lovely and restores the bloom of health and freshness to the faded cheek. The restorative powers of this grand recipe are especially noticed in the enlargement of the breasts, returning to them a fullness and firmness far beyond the most sanguine expectations."

—BEAUTY CREAM ADVERTISEMENT, 1890S

Just when you really start to believe that we have, indeed, come a long way, baby, something like this advertisement comes across your desk to point out how the more things change, the more they stay the same. Compare the advertising language above with the following excerpt from the package insert of a product sold today.

Wake to a visibly fresher appearance in the morning. A smoother skin texture. Firmer skin tone. Maximize the benefits of beauty rest with _____. This patented formulation effectively utilizes the stabilizing environment of the night (darkness, stillness, relaxation) while neutralizing free radicals, a recognized factor in the appearance of skin aging. The high performance ingredient is encapsulated for progressive release up to eight hours, safeguarding skin's beauty from free

radicals through the night. The result: skin achieves maximum benefits of unaltered rest.

I've left out the name of the product, because this company
makes no more grandiose claims than many other companies. My
point here is not to embarrass anyone, but simply to illustrate that
companies have been wooing us for more than a century with unrealistic, even silly, claims about their beauty products. The skin creams of
today can actually improve the appearance of wrinkles and help fade
freckles. They won't increase your bustline, as the 1890s product
promised, but that can be taken care of surgically if necessary.

We all know that avoiding the sun is the only surefire way to
keep from drying up like a raisin, but a growing number of products
can remove or reduce wrinkles once they appear. For information on
cosmetic services such as laser and acid peels, as well as surgical
choices such as lifts, tucks, and liposuctions, please see Chapter 5.

MY PERSONAL QUEST FOR
THE FOUNTAIN OF YOUTH

For the last twenty-five years or so, I've been on a mission to preserve my looks and have tried nearly every product that's come on
the market from Lowila and Dove soaps and Cetaphil lotion to Capture by Christian Dior and La Prairie cleansers and lotions. Along the
way, I've used Ponds, Ethocyn, Neutrogena, Alpha Hydrox, Exuviance, and Avon. I've also tried products my dermatologist recommended, and something from nearly every line of physician-dispensed
products from glycolic acid pads, Lac-Hydrin 12 percent, and Neo-
Strata. Like many people, I'm convinced that one day someone is
going to develop the cream that really is the answer to my skin-care
prayers.

More realistically, I know that a large part of the reason that my
skin looks so good is that I've been religious about protecting myself
from the sun and I have good genes. Being faithful about cleansing
and moisturizing my skin is another significant factor, too. I'm not
sure how much of a role any particular product has played in my
young-looking skin, but you can bet your last dollar that I'm going to
stick with what's worked so far and continue to experiment with
new products, avoid the sun, and tend to my skin like a devoted
lover.

PLANET COSMECEUTICAL

My quest for eternal youth has recently led me to a place I call Planet Cosmeceutical. It wasn't long ago that the world of skin care included little more than moisturizers, cleansers, toners, and eye creams. Today, mapping a course through the cosmetics aisle is like charting virgin territory in outer space.

On this new planet, the rulers talk about delivery systems and they don't mean UPS or Federal Express. They sell time capsules, but they don't intend for you to bury them in the ground for unearthing in fifty years and they claim they can erase the signs of aging. Some days I feel like I got stuck in an episode of "Star Trek" and that somebody is going to beam me up any minute.

The research and development labs of every major cosmetics company have been operating on overdrive to create products that actually improve the skin and the billions of dollars invested have paid off in products that really work. Many of them do erase fine lines, firm up facial skin, speed up cell turnover, improve complexions, and fade brown spots to some degree or another.

Common sense has always told you that if something seems too good to be true, it probably is, but I'm happy to report that women everywhere are getting great results from all different kinds of products. Whether it's a $12 jar of Avon's Anew or a $75 bottle of vitamin C serum, many of these products work well and are part of the growing category of cosmetics that are more properly called "cosmeceuticals." They work like a pharmaceutical product to deliver cosmetic effects.

Pharmaceuticals, of course, are the business of the Food and Drug Administration. So, you might ask, why hasn't the FDA begun to regulate these products? According to Dr. Gary Grove of the Skin Study Center in Pennsylvania, the simple fact of the matter is that every major FDA crackdown or regulation has come in the aftermath of a major catastrophe. Since no one's been hurt using wrinkle cream, the FDA hasn't been in much of a hurry to increase its workload. In addition, the cosmetics companies are certainly not interested in spending the extra time and money needed to have their products approved and tested by the FDA, so they scrupulously avoid creating a catastrophe.

Furthermore, Dr. Nicholas Perricone, who has conducted a great deal of research on antiaging ingredients, points out that the ingredients that are getting results are derived from common, natural products like milk and fruit that aren't normally regulated by the FDA.

Before we get further into this discussion of the FDA and cosmetics, it is important to understand how they define and regulate drugs. In order to be a drug, the *purpose* of the product must be to alter the body's function. While wrinkle creams clearly intend to alter body function, as long as their *stated* purpose is cosmetic, or superficial improvement, the product is not *intending* to be a pharmaceutical and is therefore considered to be cosmetic.

All of this legal, bureaucratic stuff aside, the good news for consumers is that good products cost much less than we would pay if cosmetics companies had to seek FDA approval before bringing them to market. Just as new drugs are expensive when they are first introduced, it is reasonable to expect that FDA-approved wrinkle creams would be slow to reach store shelves and beyond the pocketbooks of most consumers.

The bad news is that little independent research is done on these products. Long-term safety and efficacy studies are simply not performed. Can we be certain that long-term use of any particular ingredient doesn't cause cancer? Is there a limit to how much exfoliation the skin can handle? We don't know for sure.

But that's the problem. Everyone wants to know if wrinkle creams really work, and companies spend a fortune trying to convince you that they do. If you believe the advertising, these products will not only smooth your skin, they'll iron your husband's shirt and start the coffee in the morning.

In the United States, we turn to the FDA to assure us that products are safe and effective. Because the FDA is considered a reliable watchdog, many people have been wondering when the FDA was going to give its blessing on the new wrinkle creams and moisturizing products that appear to work and work safely. But, the FDA is in the business of approving drugs—products that treat diseases. Much as we might consider wrinkles to be a pox on humanity, they're really not an illness and certainly no one ever died from terminal wrinkles. In addition, products that merely change the appearance of the skin are considered cosmetics because the results of using the product are superficial.

Until recently, that kind of separation between government and the cosmetics industry has been appropriate and reasonable; and for most products, it continues to make sense because the products don't cross one very important line: They don't alter body function. Moisturizing skin or sloughing off dead cells does not qualify as altering the body's function. Essentially, that's why the FDA has not gotten involved in skin care. Not to mention that the FDA's cosmetics division has a $4 million budget to regulate a $20 billion industry.

Now, however, we have products that deliver active ingredients like alpha hydroxy acids (AHAs) in strong enough concentrations that researchers say they thicken the skin or boost collagen production, for example. If a product can cause the skin to increase collagen production, isn't that altering the normal functioning of the body?

"Past policy has been for the FDA to only look at the claims made on the package labeling," said the FDA's John Bailey. "If you look at the labels, companies are very careful to avoid making drug claims. We're currently deciding if it is appropriate to look at the other ways companies communicate with consumers, like their advertising, and infomercials." Bailey points out that although the package labeling may avoid drug claims, published articles, published research, advertising, and infomercials build up the public perception of what a product can do.

This explains why you won't hear cosmetics companies talk in truly scientific terms. They can't, legally. They stick to the "younger-*looking* skin" claim that won't bring the FDA into their labs. As long as they only claim a superficial intent, they are not claiming to be a drug and the FDA has no business in their business. It's kind of like regulatory hide 'n' seek, but now consumers are calling olley, olley oxenfree. It's time for everyone to come in and start the game over.

According to Bailey, the FDA has received only one hundred or so complaints regarding alpha hydroxy acid (AHA) products over the past three years, a number that is statistically insignificant given the enormous amount of product sold each year. As long as there is not a major safety issue, the FDA will probably not feel a need to devote its time and resources determining whether or not fruit acids actually smooth wrinkles.

Bailey and his colleagues at the Cosmetics Ingredient Review (CIR) Board are, however, interested in the high-potency AHA products that are sold through doctors' offices and 800 numbers because no one knows for sure what other effects (besides exfoliation and collagen production) they may have on the skin. The FDA is examining

AHAs to determine if their use causes the skin to become a less-effective barrier to other chemicals. For example, they want to know if the use of AHAs causes the skin to absorb more sunlight, or if topical drugs pass into the skin more readily when AHAs are also used. Both the CIR and the FDA are concerned about increased photosensitivity with AHA use, but a Connecticut dermatologist may have already resolved that issue.

In an article in the May 1996 issue of *Dermatologic Surgery,* Dr. Nicholas Perricone, a well-known researcher and clinical professor at Yale Medical School, points to research that indicates that glycolic acid, the most commonly used AHA, has a photo-*protective* effect on the skin. In his study, Dr. Perricone showed that skin treated with glycolic acid had a sun-protection factor of 2.4 compared with untreated skin. Studies, of course, are ongoing and the photo-protective effect is small, so don't take that piece of information as license to go without sunscreen.

While every company would like to be able to legitimately and legally claim to stop wrinkles or create younger skin, most companies don't want to finance the scrutiny of the FDA in order to make that claim. That doesn't mean that the companies are making unsafe products or doing something illegal. It's just that FDA approval for a product involves so much time, red tape, and expensive research that a $35 jar of alpha hydroxy moisturizing wrinkle cream would become a $135 jar of FDA-approved wrinkle cream that does the same thing. That's an endorsement cosmetics companies don't want to pay for and its fairly safe to say that consumers aren't interested in paying for it either.

Dr. Grove points out that companies like Avon, Dior, Estee Lauder, and the like have billions invested in their good names and their research, and they have far too much to lose by hastily bringing something to market that might hurt people. "A product from a reputable company is not likely to hurt you," says Dr. Grove, although it may or may not work as well as you'd like.

This sort of regulatory fan dance will probably go on as long as consumers don't complain. Since most people are relatively pleased with the products, and others think they are manna from heaven, don't look for any official proclamations any time soon.

This desire to avoid government scrutiny is not an altogether bad thing for consumers. Cosmetics companies have more to gain by making safe, quality products then by making ineffective potions that will never generate repeat business and could compel the government to regulate them. Consumers get good products at a price that doesn't include legal fees, extensive clinical trials, and the cost of regulation.

THE EXCEPTION TO THE RULE

There is one product, and only one product, that has proven its safety and efficacy to the FDA: Renova. Ortho Pharmaceuticals actually conducted the research and proved to the FDA that tretinoin, the active ingredient in Renova and its sister product Retin-A, actually reduces fine lines, surface roughness, and age spots. Ortho spent billions to accomplish this, but they now have the patent on the only FDA-approved wrinkle cream.

Experts disagree on whether Renova, which is only available by prescription, does anything more than a strong AHA product, but many women like the idea of having a prescription wrinkle cream. Ortho has a captive audience in those consumers—some experts estimate that audience to be worth $175 million in first-year sales alone.

Before Renova burst on the scene, however, Retin-A was the unofficial prescription wrinkle cream with a somewhat controversial past.

Retin-A

Discovered by the University of Pennsylvania School of Medicine's Dr. Albert M. Kligman, Retin-A is a compound whose active ingredient is tretinoin, or all-trans-retinoic acid, a vitamin A metabolite that occurs naturally in the body. Retin-A has been used since the seventies to treat acne topically, while its sister product, Accutane (isotretinoin), is the oral alternative. Dr. Kligman discovered Retin-A's usefulness in treating wrinkles and sun-damaged skin based on the feedback from his acne patients, who in addition to becoming blemish-free also had smoother, more elastic skin as a result of using the drug.

Those results prompted doctors to prescribe Retin-A for what's known as "off-label" use. Doctors are legally permitted to prescribe a drug for any beneficial purpose even if the use is not listed on the product's label. Doctors and patients agreed that even though the FDA had not approved Retin-A for wrinkles, as long as it worked, and worked safely, it didn't matter.

That's where the Retin-A story gets juicy.

In 1988, Johnson & Johnson, the parent company of Ortho, which manufactures Retin-A, announced in the *Journal of the American Medical Association* that researchers had proven Retin-A to be the cure for the common wrinkle. While it was approved by the FDA to treat acne, and doctors could legally prescribe it for "off-label" uses such as treating wrinkles, Retin-A was not approved by the FDA for *marketing* as a wrinkle cream and that legal detail prompted an FDA inquiry that was later turned over to the Justice Department.

In 1991, as the Justice Department was requesting documentation from Ortho's dermatology and public relations departments, company officials pulled a Fawn Hall and shredded incriminating records. Four years later, Ortho admitted to shredding documents from the dermatology and public relations departments and agreed to a $5 million fine plus $2.5 million to cover the cost of the government's investigation. In exchange, the company can legitimately say that it was never charged with the illegal promotion of Retin-A.

Retin-A is still widely used for the treatment of wrinkles, surface roughness, and pigmentation problems, with good results. It comes in gel, cream, and liquid forms in several concentrations ranging from .01 to .1 percent. Its base is oil in water, so it tends to be rather drying, which makes sense since it was developed to treat acne. Furthermore, patients must be vigilant about using sunscreen or avoiding the sun altogether when using Retin-A because the drug does increase sun sensitivity.

Darkly pigmented women can safely use Retin-A, according to dermatologist Barnett Johnson, but patients should start at the lowest possible concentration, using the drug every other night to avoid hypopigmentation.

Renova

In January 1996, one year after Johnson & Johnson pleaded guilty to destroying documents, the FDA gave the company the go-ahead to market Renova, an emollient cream with tretinoin, Retin-A's active ingredient, that had been undergoing clinical trials for several years. The approval made Renova the first prescription skin cream proven to reduce fine wrinkles, brown spots, and surface roughness.

While AHAs work on the top layers of the skin, according to one of its clinical investigators, Dr. James Leyden of the University of Pennsylvania, Renova works on all layers of the skin, including the dermis where pigmentary changes occur and fine wrinkling begins.

In the clinical studies of Renova, 78 percent of the patients treated with the drug experienced some improvement in fine wrinkling, 65 percent showed reduction in brown spots, and 51 percent showed smoothing of surface roughness.

That's the good news.

The bad news is that after twenty-four weeks, only 30 percent of the patients who used Renova for brown spots or fine wrinkling saw moderate improvement and 35 percent had minimal improvement. Of the patients who used Renova for rough skin, only 16 percent had moderate improvement and 35 percent had minimal improvement. Close to 50 percent had no improvement at all.

The press material that accompanied the release of Renova was full of caveats and cautions that Johnson & Johnson's legal department and/or the FDA undoubtedly require. For example, the literature clearly states that Renova may help *treat*, but will not cure fine wrinkles, etc., and that the efficacy of Renova on patients over fifty was unknown because they were not included in the study. That doesn't mean that doctors cannot prescribe Renova for patients over age fifty, only that those people with the most to gain were not included in the study. The studies did not include women with dark skin either, and there is a risk that Renova could alter their pigmentation. In addition, Renova can cause dryness, itching, peeling, etc. Pregnant and lactating women should not use Renova because of the risk of birth defects from the unusually high dosage of vitamin A.

It's interesting to me that because Renova applied for and received FDA approval as a drug to treat wrinkles, its package labeling and accompanying literature are more carefully scrutinized and restricted than over-the-counter products that don't have to prove anything. Renova can only claim to do what the controlled clinical trials actually proved, despite mountains of anecdotal evidence from devoted Retin-A users.

Renova, which is formulated in a water-in-oil emollient base, is available by prescription for about $60 for a four- to six-month supply. Because it was designed to treat wrinkles, the emollient base is important for mature, dry skin. Some people, however, who switched from Retin-A to Renova because of Retin-A's drying effects found that Renova caused them to break out.

Like Retin-A, Renova only works as long as you continue to use it. Furthermore, using Retin-A or Renova means a self-imposed exile from the sun. Ironically, these products, which correct sun damage, make the skin more sun-sensitive. Exposure to the sun while using either of these products without ample sunscreen or a sunblock can do far more damage than you'll ever reverse by using the product.

Finally, keep in mind that even though Renova is a prescription drug, approved by the FDA, there is no guarantee that it will work for you.

FUTURE APPLICATIONS

Now that Renova is approved for wrinkles, experts believe it won't be long before tretinoin-based products will be available over the counter. In fact, some over-the-counter products, in an apparent attempt to capture some of the prescription spotlight, are advertising the use of an ingredient called Pro-Retinol A, or retinol palmitate, which sounds like Retin-A, but is actually a cheap imitator. Don't be fooled into thinking those ingredients do anything special.

Research also continues on the efficacy of tretinoin in treating and preventing some kinds of cancer, and while the research is certainly far from conclusive, it does appear to be promising. It seems that tretinoin's cell-sloughing ability may enable it to whisk away cancerous and precancerous cells. Renova studies conducted by Johnson & Johnson, however, specifically excluded patients with a history of skin cancer.

Elaine's Exclusive

BEWARE OF CHEAP IMITATORS

There are a lot of skin-care products masquerading as antiaging products. Their labels announce ingredients that are deceptively invented to sound like an alpha hydroxy acid or Retin-A. They'll claim to have alpha-something or retin-whatever as a secret ingredient. Read the list of ingredients. If you don't see glycolic, lactic, malic, citric, or tartaric acid, or fruit or sugar cane derivatives listed among the first few ingredients, assume the product is simply a moisturizer. The only way to get Retin-A is by prescription.

GETTING WHAT YOU PAID FOR

Aside from our two prescription wrinkle fighters, there are hundreds of products on the market that claim to help reduce surface wrinkles and many of them work pretty well. As a consumer advocate, I wanted to be able to tell you how to read a label so that you would be able to make educated choices. But the truth of the matter is that the science of skin care has become too complex and the average person can draw precious few conclusions from reading a label these days. Judging the quality of skin-care products isn't as simple as reading a spaghetti sauce label and choosing one product over another based upon how far down water is on the list of ingredients.

As with food labels, skin-care ingredients are also listed in order of weight, so the top five or seven ingredients make up the bulk of the product. But that isn't the whole story because other ingredients can dramatically affect the formulation as well. The pH of a product has a tremendous impact on how well an AHA product works, but without a Ph.D. in chemistry you can't discern that information from the package label. For example, a product with 5 percent glycolic acid and a pH of 3.5 would be more potent than one with 15 percent glycolic acid and a pH of 5.

Given that, my best recommendation is to ask for product samples before you buy. To narrow the field, check the charts at the end of this chapter. The products listed are the ones I recommend to my friends based upon consultation with chemists, dermatologists, and personal trial and error. Once you find something you like, stick with it until the next wave of products comes along and you want to try something else.

ALPHA HYDROXY ACIDS

When I was writing *Take Care of Your Skin* back in 1988, alpha hydroxy acids (AHAs) were relatively new on the market. While they held a lot of promise, they were certainly not a household word and only department store brands included this age-erasing fluid.

Since then, a lot has changed and every company from Avon to Prescriptives now offers some sort of alpha hydroxy product. Although we touched on the topic briefly in skin care, I want to tell you a little more about alpha hydroxy acids and their wrinkle-removing ways.

There are several kinds of alpha hydroxy acids: lactic acid, derived from sour milk; malic acid, made from fruit juice; glycolic acid, which comes from sugar; citric acid, derived from citrus fruits; and tartaric acid, made from wine. These acids are essentially why women have been whipping up refrigerator cosmetics for years. Although no one was certain why lemon juice seemed to help fade freckles, or why honey made for a good facial mask, we knew it worked—at least a little. Now you know why Cleopatra, whose beautiful skin made her a legend in her own time, took milk baths.

Essentially, these acids, in their more refined, cosmetic form, work to encourage cell turnover, which slows down as we age. They do this by dissolving the "glue" that holds cells together. (Think of skin cells as bricks. AHAs dissolve the cellular mortar that binds the cells to one another.) Just as cutting dead flowers from a plant encourages new blooms, sloughing off dead skin cells helps new cells emerge. That's what all the ad hype about cell renewal and revealing younger skin is all about. In fact, according to the Cleveland Clinic's Dr. Wilma Bergfeld, products containing these active ingredients can improve skin quality by as much as 40 percent, while moisturizing alone will yield improvements of approximately 16 percent.

For the sake of description only, imagine that your skin is a nine-layer cake and an excited four year old came along just after you finished assembling and icing it and stuck her fingers in the top of it. Now the top two layers have an unmistakable dent in them. If you remove the top two layers of the cake, you'll again have an unblemished dessert. AHAs work by helping your body gradually shed the damaged, wrinkled skin to bring undamaged skin to the surface.

Companies also boast that AHAs will "revitalize your complexion" or "give your skin a rosy glow." That's because AHAs increase collagen and elastin production and blood flow to the skin.

Some dermatologists offer AHA products with as much as 20 percent acid. These products are being offered as an alternative to Retin-A because they are safe for pregnant women (high doses of vitamin A have been known to cause birth defects) and do not create the severe sun sensitivity that Retin-A is famous for. Additionally, women of color find AHA products to cause less pigmentation alteration.

For patients who want aggressive skin-care treatment, many physicians prescribe a combination of Retin-A in the evening and a 12-percent AHA product during the day. While the results are effective, I would caution anyone reading this to work closely with their dermatologist on a skin-care program that is this aggressive. Don't skip off to the pharmacy with your prescription in hand and dial up the 800 number of the recommended AHA product and never return to the doctor for follow-up. By the same token, don't assume that if one dab of a product is good, two dabs are better. You could develop a case of "too much of a good thing."

In the not too distant future, you'll begin to hear companies advertising beta hydroxy acids (BHAs), which are kissing cousins of the alphas and essentially do the same thing. Salicylic acid, used in acne products, is one BHA. NuSkin is among the companies pioneering work with these acids and I expect that they'll be in stores before long. NuSkin's MHA (multi-hydroxy acid) Revitalizing Lotion products are reasonably priced and formulated with SPF 15 for daytime use and without SPF for nighttime use. Also, the newest formulation of Estee Lauder's popular potion, Fruition Extra, boasts three AHAs and one BHA in its formulation.

Elaine's Exclusive

CHICKEN AGAIN?

Just as your family gets bored eating chicken six nights a week, so too does your skin fail to respond to the same old skin-care products week after week. If you're using AHA products, consider buying two or three different products and rotating them every month. Read the labels and select one that is primarily glycolic acid and a second product that is primarily lactic or some other acid for best variety. NuSkin scientist Dr. Walter Smith suggests four weeks of an acid product, followed by four weeks of a gentle facial scrub.

Studies are conclusive that AHAs not only stimulate cell turnover, but that they act as antioxidants and can have anti-inflammatory effects as well. When you begin using them should depend almost entirely on the quality of your skin. People with acne or heavy sun damage may want to begin using them sooner than the average woman who hopes to use them to address fine lines and complexion roughness. Given that the FDA has had practically no complaints, I can see no reason not to use good AHA products. They do get results and even if you stop using AHA products, you are likely to find that the improvements will last. Keep in mind, though, that your skin won't stop aging altogether and that new lines and new photodamage will eventually appear.

Knowing which products are good, however, is tricky business.

AHA!—SEEKING OUT THE AHA
PRODUCTS THAT WORK

Back in the good old days, when cosmetics companies sold hope-in-a-jar, everyone understood, even if their spending habits indicated otherwise, that there were no miracles and that skin-care products really didn't do much for wrinkles or other signs of aging.

Today many of these products do work. They're not little jars full of miracles, but they can improve the look of the skin. This progress has raised consumers' expectations at a time when we try to quantify almost everything. We have SPF numbers for sunscreen, and numeric ratings for wine, our food labels quantify fat grams and calories, the octane of gasoline is listed on the pump, and movies get four stars if they're good. You would think that someone would come up with a simple way to rate the efficacy of skin-care products. It could be a simple system, like: four crow's-feet mean that your wrinkles will be gone overnight, and one crow's-foot means that the product comes with the phone number of a plastic surgeon in your area. Is that too much to ask?

Actually, it is too much to ask, but cosmetics companies are attempting to accommodate in a somewhat deceptive way. You may have noticed that some products will boast claims like—8 percent alpha hydroxy acid, 5 percent fruit acid, and so forth. That's somewhat interesting and helpful, but unfortunately, it doesn't tell the whole story. If it were that simple, we'd know that an 8 percent product was more potent than a 5-percent product and we'd work our way up the scale, starting with a 2-percent in our twenties and slowly increasing the concentration as our skin needed more attention. Wouldn't that be nice?

The trouble is that the efficacy of an AHA product has as much to do with the pH of the product and its formulation as it does with the concentration of acid. The ideal pH for a skin-care product is between 2.8 and 3.5. At this pH, the acid is not neutralized as it would be if the pH were higher, and the product is not too irritating as it would be if the pH were lower.

Elaine's Exclusive

HURTS SO GOOD

You'll know an AHA product is working if you experience a *slight* stinging or tingly sensation when you first apply it. If the stinging is severe or persists, or if the skin turns especially red, gently wash your face, apply a soothing, non-AHA moisturizer, and buy a new antiaging product. The product you've chosen is probably too strong for your skin.

So, in reality, if a product has a high pH, the 8-percent acid may be only as effective as a 2-percent acid product. Conversely, a well-formulated 4-percent acid product could be more potent than a poorly formulated 7-percent solution. See why this is so complicated?

Unfortunately, sampling products is the only real way to find something that works for you. As a rule of thumb, you can assume that anything you buy in a department store will have a small amount of acid in it, but it will be sufficiently neutralized to prevent any problems. These products are formulated for mass marketing and you can be sure that Estee Lauder is not interested in selling products that irritate the facial skin of thousands of customers. The exception to the rule is Exuviance, the new prestige line by NeoStrata, which is similar in formulation to the professional line (8-percent AHA) that is sold by doctors and estheticians. To the best of my knowledge, this is the only department store brand that can make such a claim. What's more, the lotions contain sunscreen, too, making them great all-in-one products.

Be sure to ask the salesclerk if the product actually contains an AHA. Many of the "firming or refirming" products have no AHAs at all. They're simply very good moisturizers and, in plumping up the outermost layer of the skin, create the appearance of additional firmness. Also take note of the items listed under "Active Ingredients" on the labels of antiaging products. In most cases, the active ingredient is sunscreen, which will only protect against future damage, not correct current damage.

If you haven't been using an AHA product thus far, I'd suggest that you avoid any of the products that promote themselves as having 10- or 12-percent acid. Start out with something less potent for a few months.

Just as you start out walking around the block and build up from there, you should not introduce your skin to AHA products starting with a 12-percent formulation and not expect some problems with irritation.

If I were in charge of the cosmetics world, every company would be required to specify the percentage of acid and the pH of the formulation on the product's label. That way consumers would know what they were getting. But since no one's asked me to take over yet, I hope these suggestions are helpful.

One Word of Caution

Everyone is in agreement that stimulating cell turnover will help skin look younger, but truly, no one knows for sure if there is a limit to how much the skin can proliferate. Dr. Lorraine Meisner from the University of Wisconsin notes that every time a cell divides it loses a small part of the tip of its chromosome. Without this telomere tip, chromosomes stick together and die, suggesting that normal cells cannot turn over indefinitely. It's interesting to note that cancer cells make their own telomeres, which is why they can proliferate so quickly and easily.

Now, don't take this piece of information and conclude that AHAs are going to kill your skin, just understand that future research may prove that we should exercise a little restraint in our use of AHA products.

Elaine's Exclusive

A PICTURE'S WORTH A THOUSAND WORDS— OR AT LEAST A REFUND

If you're planning to buy an antiaging product, take a close-up picture of your face without any makeup prior to using the product. Use whatever product you select for thirty days. If you're not happy with the results, take another picture of yourself and take both pictures with you when you return your purchases. This way you've got proof that the product didn't perform and the salesperson will be less likely to try and schmooze you into believing that they can see an improvement because they remember you from when you came in.

ANTIAGERS

The following recommended products contain the ingredients to support the label claims. Each of these products are absorbed quickly. The women who sampled these products found that they delivered reasonably good results. Keep in mind that the drugstore and department store brands neutralize a good bit of the AHA to ensure that the product does not cause any irritation. For heavy-duty AHA products, get the physician-dispensed antiagers or the specialty products listed below.

Skin Type Key: N normal; D dry; VD very dry; S sensitive; O oily; C combination

Price Key: $ under $10; $$ $11–$20; $$$ $21–$30; $$$$ $31–$40; $$$$$ $41–$50; $$$$$$ over $50

DRUGSTORE BRANDS

PRODUCT	AHA (%)	PH	SIZE (OZ)	PRICE
Aqua Glycolic Face Cream	10	4.4	2	$$
Pond's Age Defying Complex for Delicate Skin	8	3.8	2	$$
Pond's Age Defying Lotion	8	3.8	3	$$
Pond's Age Defying System Prevent & Correct Correct formula	4	3.8	2.5	$$
Pond's Age Defying System Prevent & Correct Prevention formula (SPF 8)	2	3.8	2.5	$$

HOME SALES/SALON PRODUCTS

PRODUCT	AHA (%)	PH	SIZE (OZ)	PRICE
Avon Anew All-In-One Intensive Complex	8	*	15	$$
Avon Anew All-In-One Perfecting Complex	4	*	15	$$
Avon Anew All-In-One Perfecting Lotion for Problem Skin	2	*	8	$$

* Manufacturer declined to provide information.

Department Store Brands

The following products received great reviews from the women who sampled them and they contain quality ingredients that make them excellent moisturizers. These products claim to firm the skin or give it a little lift, which is accomplished mainly by plumping up the stratum corneum. They will not eliminate wrinkles through exfoliation, but they do not claim to provide that kind of benefit either.

PRODUCT	SKIN TYPE	SIZE (OZ)	PRICE
Chanel Lift Serum Extreme Advance Corrective Complex	all	1	$$$$$$
Christian Dior Capture Lift Firming Night Treatment	N/V D	1	$$$$$
Estee Lauder Advanced Night Repair	all	1	$$$$$
Estee Lauder Resilience Elastin Refirming Creme	N/V D	1	$$$$$
Estee Lauder Resilience Elastin Refirming Lotion	N/V D	1	$$$$$
Montiel Energy Concentrate	N/V D	1	$$$$$
Princess Marcella Borghese Spa Energia Skin Energy Source	N/V D	1.5	$$$$

Samplers also liked these department store AHA products. With the few exceptions noted, the manufacturers would not give out information concerning the percentage of acids or the pH, which makes it impossible for me to give them a full recommendation. What I can tell you is that the products feel nice, absorb well, and women who tried them were pleased with the results. If you don't find that the products perform up to your expectations within thirty days, take the product back to the store for a refund. (Don't forget your receipt.)

PRODUCT	SKIN TYPE	SIZE (OZ)	PRICE
Chanel Creme Parfaite Night Lift Plus	N/V D	1.7	$$$$$$
Decleor Timecare Serum (1% AHA, pH 5)	all	.8	$$$$$$
Elizabeth Arden Ceramide Time Complex Moisture Cream	N/D	1.7	$$$$$
Estee Lauder Fruition (1% glycolic)	N/D	1.7	$$$$$
Lancôme Primordiale Visibly Revitalizing Solution	N/V D	1	$$$$
La Prairie Age Management Serum (5% lactic acid)	N/D	1	$$$$$$
Origins Starting Over	D	1	$$$
Prescriptives All You Need	N/D	1.7	$$$
Princess Marcella Borghese Cura Notte	C/D	1.7	$$$$

PHYSICIAN-DISPENSED PRODUCTS

There are a number of well-formulated high-potency AHA and vitamin products available from dermatologists and some doctors are putting their own names on private-label AHA products as well. But do not assume that these products are drugs just because your doctor recommends or sells them. They are not. They do, however, have a higher concentration of AHA or a special molecule that makes them more potent than products you might find in a department store. Because they are more potent, some patients experience stinging, peeling, or scaling, which is why the manufacturer *prefers* that customers use these products under a doctor's supervision.

Some consumers and physicians are uncomfortable with the idea of doctors selling products and rightfully question a doctor's objectivity when they are making money selling skin-care products like highly educated Avon ladies and gentlemen. I think that's a legitimate concern that can only be resolved individually. Do you have a good relationship with your doctor? Do you trust him or her to give you sound advice? Does the doctor also suggest products that are not sold in his or her office? Did your doctor actually formulate the product, or is it something made by a private label company that anyone can slap their own label on?

I can't tell you whether or not you should buy skin-care products from your doctor, because that really is a personal choice. I have, however, recommended what I feel are the best products in this category of physician-dispensed skin care.

Before you buy products from your doctor, check the back of this book for the 800 numbers of the best-known physician-dispensed cosmetics companies. Often you can buy directly from the company and save yourself a few dollars. Again, be careful because these products tend to be well-formulated and have a much higher percentage of acid than you would get from any department store product.

PHYSICIAN-DISPENSED ANTIAGERS

*Products listed in **bold type** are only available from a dermatologist or plastic surgeon; others are available through the company's 800 number.*

PRODUCT	AHA (%)	PH	SIZE (OZ)	PRICE
Biomedic Conditioning Gel Plus	15	2.2	2	$$$
Biomedic Conditioning Gel	8	2.2	2	$$$

PRODUCT	AHA (%)	PH	SIZE (OZ)	PRICE
Biomedic Conditioning Solution	10	2.0	6	$$$
Glyderm Cream	5, 10, 12*	1.5–1.8	.5–1.0	$$$
Glyderm Lotion, Lotion Plus, Lotion Lite (12% lotion and cream cost a few dollars more)	5, 10, 12	1.5–1.9	2–3.3	$$$
Glyderm Solution	5, 10, 12	2.0–2.5	2–3.3	$$$
Jan Marini Bioglycolic Facial Lotion	12	3.25	2	$$$$$
Jan Marini Bioglycolic Night Cream	14	3.25	2	$$$$$$
MD Formulations Facial Cream	14	3.25	2	$$$$$$
MD Formulations Glycare Alcohol Based Facial Lotion	5, 10	4.0	4	$$$$
MD Formulations Oil-free Facial Lotion	12	3.25	2	$$$$$
MD Formulations Smoothing Complex	10	3.25	.5	$$$$
MD Forte Facial Cream	15, 20	3.8	1	$$$$
MD Forte Facial Lotion	15, 20	3.8	2	$$$$$
MD Forte Glycare	15, 20	4.5	2	$$$
MD Forte Skin Bleaching Gel (with 2% hydroquinone)	10	3.8	1.5	$$$
Murad Advanced Combination Skin Formula	8–12*	4.5	3.3	$$$$$
Murad Age Spot & Pigment Lightening Gel with 2% hydroquinone	8–12*	3.5	1.4	$$$$$
NeoStrata AHA gel for Age Spots and Skin Lightening	10	4	1.6	$$
NeoStrata AHA Solution for Oily Skin	8	4	4.0	$$
NeoStrata Enhanced Body Lotion	15	3.6	6.8	$$
NeoStrata Enhanced Cream	15	3.6	1.75	$$
NeoStrata Enhanced Gel	15	4	4	$$$
NeoStrata Sensitive Skin AHA Face Cream	4	3.5	1.75	$$
NeoStrata Skin Smoothing Cream	8	3.5	1.75	$$
NeoStrata Skin Smoothing Lotion	10	3.8	5.8	$$
Nova Skin Facial Lotion	12	3.8	2	$$$$

*Indicates approximation. Company would not share specific details.

OTHER PRODUCTS WITH PROMISE

While many antiaging products currently on the market have one kind of AHA or another as their main wrinkle-reducing ingredient, there are a few other products available that are unique and seem to have real promise. Because they are somewhat unusual, I felt they deserved special attention here.

Cellex-C

Cellex-C is the granddaddy of the topically applied vitamin C products and, interestingly enough, it was developed in response to the widespread use of Retin-A on mature skin.

Dr. Lorraine Meisner, a professor of preventive medicine and pathology at the University of Wisconsin, was concerned about older women using Retin-A on an ongoing basis. She believed that the better way to fight wrinkles would be to "build up the collagen mattress" under the epidermis. Knowing that vitamin C stimulates collagen growth, she and a colleague, Dr. Schinitsky, developed a technology that combined ascorbic acid with zinc and tyrosine in a skin cream. They tried to sell the system to established cosmetics companies but had no takers. Then along came Dr. Sheldon Pinnell of Duke University, who was thinking along the same lines and had patented a way to stabilize vitamin C. The three teamed up and licensed their technology to Megan McLellan, a Canadian cosmetic researcher and entrepreneur, who successfully brought Cellex-C to market.

Cellex-C is the first product to deliver 10-percent vitamin C straight to the skin. In this strength, vitamin C is credited with reversing the signs of sun damage by reducing present wrinkles, preventing future wrinkles, scooping up free radicals on the skin, lightening age spots, and boosting collagen production. Rosacea patients have also found that Cellex-C eases this condition because of vitamin C's anti-inflammatory properties.

Since vitamin C is known to build collagen, Cellex-C is recommended for use on the backs of hands, too. Thinning skin shows protruding veins and bony knuckles, making the hands look old. Cellex-C has been shown to thicken skin by increasing collagen.

Cellex-C uses L-ascorbic acid, the simplest form of vitamin C and the only form that the body can actually recognize and use. Unfortunately, L-ascorbic acid tends to be unstable (it degrades quickly when exposed to the air) and it is only soluble in water, which cannot penetrate the skin. Furthermore, acid in water can be drying or irritating. That's where the zinc and tyrosine come in. Tyrosine and zinc act as escorts for the vitamin C and usher it into the skin—that's what's known as a delivery system.

While it seems as though it would be simpler to swallow vitamin C in tablet form, researchers know that the body distributes ingested vitamin C equally to all cells, making it impossible to specifically target the skin with oral vitamin supplements.

In his patent application, Dr. Pinnell proved that he had successfully stabilized vitamin C for seven weeks, which is an incredible accomplishment. Unfortunately, seven weeks isn't much of a shelf life for a cosmetic product and that has been the biggest complaint with Cellex-C. After a comparatively short amount of time, the product begins to turn color, indicating that the vitamin C has begun to oxidize. That doesn't mean that the product has spoiled, only that you may not be getting the full 10 percent promised on the serum's label. According to Dr. Meisner, however, it only takes a small amount of oxidized vitamin C to turn any product orange, so discolored Cellex-C could still deliver the full 10 percent.

According to Megan McLellan, Cellex-C products are good for a year (the cream will last for eighteen months), but it is best used within three months of purchase for optimum results. As she pointed out, when you're spending $75 for a 1-ounce bottle of serum, you should use it as directed and not let it sit on your night table where it is guaranteed not to fix a single wrinkle.

Because Cellex-C serum is formulated in a water base, it is "less elegant" than some of the other vitamin C products that are being sold. But Cellex-C's supporters say who cares if it is not a luxurious product that feels like whipped cream, it works. Because it is an acid and can sting, wait fifteen minutes after cleansing before applying Cellex-C. And, because it can make the skin feel dry, be sure to apply a moisturizing sunscreen after the Cellex-C dries. Cellex-C can be used in the same regimen as AHA products, but company information suggests using Cellex-C in the morning and the AHA at night to minimize irritation.

Research continues on topically applied vitamin C and according to Dr. Pinnell, studies that are currently underway or recently completed will help investigators to better understand the role vitamin C plays in preventing and correcting wrinkles and protecting against UV exposure.

A third study will look at vitamin C as an immunosuppression inhibitor. When many people are exposed to UV light, their skin's natural immunity becomes temporarily suppressed, making them more susceptible to other stimuli, like poison ivy, for example. This characteristic seems to be a marker for skin cancer. Even the application of sunscreen, which will prevent sunburn, will not totally prevent the immune system from becoming suppressed. Researchers have shown that topically applied vitamin C can prevent the suppression of the immune system in mice and they hypothesize that vitamin C could provide humans with the same protective benefits and therefore could help prevent skin cancer.

Let's be clear here. This is a possibility that researchers are investigating. Neither Cellex-C or any other vitamin C product claims to prevent skin cancer, but research is promising and ongoing. If proven, says Dr. Doren Pinnell, Director of Public Relations for Cellex-C, vitamin C skin creams could do for skin care what fluoride did for dentistry.

The results of these studies may be the basis for an over-the-counter drug application for a modified version of Cellex-C, but the clinical trials needed to accomplish that will take anywhere from eighteen months to five years.

Cellex-C is available from physicians or by calling 800-423-5539.

C-ESTA, Factor A, and Factor-A Plus

Jan Marini Research of San Diego applies Dr. Nicholas Perricone's vitamin C technology to a product that is similar to Cellex-C but has one important difference: C-ESTA utilizes ascorbal palmitate, which is L-ascorbic acid linked to a lipid so that it remains stable and can penetrate the top layer of the skin. Supporters say this is the best way to get vitamin C into the skin. Detractors say that the body must separate the molecule into its L-ascorbic acid and lipid components to actually make use of the vitamin C — not a difficult task for the body, but another step in the process. C-ESTA products also boast DAE Complex, which aids in the absorption of vitamin C and stimulates neurotransmitters to firm up sagging skin — the truly exciting part of the C-ESTA story.

The DAE complex, which includes the ascorbal palmitate, zinc, vitamin B6, tyrosine, and a delivery agent, stimulates neurotransmitters to eventually shorten muscles at the neuromuscular junction. (I told you this stuff sounded like science fiction.) The visible result is tighter skin around the eyes, jawline, and nasolabial folds, and it could help to postpone cosmetic surgery, as company before-and-after photos suggest.

Over the next few years, you will probably hear a lot more about stabilizing and absorbing vitamin C, but for now Cellex-C and C-ESTA are the two big players in the game.

C-ESTA is available only from physicians and is compatible with Renova, Retin-A, and AHA products. Call 800-347-2223 to find a physician in your area who offers Jan Marini products.

Factor-A and Factor-A Plus are two other Jan Marini products that dermatologist Toby Shawe says work just as well as Retin-A in removing wrinkles. These products combine vitamin A propionate with glycolic acid, which combine to help resurface skin. According to product literature, these products are particularly good for people with acne.

Jan Marini also makes a line of products for use before and after laser resurfacing. Using vitamins, glycolic acids, kojic acid for lightening the skin, and Transforming Growth Factor (TGF) Beta, a new technology used in advanced wound care, these products are intended to help laser-peel patients get optimum results and heal more quickly following the procedure. Naturally, they are only available through a physician.

Although some of the more advanced skin-care systems are also available to the consumer without the benefit of physician guidance, Marini feels that consumers get better results when they are guided by a physician who can recommend specific products for specific skin problems. Jan Marini products, including the C-ESTA line, the Pre & Post-Op Home Care Products, Factor A-Plus, Even Tone Pigment Lightening Gel, Transformation Cream, and Bioglycolic products are priced between $25 and $75.

Glycolic Acid and Vitamin C Pads

Topix Pharmaceuticals, a Bohemia, New York, company, is on to something really great. In addition to a traditional line of creams, lotions, gels, cleansers, etc., they sell glycolic acid pads, like Stridex medicated pads for acne. The pads come in two strengths, 5- or 10-percent glycolic acid, for twice-daily use. The acid is formulated with a pH of 4.5 so it is not irritating. You just wipe them across the area to be exfoliated and discard the pad.

The company also offers an SPF 15 sunblock that's sold the same way, and they have just introduced a vitamin C pad to complement their line of vitamin C lotions and creams that are sold under the Citrix name.

According to Technical Director Steven Hernandez, the Citrix Facial Complex provides 10-percent stabilized L-ascorbic acid, and the hand-and-body product has 12-percent vitamin C. He says the products will last for two years, but to play it safe the company advertises potency for one year.

Topix products are available primarily through physicians' offices, and you can call 800-445-2595 for the name of a dispensing doctor near you. If there is not a physician near you who sells the products, the company will mail products to you, so have a credit card ready when you call them.

Vitamin C Derms

Osmotics is a very elegant line of skin-care products whose centerpiece is vitamin C derms, adhesive patches like transdermal estrogen or nicotine patches that contain powdered ascorbic acid and sodium ascorbate. Women who use the derms apply one over a particular wrinkle before going to bed. During the night, moisture from the skin interacts with the powdered vitamin C, which is then absorbed by the skin to improve the wrinkle. Knowing that ascorbic acid degrades quickly when exposed to oxygen and sunlight, Francine and Steven Porter, the creators of Osmotics, decided to prevent the vitamins from ever seeing the light of day by putting the antioxidant in the patch. For best results they suggest wearing the patches to bed three nights a week for two months, followed by a one-month break.

According to Porter, the skin tends to relax a little when it is occluded by something like a Band-Aid. It seems to know that another substance is doing its job of protecting the body and takes a break. During that break period, the skin is better able to receive the healing benefits of, in this case, vitamin C, but also, for example, an antibiotic cream on a paper cut.

While the skin-care products in this line are truly luxurious, the derms are a little awkward—who wants to sleep with vitamin-C laced tape on their face three nights a week? And, at $125 for a three-month supply of derms (two months on plus one month off equals a three-month supply!), I'm not sure the benefits of derms are any greater than the high-potency vitamin C creams and serums that cost much less for the same three-month supply (that is actually used for three whole months).

On the other hand, transdermal delivery is a popular and effective method of administering other drugs and just may prove to be a breakthrough in the topical application of antioxidants as well. People who use them swear by the derms and Porter has used herself in the company's before-and-after pictures, which display significant improvement.

Until the fall of 1996, Osmotics products were sold exclusively at Saks, but they are now also at Nordstrom's and a few other high-end department stores.

Ethocyn

By now you've seen the television commercials that show the woman who has applied Ethocyn to half of her face and achieved dramatic results, and I must say that the women who have sampled Ethocyn to help me research this book have also seen improvements in their skin. If seeing is believing then you have to believe in Ethocyn. I'm really astounded by the results.

Ethocyn is a product of Chantal Pharmaceuticals of Los Angeles that has been on the market since 1995. Unlike other wrinkle products that are using vitamins or AHAs, the key ingredient in these products is the patented ethocyn molecule, a synthetic compound that blocks hormone receptors in the skin.

Company information says that ethocyn stimulates elastin production by preventing dihydrotestosterone (DHT) receptor-binding. These hormone receptors are known to limit elastin production, and by blocking them, ethocyn can bring elastin fiber levels up to those of someone in their twenties. The increase in elastin makes the skin smoother and more supple.

While this may sound like science fiction, Ethocyn has a lot of believers among the staff and patients of Manhattan facial plastic surgeon Norman Pastorek, a past president of the American Academy of Facial Plastic Surgery. His wife, Janice, who is a nurse and esthetician in his office, tried Ethocyn on herself before giving it to patients and staff. She says she noticed a difference in just ten days and that others noticed an improvement in her skin within a month.

While Ethocyn builds up elastin, it does not exfoliate, so Janice Pastorek recommends using the product twice a day for a month as directed, and using no AHA or Retin-A during that time. After the first month, she tells patients to use Ethocyn once a day and an AHA once a day as sort of a skin-care one-two punch.

Ethocyn is available at the pharmacy counter of many national drugstore chains, but the prices are more like department store cosmetics. Although you can buy the two 2.3-ounce vials of Ethocyn Essence for $75 (some retailers discount it to $62), the company also sells the essence, packaged along with other skin-care products that contain very small amounts of Ethocyn, for $60 and $120, depending upon the package. Physicians, who were originally the only outlet for Ethocyn, still sell the product, too.

It's interesting to note that others in the industry rejected the idea of marketing their products through mass-market drugstores because they felt no one would pay $75 for drugstore skin care. They were shocked by what they considered to be a gutsy move on the part of Chantal and are surprised by how well the gamble has paid off. Ethocyn is selling very nicely at Eckerd's, Walgreens, Walmart, etc., and developing legions of loyal repeat customers.

PRODUCTS WITH PROMISE

There are a few products that deserve special mention here because of the great results they deliver. They were discussed at length in the section on Promising Products and are listed separately here because they are not AHAs like all of the others.

PRODUCT	ACTIVE INGREDIENT	SIZE (OZ)	PRICE
C-ESTA Cream	ascorbal palmitate	.5	$40
Cellex-C Serum	L-ascorbic acid	1	$75
Citrix Facial Moisturizer	L-ascorbic acid	.5	$42
Citrix Pads	L-ascorbic acid	60 pads	not yet available for sale
Ethocyn Vials	ethocyn molecule	.46	$75
Osmotics Derms	L-ascorbic acid	2 months	$125
Topix Glycolic Pads	10% glycolic acid	60 pads	$22
Topix Glycolic Pads	5% glycolic acid	60 pads	$18

SPECIALTY ITEMS

Sudden Change Under Eye Skin Smoother*		.5	$
Sudden Change Skin Smoother*		.5	$

*These products do a nice job of temporarily concealing fine lines and work well under makeup. Unfortunately, they have an unpleasant odor.

PRESCRIPTION FOR THE FUTURE

Sooner or later, the FDA will probably end up regulating some of the more potent products like Ethocyn or Cellex-C, whose published research clearly states that the products alter body function. For example, Cellex-C says that the topically applied vitamin C "cues cells to produce collagen." Ethocyn's information says that, in clinical studies, the use of Ethocyn has been shown to significantly increase the levels of elastin tissue in the areas where the product was applied. If products cause the body to produce collagen or elastin, isn't that altering body function? After all, the body was not producing as much collagen or elastin before the product was used.

It's interesting to note that in 1988, Chantal Pharmaceuticals, the company that makes Ethocyn, prepared an FDA application for clinical trials, but withdrew the application because they didn't want to spend the money. And who can blame them? Why would a company willingly strap on the financial burden of securing the approval of an agency that doesn't require it?

I think this will eventually change. In fact, in consumer question-and-answer material distributed by Chantal, the company notes that "Ethocyn is considered a cosmetic by the FDA (at least for now) and cosmetics do not need to be approved in the same fashion as normal drugs, only safety tested, which has already been done." Chantal's earlier willingness to submit an application for clinical trials suggests the company's confidence in the product, so don't be surprised if they turn up with an FDA-approved formulation some time in the next few years.

The makers of Cellex-C have begun FDA trials for a modified version of the product that would be considered an over-the-counter drug. Cellex-C will remain on the market as a cosmetic and the modified product, if approved, will be sold as an over-the-counter drug. They have created a modified formula because if the company sought FDA approval for the current version of Cellex-C, the product would have to be withdrawn from the market for the duration of the clinical trials, which can last from eighteen months to five years.

So what's a consumer to do? How do you know if products will work and if they are safe? It's practically impossible to tell by reading labels, concedes the FDA's Bailey. "Some of these antiwrinkle claims are pure hype," he said. "If they really worked, companies would want to protect the product and get drug approval like Renova did. It's an expensive process, but it gives a high degree of protection to the sponsor." Protection, in the form of FDA approval and patents, certainly provides exclusive market access for the products, but cosmetics companies are making plenty of money without it.

On the Horizon

After talking to doctors, researchers, and cosmetics-company executives, I'm convinced that in the future you'll see more and more companies introducing vitamin C products, and that the vitamin E products will be right behind them.

Ideally, one researcher told me, companies would formulate a product that was heavy on both vitamins, but so far that's been difficult to accomplish without making a skin cream that smells like a jar of vitamins. "It's like granola," he said. "The granola bars that sell taste like candy; the ones that are really nutritious taste like birdseed. The cosmetic products that work are not very elegant and consumers don't use them as faithfully as the products that feel good."

Keep your eyes open for those products. I'm certain the researchers will find the answer soon.

DON'T BE FOOLED

Because cosmetics are not regulated, anyone can cook up face cream in their basement and sell it. There's nothing to stop them. That's why I caution consumers to only buy brands they know and trust from companies that are well known.

If you send $29.95 to a P.O. box expecting to receive miracle wrinkle cream, you could be in for a big disappointment. That post office box could be closed any day. Even a money-back guarantee is no good if you can't find the company in sixty days. I hate to knock anyone, and certainly plenty of good companies have started out with one product offered through mail order, but without the financial investment in image, name-recognition, and research, I'm concerned that some of them may be selling wrinkle cream today and carpet cleaner tomorrow. If you send $20 for the latest kitchen gadget and it doesn't work, you're only out $20. If the wrinkle cream is garbage and causes your skin to break out, you've got bigger problems than a few lost dollars.

As in all things, use your good judgment, don't expect miracles, and go with a name you trust.

Elaine's Exclusive

LISTEN CAREFULLY

The people who answer the customer relations lines for cosmetics companies say some pretty incredible things. One company's representative told me their products were FDA approved, but of course, we know that cosmetics don't require FDA approval. Another person told me that the combination of acids in their product were targeted to specific areas of the skin. Am I to believe that there's a microscopic traffic cop loaded into every dollop of moisturizer directing the fruit acids to my crow's-feet and the lactic acids to my lip lines? Yet another woman told me her company's products contained between 8 and 12 percent acid, but they weren't sure exactly how much. If a company refuses to share critical information like the ingredients, pH, percentage of acid, makes claims that defy logic, or says they don't know what's in their product, do not buy from them.

Hype, Hype Hooray: Help Is on the Way

Just as the 1890s advertisement at the front of the chapter illustrated, cosmetic products are marketed with all kinds of hyped-up claims like:

> Patented molecules "flood" between dried out layers of surface skin, rapidly renewing translucency. Skin virtually glows from within.

or

> When elastin weakens, there is a visible loss in tone and firmness. Today we know this is due to more than passing time. It is accelerated by stress, environmental factors and daily irritation. Now for the first time, you can do something to intercept the cascade of negative events that begins with these everyday effects—and ends with the loss of tone and firmness.

The first example makes it sound as though your face will look like ET's finger and the second, describing the cascade of negative effects, makes wrinkles sound like they are comparable to deteriorating peace negotiations. But, while these claims may sound ridiculous when they are isolated like this, who wouldn't want to glow from within, and who wouldn't spend a few dollars to prevent the trickle-down hazards of daily living from showing up on our faces?

Skin-care products are loaded with advertising claims that, without critical review, could lead you to believe that someone has, indeed, found the fountain of youth. While most of us are sensible enough not to expect miracles, the scientific advances in the skin-care industry have made real improvement a reality and it's sometimes hard to separate the hype from the honest possibilities. So here's the English-to-English translation for the commonly used advertising language on skin-care products.

Antiaging/prevents premature aging: Contains sunscreen. The only way to gain any significant ground on the aging of your skin is to protect it from the sun.

Cell renewal: Contains an exfoliating agent, either an alpha hydroxy acid or some cleansing grain. This sloughs off the old surface cells to make room for new surface cells.

Enhanced microcirculation: Product contains an ingredient that brings blood to the surface of your skin. As we age, circulation slows down, which makes the skin pale. Products that claim to boost microcirculation merely include witch hazel, or some plant extracts or botanicals. (Remember, witch hazel is a good toner, so it may not be right for your skin type, despite the mircoboost to your circulation.)

Free radical protection: Contains antioxidants such as vitamin E (tocopherol), beta-carotene, vitamin C (ascorbic acid), bioflavonoids, and superoxide dismutase. Free radicals have been implicated in the aging process and are commonly believed to cause wrinkles. Antioxidants neutralize free radicals.

Night repair: Contains a mucopolysaccharide such as hyaluronic acid. Mucopolysaccharides are part of the cellular structure of the dermis and can be damaged by ultraviolet light, which is why the products are touted for use beyond the light of day.

Oil-free moisturizer: Contains no emollients. Usually claimed for oily-skin products. These products usually contain humectants and silicone derivatives instead.

Hypoallergenic: Doesn't really mean much. This only means that the product has fewer allergens than other products of its type and probably contains no fragrance. This does not, however, guarantee no allergic reaction.

Natural: Most people think that "natural" means that the product contains no synthetic ingredients. However, without preservatives, most products would have a very short shelf life. Others believe that if a product is "natural" it must be mild and wholesome, but, in fact, natural ingredients can be just as irritating as synthetic ingredients. Lanolin, for example, which is derived from sheep's wool, is as natural as they come, but many women are allergic to it. The fact is the term "natural" is loosely defined and is often used as a gimmick to attract health-conscious consumers who want to buy products that are not tested on animals and are environmentally friendly. But the truth is that the product may not be much different from any other on the shelf.

Noncomedogenic: Does not contain one of many ingredients known to cause blackheads or whiteheads.

Visible results overnight: Skin will be better hydrated and therefore *appear* more plump. Lines and wrinkles cannot actually vanish without the help of cosmetic surgery.

Elaine's Exclusives

SPECIAL DELIVERY

Dimethicone and Cyclomethicone are two ingredients that are used to help get beneficial ingredients into the skin. This is what's often called a delivery system, which, along with liposomes and niosomes, help make products work.

Wrinkle Pills

Longevity magazine reports that glucosamine supplements, which are often recommended to arthritis patients, may help the skin make its own hyaluronic acid, which lubricates joints and moisturizes the skin. Participants in the few studies conducted reported significant improvements in the texture of the skin, but because glucosamine can't be patented, its wrinkle-removing possibilities probably won't be researched fully. Other wrinkle pills like Sincera, a product advertised in women's magazines, are little more than expensive vitamins with some secret "marine proteins." While the glucosamine supplements may be worth a try, Sincera, at $130 for a three-month supply of vitamins, certainly isn't.

Chapter 5

TO TUCK, OR NOT TO TUCK

"I don't plan to grow old gracefully. I plan to have face-lifts until my ears meet."

—Rita Rudner

"I arrived in Hollywood without having my nose fixed, my teeth capped, or my name changed. That is very gratifying to me."

—Barbra Streisand

Not too long ago, the only people who had cosmetic surgery were movie stars, the very rich, or the very vain. Today, four-hundred thousand men and women from all walks of life are choosing to enhance their appearance each year from a fast-growing menu of cosmetic options.

Once, a face-lift was the main course on this menu, but now you can have almost anything lifted, from your eyes to your derriere. In between, there is liposuction, tummy tucks, peels, injections, and lots more to help wipe the years right off your face and body.

There are any number of reasons people choose to have their appearance surgically improved. Some are disfigured from disease or disaster and want their faces or bodies restored. Others want to be competitive in an increasingly tight job market and they want their know-how to communicate experience to a prospective employer without their looks saying "burned out" or "too old."

Still others, especially the baby boomers with their physically fit bodies, want their faces to match their youthful physiques and hip attitudes. "I'm in good shape and dress stylishly. I like to do fun things and I'm up to date on what's happening in the world. I want my face to match my lifestyle and the way I feel," said one woman I know.

Regardless of the reasoning, Clinique's Truth & Beauty Survey reports that 97 percent of women over forty want to look as attractive as possible for their age, and more than 70 percent are happy with what they see in the mirror. For the remaining women who are not as pleased with what they see, there have never been more ways to improve their looks.

KNOW YOUR OPTIONS

I set aside this chapter to give you some general information about the variety of surgical and nonsurgical options for improving your looks. Whether or not you decide to take advantage of what's available or stick with what you've got is completely up to you, but at least you'll have good information on which you can base a decision.

In this section, you'll find a brief description of each procedure, what kinds of imperfections the procedure will correct, as well as risks and recovery times. I've also included price ranges for these procedures, but you should keep in mind that the costs will be dependent upon many factors, including the doctor you choose, where you live, the amount of work being done, hospital costs, and much more.

Careful, almost religious, sun-avoidance using a wide-brimmed hat and sunscreen is required following any of these services to achieve optimum results.

LOOK BEFORE YOU LEAP

Prior to undergoing any kind of cosmetic surgery or service, make sure you have reasonable expectations about the results of the procedure. A new nose may make you feel more confident or less conspicuous, but it's probably not going to change your life.

If you're contemplating cosmetic surgery, make sure you are doing it for yourself, not to change someone else's opinion of you. If you feel young and vigorous and want your face and body to match the way you feel inside, great. But don't jump into plastic surgery on the heels of a personal crisis. Just because your husband ran off with a younger woman doesn't mean you need a face-lift.

Make sure you are in good health both mentally and physically before heading to the doctor's office for surgery.

Finally, to get the very best results you must be candid with the doctor about your medical history, current lifestyle, etc. Don't leave out any medications, habits, or exercise regimens, no matter how embarrassing. Because so many things can impact the outcome of your surgery, you should tell the doctor everything, even if it seems irrelevant.

Among the seemingly irrelevant habits a patient should disclose is cigarette-smoking. While quitting smoking is always a good idea, doctors caution women contemplating cosmetic surgery to give up cigarettes prior to surgery because nicotine causes blood vessels to constrict and, in a surgical situation, could cause the death of some tissue. In addition, cigarette-smoking changes the quality and texture of the skin and slows healing.

Many people take an aspirin every day to help keep the blood thin, but this same habit should be stopped for a period of time before surgery because it can cause increased bleeding.

Before you have any procedure, help yourself as much as possible by getting into a good skin-care routine. Healthy skin will respond better to the procedure and heal faster. Get the rest of yourself in good shape, too. If you're exercising and eating right, you'll bounce back more quickly after surgery and run fewer risks of complications.

CHOOSING A DOCTOR

Selecting a capable, qualified physician is the most important thing you can do to assure a successful procedure. Before settling on a physician, ask your friends who they recommend and then ask the doctors you interview for more referrals. Once you've narrowed down your choice, check the physician's certification.

Credential-checking is important because not all doctors are board certified and many physicians, who are not plastic surgeons, perform some kinds of cosmetic surgeries or services.

As long as a doctor is licensed in their field of expertise and trained in a particular procedure, it is perfectly *legal* to offer the treatment. It is also legal in most states for a person with a medical degree and no specialized training to hang a shingle and call him or herself a cardiologist. It may be legal, but do you really want to trust your heart to that person?

Since 1934, the American Board of Medical Specialties (ABMS) has established quality control standards for the education, evaluation, and certification of specialists. They recognize twenty-four specialty boards, among them dermatology and plastic surgery.

In order to be certified by one of the boards that is recognized by ABMS, a physician must have graduated from an accredited medical school and completed residency training before taking the board examination. In the case of plastic surgeons, the doctor completes a three-year residency in general surgery, followed by a two-year residency in plastic surgery. Then, after practicing for another two years, a surgeon can take the final qualifying exams for board certification in plastic surgery. Some specialties allow doctors to sit for the exam after completing the residency program.

What makes matters confusing is that there are 126 other boards that are not recognized by the ABMS. Some, like the American Board of Cosmetic Surgery, also certify physicians against very rigorous standards. In fact, to be certified by the ABCS, a cosmetic surgeon must first be certified in a medical discipline that is recognized by the ABMS. Although the ABMS does not recognize the cosmetics board, ABCS-certified doctors work primarily in cosmetic procedures, while someone who is a certified plastic surgeon could do mostly reconstruction work.

To make matters even more complicated, board certification is a voluntary rite of passage but not a licensing requirement. In 1973, less than half of all licensed physicians were board certified; today approximately 70 percent are. Managed-care programs are now demanding certification and most hospitals will not grant privileges to new doctors who are not board certified, but there are plenty of excellent older physicians who simply never took the test because it wasn't necessary.

Who Does What?

A plastic surgeon is a surgeon who specializes in the field of plastics, which includes repairing congenital defects, reconstructing the body after injury and disease, as well as making cosmetic improvements. Some, but not all, doctors who advertise as cosmetic surgeons are indeed plastic surgeons who have chosen to specialize in cosmetic work instead of correcting birth defects, for example.

Dermatologists are trained to treat the skin. Dermatologic surgeons are dermatologists who have focused their practice in surgery. And because dermatologists and dermatologic surgeons have pioneered the development of laser surgeries, peels, fills, and liposuction, they may be better choices for those kinds of procedures than plastic surgeons. By the same token, an occuloplastic surgeon—an ophthalmologist who has been trained in plastics—may be the very best choice for eyelid work.

Because these titles and certifications are so confusing, contacting

professional associations is a good way to start your search for a qualified physician. The following groups will provide the names of ABMS
board-certified specialists in your area as well as information about
any procedure you are considering. State and county medical boards
are also good resources.

American Society of Plastic and Reconstructive Surgeons
800-635-0635

American Society for Aesthetic Plastic Surgery
888-ASAPS-11

American Academy of Facial Plastic
and Reconstructive Surgery
800-332-FACE

American Society of Dermatologic Surgery
800-441-2737

American Academy of Dermatology
930 N. Meacham Rd. Schaumberg, IL 60173

American Academy of Cosmetic Surgeons
800-A NEW YOU

The American Board of Medical Specialities also has a toll-free
number (800-776-2378) that you can call to verify certification without quizzing the doctor about whether or not their board certification comes from an ABMS board or one of the others.

Because of the politics involved in medicine, board certification is
overly complicated by too many boards. What's more, it is not the
only measure of medical training and professional expertise. Some
people simply don't test well, despite the fact that they might be bril-
liant in their field. Additionally, some doctors with years of experience
simply never took the test. After all, people perform surgery, not
diplomas.

All of this aside, however, we all want to be assured that we are
going to have good results from our experiences with the medical
profession—at the very least, that we'll be no worse off than when
we started. Given that, I think that board certification and good referrals are the best basis for selecting a physician for cosmetic work.

And keep in mind that the best-known doctors are not always the best surgeons. Sometimes they just have good public relations firms working for them.

Always remember: There are no guarantees in medicine; that's why they call it a "practice."

Doing Your Homework

1. Just as you would not choose a brain surgeon from the Yellow Pages, don't choose someone to alter your face that way either. Ask around for referrals and let the doctor know who referred you. (Your hairdresser, who knows everyone's secrets and sees plastic surgery scars up close, may be a great source of referrals.)
2. When you call for an initial consultation, ask the receptionist to send you information about the procedures you are contemplating. That way you can read up before seeing the doctor.
3. Write down all of your questions and bring the list with you so you don't forget to ask anything.
4. Don't choose a doctor who doesn't make you feel comfortable. If the doctor is offended by direct questions about his or her experience and certifications, choose someone else.
5. If you notice that someone has had work done and you think they look great, discreetly inquire about their doctor or procedure. Keep in mind that some people don't want anyone to know about their surgery, so be sure to handle the inquiry gently if you don't know the person well.

Questions to Ask When Interviewing a Physician

1. Are you certified by an ABMS-recognized board? In what specialty?
2. Will *you* be performing the procedure? (Sometimes the physician will allow someone else in the practice to perform the procedure. Make sure you meet with the person who will be doing your work.)
3. How many of these procedures have you done in the past? (With newer technology such as laser resurfacing, choose someone who has done at least twenty to forty procedures already.)

4. Can you give me the name and number of a few of your patients who have had this procedure?
5. Do you have admitting privileges at a nearby hospital? (If the procedure is being done in the office or in a nonhospital setting.)
6. What kind of anesthesia will you use?
7. Who will be administering the anesthesia? Is that person board certified?
8. How much experience do you have treating someone with my complexion? (This is primarily for dark-skinned women.)
9. What will the procedure cost? Does that price include everything or just your fee?
10. How long is the recovery time? When will I be presentable? How soon before I can wear makeup?

Extra Precautions

Dr. Thomas Romo III, president of the New York Academy of Facial Plastic and Reconstructive Surgery, requires that his patients obtain clearance from their family doctors or internists prior to performing surgery. "The patient's internist knows about specifics in the patient's history that might cause a complication during surgery," he said. The internist's report guides Dr. Romo's choice of location—either hospital or his own Park Avenue operating suite—for the surgery.

"This isn't a salon, this is surgery," he emphasized, adding that the same pre-op testing that is required for procedures done in hospitals should also be done prior to having surgery at an outpatient center.

Outpatient Surgical Centers

Cosmetic surgery centers are cropping up all over, providing comfortable, private, cost-effective alternatives to hospital visits. These facilities tend to charge set amounts for procedures performed at their facilities and, generally speaking, the expense for a procedure is less at a same-day surgery center than in a hospital.

The American Association for Accreditation of Ambulatory Plastic Surgery Facilities inspects and accredits these facilities, provided they are owned or directed by board-certified surgeons. The facilities are categorized as Class A, B, or C depending on the kind of anesthesia they are certified to administer. Only local anesthesia and medication to relieve tension may be used in Class A facilities. Both Class B and C facilities have life-support equipment should it become necessary.

Class B centers, however, use intravenous sedation and Class C uses general anesthesia, allowing the patient to sleep through the entire procedure.

If you are having a procedure done at an outpatient surgical center, you may want to call one of the three organizations that accredit these facilities:

The American Association for Accreditation of Ambulatory
Plastic Surgery Facilities
708-949-6058

The Joint Commission on Accreditation of Healthcare
Organizations
708-916-5600

The Accreditation Association for Ambulatory Health Care
708-676-9610

Prior to your procedure, find out if the doctor has admitting privileges at a nearby hospital in case there is an emergency that the center can't handle. Also, be sure to arrange for someone to take you home following the procedure.

TO TELL OR NOT TO TELL

Even though Phyllis Diller supplies anyone who asks with a complete list of her cosmetic surgeries and the surgeons' names, not everyone is as willing to tell the world that they've "had some work done."

The fact is that choosing cosmetic surgery or services is a very personal choice that only you can make. If looking younger will make you feel better about yourself, who cares if your mother thinks you look just fine and don't need it? What difference does it make if your best friend thinks you're vain? If you can afford it, have weighed the dangers of elective surgery, and you think cosmetic surgery will make you happier, then do it. On the other hand, just because a service is available and affordable, doesn't mean you have to have it. It's a purely personal choice.

Whatever you decide to do, or not to do, there are certainly plenty of good reasons for not choosing to share that kind of personal information with anyone — the best being that it's nobody else's business.

PEELS AND FACIAL RESURFACING

If you're bothered by wrinkles—and who isn't—you may want to consider one of the latest weapons in the war on wrinkles, which is a variation on one of the oldest weapons in the arsenal, the peel. While the idea of having the top layer of your skin removed may seem a little unsettling, a peel is less invasive than plastic surgery, promises less recovery time, and certainly costs considerably less. Although the effects don't last forever, women and men are having peels on their lunch break, and often undergo the procedures on a regular basis, because they are easy to endure and the results are good.

According to Dr. Mark Solomon, formerly the cochief of plastic surgery at Hahneman University Hospital and Medical College of Pennsylvania in Philadelphia, and now in private practice, a woman can keep wrinkles at bay with a combination of regular peels and aggressive skin care.

Alpha hydroxy acid peels can be done by almost anyone—estheticians, dermatologists, cosmetic surgeons. Even your obstetrician could, technically, perform a peel if he or she went to the training class. For my money, I'd choose a dermatologist or a plastic surgeon.

Fair-skinned women of European descent are the best candidates for all types of peels because there is little risk of pigmentation problems. Doctors peeling dark-skinned (Mediterranean, Hispanic, Asian, and Black) women should exercise extra care, says Dr. Gustave Colon, a New Orleans plastic surgeon, because there is always the risk of hyper- (excess) or hypo- (loss of) pigmentation. Although the change in pigmentation is not usually dramatic, it can be noticeable, so be sure to ask the doctor pointed questions about his or her experience treating women with darker skin.

While dark pigmentation may make someone less of a candidate for a peel, the extra pigmentation also makes a person less likely to wrinkle, says Dr. John Skouge, an assistant professor at Johns Hopkins and president of the Center for Dermatologic Surgery in Baltimore. "Darkly pigmented people just don't get the kind of wrinkles that these modalities treat best." Dark-skinned individuals do, however, get acne scarring and melasma, abnormal pigmentation problems that can be addressed through laser treatment and peeling.

Dr. Ferdinand Ofodile, the director of plastic surgery at Harlem Hospital and an associate clinical professor at Columbia University, points out that Black people are especially prone to hypertrophic scars and keloids, although no one knows why. For that reason, he recommends that Black women, in need of more aggressive treatment for acne scars, etc., choose a laser surgeon with a great deal of experience.

Although there are exceptions — such as acne-scarring mentioned above — as a rule of thumb, TCA, phenol, laser resurfacing, and dermabrasion are not recommended for dark-skinned (Black, Hispanic, Asian, and Mediterranean) women.

AHA Peels

Paying someone to put acid on your face may sound like the opening scene from *The Invisible Man,* but the truth is that people do it everyday to improve the look of their skin.

Alpha hydroxy acid peels, at concentrations of as much as 70 percent, are offered by many physicians. In effect, application of a 20, 30, 50, or 70 percent glycolic acid solution loosens the top layer of skin, revealing new, pink, but possibly slightly irritated, skin underneath.

If you think of your skin's cells as bricks that are held together by mortar, you'll get a good picture of what AHAs do. AHAs dissolve the cells' mortar so that the old, dead cells can be sloughed away.

In researching this book, I had a peel done by Toby Shawe, a wonderful dermatologist near my home in Pennsylvania. She performed a 20-percent peel, which did sting, but I could immediately see the improvement in my skin.

The peel process is quick and simple. First the hair is pulled away from your face and the doctor cleans your face thoroughly. The acid is then applied with a paintbrush and a fan is directed at the treated area. The doctor watches carefully for the first signs of pinkness and then neutralizes the acid. A facial immediately following the procedure soothed the burning sensation and left my face feeling like the proverbial baby's behind.

Although I could have put on makeup only one hour after the peel, my complexion was so fresh and my skin looked so great that I brushed lipstick across my lips, put on a little mascara, and spent the rest of the day barefaced for the first time in thirty years. It reminded me of the clean, fresh feeling you have after having your teeth cleaned. I'm really pleased with the results and will definitely do it on a regular basis now, because Dr. Shawe says it can truly help keep wrinkles away.

Just as you would prior to having minor surgery or scheduled testing, you should follow your doctor's instructions carefully prior to having a peel. Typically a patient will have a consultation with the physician a week or two before the peel, at which time the physician will recommend an appropriate skin-care regimen and caution the patient about things to do and things to avoid both before and after a peel to get optimum results.

For example, the physician guidelines that accompany NeoStrata's peel products specifically require two weeks of pretreatment, a week of post-peel treatment, and also recommend starting with the lowest concentration for only one or two minutes for the first peel. In addition, the company advises patients to stop waxing, electrolysis, and the use of masks, loofahs, Retin-A, hair color, and much more one week prior to the peel. These are safety precautions designed to reduce the risk of scarring or bad results.

Doctors are also advised to gradually work up to stronger peels as the patient develops a tolerance, so don't feel you are not getting your money's worth when your doctor suggests a one-minute peel with a 20-percent solution for your first treatment.

Regardless of the percentage, the AHA peels are light, superficial treatments intended to reduce fine lines and improve the texture of the skin. Keep in mind that AHA peels cannot eliminate deep acne scars, wrinkles, or sagging skin and jowls.

Typically dermatologists recommend a series of six peels over the course of three to six months. Depending on the way your skin responds, the doctor will increase the duration of the peel, the concentration of the acid, or both. Following the initial six treatments, refresher peels are suggested two or three times a year, but with continued use of AHA skin-care products, and sun avoidance, the results can last as long as nine months. Don't be taken in by doctors who recommend peels every six weeks. According to Dr. Shawe that's a waste of money and totally unnecessary. Dermatologists charge between $50 and $125 per peel. The facial is an extra $50 and should only be done when a short-duration, low-concentration peel is performed, otherwise even the gentle facial products can be irritating.

According to Dr. Aaron Shapiro, a Philadelphia-based plastic surgeon, almost anyone is a good candidate for a peel; from seventeen year olds with acne to fifty year olds with sun-damaged skin.

Skin type is not a factor in a peel's effectiveness, but darker-skinned individuals, Blacks, Hispanics, and Asians would be well advised to insist that the doctor or esthetician do a test patch behind the ear or on the arm prior to peeling the face. Dr. Shawe recommends a low concentration peel for no more than two minutes for darkly pigmented skin.

When you are scheduling a peel, be sure to ask who will be doing the treatment. Many physicians have estheticians or physician's assistants on staff who perform the peels under the doctor's supervision.

Beauty Salons, Nail Salons, Spas

Beauty salons and spas offer AHA peels up to a concentration of 40 percent. (Anything over 40-percent solution must be administered by a physician.) They'll recommend using a glycolic acid preparation for a few weeks before the peel, and then do as many as six treatments over the course of two to four months. Some estheticians do the peels weekly, others recommend treatments every other week. The cost of approximately $200 for a series of six peels is pretty affordable and many places offer a peel with a facial for a reduced price.

Because the peels are superficial, at low concentrations, they do a nice job of refreshing the skin, but are not likely to cause any harm. Even so, I would still recommend that women with dark skin see a doctor instead. Practically every day spa in the country offers alpha hydroxy acid peels along with facials and other services.

Estheticians are licensed by the state in which they operate, but an esthetician's license means the state has trained the operator in waxing and skin care only. The product manufacturer trains estheticians in the use of the peeling products. According to Marlene Cahill, product manager for MD Formulations, estheticians are given a detailed procedure manual, a training video, and in-person training at the salon and at seminars offered around the country.

Just as you would ask your friends for physician referrals, ask around for a good esthetician. Before you schedule the appointment, meet with her and ask about her training and experience doing peels.

Chemical Peels

While AHA peels require virtually no downtime, you can obtain a deeper, more lasting peel from the use of one of two commonly used chemicals, trichloroacetic (TCA) acid or phenolic acid. Like alpha hydroxy acid peels, these too can be done in a doctor's office, depending on the depth of the peel, and the results are far more dramatic but, naturally, so are the risks.

With either of the chemical peels, the physician creates a controlled injury by applying TCA or phenol to burn away the top layers of skin. What's left behind is red, sometimes blistering, seeping skin. Once it heals, the skin that emerges is more elastic and evenly textured, but the risks of infection and scarring are far greater with this kind of peel because of the open wounds it initially creates.

As I mentioned earlier in this chapter, it is important to thoroughly chronicle your medical history for a new doctor planning cosmetic work and here is another good reason why. Patients with acne or acne scars often seek out peels to improve the scarred areas. Patients who have taken Accutane, however, should not have a TCA or phenol peel within one year of stopping the drug because the risk of scarring is very great.

Doctors differ on how they use peeling chemicals. Some like TCA for a peel, but others find it difficult to control the depth. Some doctors like phenol for certain areas, such as under the eyes or around the lips, but others prefer the laser for those areas because phenol can bleach the skin. Because these chemicals are weapons in the doctor's arsenal, you'll find many different approaches for resolving the same problem.

With that in mind, you may want to consult with more than one doctor before deciding how to address a particular trouble spot. Be sure to ask the doctor why they are recommending one course of treatment over another and then choose the doctor and the treatment that gives you the most desirable combination of results, recovery time, and cost.

You can expect doctors' fees in the range of $1,300 to $1,800 for a full face peel and $550 to $925 for spot treatments. Some day spas, like the Beauty Spa at the Dermatology Center in Englewood, New Jersey, are linked with a medical practice, so clients can get chemical peels at the same facility where they get a facial or an AHA peel. The chemical peels in these facilities must still be done by physicians.

Phenol
Phenol peels were first used by nonmedical or lay peelers who started out doing Hollywood starlets like Mae West. Even though the

lion's share of publicity has been about lasers and AHAs lately, phenol is still used by many doctors for deep peels and for spot peeling around the mouth in conjunction with a face-lift.

Phenol provides a deep peel and is applied under heavy anesthetic. Once the chemical is applied and then removed, an antibiotic ointment, Vaseline, or waterproof adhesive tape strips are applied and left in place for twenty-four to forty-eight hours. (The first sixteen hours can be very painful.) The face will be red for as long as six months after the peel and patients are advised to diligently avoid the sun following a phenol peel. Phenol can leave skin looking white and shiny, kind of ghostly. It can be toxic, and there is the risk of keloids, which are thick, red, raised scars that must be treated over a period of time with cortisone injections.

Plan on two to three weeks recovery from a phenol peel, although the peeling crustiness should be through in two weeks, at which time the patient can begin wearing makeup.

The results of a deep phenol peel can last from five to seven years. Phenol also leaves a clear line of demarcation between peeled and unpeeled areas, which is why some doctors consider it to be a less than desirable alternative for spot treatments.

Trichloroacetic Acid

A trichloroacetic (TCA) peel is the chemical commonly used for a medium-depth peel that is intended to revive dull, weathered skin, improve acne scars, and to correct pigmentation problems or age spots.

TCA peels can be done in the doctor's office. Usually the skin is very red for the first twenty-four to forty-eight hours following the peel. After the first two days, the patient will look deeply tanned. That darkly tanned look will peel off just as sunburn peels and the patient can usually wear makeup five days after the peel. The patient should keep the peeled area dressed with an appropriate cream, like Polysporin ointment, to promote healing.

If a TCA peel is done to eliminate age spots, the results can be permanent as long as the patient practices diligent sun avoidance. The removal of fine lines will last for one to two years. Many doctors prefer TCA for spot treatments because it does not leave the same lines of demarcation for which phenol is known.

Dermabrasion

Just as construction workers can sandblast crusty rust and corrosion off of a steel structure, so too can doctors smooth away your wrinkles with a high-speed instrument that's attached to surgical sandpaper. It's called dermabrasion and it is performed under a local anesthetic — although some people prefer general anesthesia — on large areas like the forehead or cheeks.

Once again the top layer of skin is removed to reveal new, pink skin underneath, and once again there is the risk of infection or scarring and the possibility of uneven pigmentation. There is also some bleeding involved, though not the blisters sometimes associated with chemically peeled skin. Dermabraded skin can resemble a scraped knee or elbow and the doctor will dress the abraded area with Vaseline gauze and dry gauze to prevent crusting. Once the abraded area is healed, usually within ten days, the patient can wear makeup to hide the redness, which can last for months.

While the wrinkles will be gone for as many as ten and as few as two years, the six weeks to six months of recovery time is the longest for any of the peels. For the six weeks following dermabrasion, the patient should practice diligent sun avoidance because if the area is exposed to the sun too soon, spotty pigmentation could result. Dermabrasion is particularly useful for treating acne scars and the fine lines above the upper lip, but because estrogen levels can affect the pigmentation of the skin, dermabrasion is not a good option for women taking birth control pills or estrogen replacement therapy.

The price range is similar to a chemical peel ($1,325 to $1,800) but dermabrasion is regarded as far more risky. When you consider the great success doctors are having with laser peels, it is fairly safe to predict that dermabrasion will soon be used only for major scarring and pitting and will eventually be supplanted by lasers altogether.

Star Wars: Laser Resurfacing

Laser peels are the latest and greatest thing to hit the aesthetics circuit in years. Just as lasers are being used to remove warts and tattoos and to make procedures like gall bladder surgery much less invasive, doctors can now use lasers to zap away your wrinkles.

The technique sounds like something straight out of *Star Trek*: Carbon dioxide lasers are aimed at your face and vaporize the top layer of skin. The procedure has had extensive publicity, as when Geraldo Rivera had his wrinkles done in front of his program's live audience in March 1995. As a result there is a common misconception that laser resurfacing is like waving a magic wand over the face, according to Dr. Thomas Rohrer, the medical director of Candela Skin Care Centers and the director of dermatologic surgery at Boston University. "People don't realize that there is healing involved and that they'll look worse before they'll look better."

Two different carbon dioxide lasers are currently in use for wrinkles. One provides a rapid pulse and the other a swirling laser beam. Both are designed to keep the laser from hitting any one spot too long, but they are too new for any definitive proof as to which is better.

Most patients report some discomfort rather than pain immediately following a laser peel. (The lasering itself feels like a snapping rubber band.) The first pass of the laser removes the outer layer of the epidermis. Subsequent passes go deeper into the epidermis, tightening the collagen a little more every time the laser passes over the skin. I've read about doctors who say they can see the collagen fibers tightening before their eyes.

With a laser peel, the patient will be a little red immediately following the treatment, but over the next few days following the peel, the skin will become more red, swollen, and weepy. To prevent scarring and infection, it is important to continually apply the dressing prescribed by the doctor for eight days. Full recovery will take two to three weeks following a laser resurfacing, but makeup can be applied after only eight days. Pinkness, however, can persist for a few months.

A laser resurfacing will provide dramatic results that can last ten to twelve years. A full face resurfacing will cost between $1,500 and $4,000, which compares favorably with the other procedures when you consider the low rate of pain, infection, and scarring. Doctors can also do spot treatments with lasers, using a feathering technique so that the laser-treated areas blend in with the untreated areas. (The cost for a spot treatment, around the mouth for example, will cost between $500 and $900.)

Many think that the laser peel will soon replace chemical peels and dermabrasion altogether because the laser is nontoxic, the recovery time is usually brief, and the problems are relatively few. Others feel that because lasers are so expensive there will always be a place for chemical peels, even though they offer much less control.

That doesn't mean, however, that the fountain of youth is actually a laser beam. There have been some reported cases of infections and scarring. Also, the medical community is still trying out the machines and as yet has done little reporting for peer review because laser resurfacing has only been FDA-approved since 1994.

In addition, according to Dr. Rohrer, laser resurfacing is contraindicated for dark skin because of the risk of hyperpigmentation. "Anything deeper than one or two passes puts the doctor and the patient on a slippery slope," says Dr. Ofodile.

The best advice I can give you, if you want to run out for a laser peel, is to select a physician who has already done many procedures. You may even want to consider a laser center.

Laser Centers
Because it can cost more than $1 million to fully equip a facility with all of the lasers needed to do wrinkles, tattoos, scars, hair removal, spider veins, etc. companies like Candela Corp., that manufacture a number of lasers, are opening one-stop laser centers to offer all of the treatments. At Candela's Framingham, Massachusetts, center, Dr. Rohrer trains private practitioners on the use of the equipment. Newly trained physicians are then qualified to treat patients at the center.

The next Candela center, which will be in Dallas, will incorporate a fitness center with workout equipment and salon services in addition to the laser center, leading the way in a growing trend to blend medicine and aesthetics.

Whether you go to a private practitioner with a laser or choose the laser center option, look at the doctor's before and after pictures, understanding that they are showing you their best work, and ask pointed questions about their successes and their failures, and the number of treatments they've performed.

Laser Training
Because the technology is so new, but easily available, there are plenty of doctors who can be considered armed and possibly dangerous—since there is not a whole lot of training *required* to go with the $100,000 machines. Physicians who use hospital-provided lasers must prove that they have attended the requisite training, but certainly laser companies will sell a laser to any doctor with an open checkbook.

Coherent Medical, the first company to receive FDA approval for their laser resurfacing machine, establishes a $3,000 training account for each doctor who purchases the UltraPulse. With the money set aside, doctors are encouraged to attend one workshop in addition to a preceptorship (one-on-one training), both of which are conducted by other doctors who have been approved by Coherent. In the workshop, the doctors spend a half day in classroom training learning the physics of the laser as well as pre- and post-operative skin care. The rest of the day is spent observing surgery or practicing with the laser on tomatoes or chicken. During the one-on-one training, the new laser doc will see at least five procedures. Additional training is, of course, made available, but doctors are not required to take the courses.

Dr. Colon, who teaches other doctors to use lasers, reminds consumers that like a scalpel or a pair of scissors, a laser is only as good as the hand that guides it.

According to Dr. Rohrer, because lasers are so new and there is such great public awareness of them, doctors are being particularly conscientious about getting appropriate training before picking up the wand.

In 1996, industry experts estimated that there were one thousand carbon dioxide lasers in use around the country, which seems like a small number considering how many cosmetic dermatology centers are advertising laser peels. Because the lasers are easily portable, many doctors rent the equipment and have it brought to their office a few times a month. That way they get to become comfortable with the laser and build their business before having to spend $100,000 to $125,000 for a piece of equipment.

Other Laser Treatments

VASCULAR LESIONS Pulsed dye or vascular lasers are currently the best way to treat both small spider veins on the face and larger veins on the legs, although different machines are used for each area. Removal of leg veins will cost less than $1,000. The pulse dye laser is also good for removing warts, scars, rosacea, stretch marks, and port-wine stains and other hemangiomae (purple or red birthmarks).

These lasers work because hemoglobin in the blood absorbs the laser light and then converts into heat, which damages and seals the blood vessels, causing them to disintegrate and disappear permanently. There may be some discomfort associated with the treatment, similar to a rubber band snapping at the site. Following treatment the area may be slightly swollen, sensitive, or even warm.

Patients are likely to experience some blue/gray discoloration around the treatment site, but that will pass in a week to ten days. Patients are advised not to tan areas to be lasered as the additional pigment may absorb the laser's energy, making it more difficult for the laser to reach the lesion. Obviously, that means that dark-skinned individuals may also get less than satisfactory results from this kind of treatment.

PIGMENTED LESIONS The Q-Switched-ruby, YAG laser, alexandrite, and cooper vapor lasers are all used to "smart bomb" pigmented lesions such as tattoos, liver or age spots, freckles, broken blood vessels, and some birthmarks. The pigmented area absorbs the laser light, but the rapid absorption of the light destroys the melanin, leaving the skin looking uniform in color and texture. Removal of a three-inch tattoo will cost around $325.

Following these laser treatments, an ice pack or antibiotic ointment may be soothing and patients are advised to avoid scrubbing the area with anything abrasive. Occasionally anesthetic is applied prior to the procedure, depending on the area to be treated.

HAIR REMOVAL ThermoLase recently received FDA clearance to market its hair-removal laser, and has begun opening Spa Thira salons around the country that offer the hair-removal service. It's a quicker and less painful alternative to electrolysis, but multiple treatments are needed to get near-permanent results.

The area to be treated is waxed first and then a black, carbon-based cream is massaged into the area. When the laser is passed over the area, the carbon absorbs the energy, disabling the hair follicle. Laser treatment to remove hair on the upper lip will cost approximately $1,400. For that price, the spa will keep the upper lip hair-free for one year, regardless of how many treatments it takes. (Usually three or four treatments are needed to permanently disable the follicles, but chin hairs tend to be more stubborn and sometimes take eight or nine treatments.)

In addition to its Spa Thira hair-removal salons, ThermoLase trains and licenses physicians for in-office use of the laser, but instead of selling the equipment to the doctors, ThermoLase provides the laser and the doctors pay ThermoLase a per-procedure fee. This arrangement makes the technology available to doctors without a huge cash outlay and ensures that the physicians are properly trained.

To find a Spa Thira near you, or a physician with a ThermoLase laser, call 800-76-THIRA.

OUT-OF-THIS-WORLD PRICES FOR SPACE-AGE TECHNOLOGY Buying laser equipment is an expensive proposition for doctors, which is why the price of treatment may seem high. The laser that treats spider veins has a price tag of $90,000; the laser that treats tattoos is an $80,000 piece of equipment; the carbon dioxide laser that treats wrinkles goes for $100,000 to $125,000. New technology is always expensive, but you can safely anticipate that the prices will begin to fall as the technology becomes more available.

INFILTRATING ENEMY LINES: FILLS AND INJECTIONS

While peels can handle the surface lines and wrinkles, treating the deeper creases requires heavier artillery. It stands to reason that if wrinkles are merely crevices in the dermis, they could be filled in with the medical equivalent of spackle.

That thinking has been the driving force behind all kinds of fill-in technologies that have evolved over the years. The fill-in craze started with collagen and fat, things already produced by the body, and silicone was once widely injected, although now it is illegal as its safety and effectiveness has not been determined by the FDA. Even though it is illegal, some doctors still inject silicone because they think it is the best way to address certain problems. I wouldn't recommend it since silicone can migrate and create lumps where you don't want them.

As the science developed, however, new products have evolved to fill in the cracks. You'll be amazed, as I was, to read about some of these procedures. Sometimes truth really is stranger than fiction.

Collagen Injections

Collagen is the substance that has been injected into the wrinkles of more than one million people around the world. Collagen is a natural part of the dermis; the commercial product is harvested from cow hides and then purified. Most people tolerate it very well, but approximately 5 percent have adverse reactions, which is why a physician will want to perform two patch tests on the arm prior to injecting facial wrinkles. If after the two patch tests, done two weeks apart, the patient is showing no signs of allergic reaction, the doctor will then inject the facial wrinkles with collagen.

The injections themselves are relatively painless and, unlike peels, have virtually no recovery time. They are useful for some of the deeper frown lines that tend to crease the forehead and are too deep to be rectified by a peel. They are also good for brow furrows and some of the heavier creases around the mouth. A 1 cc vial, costing between $250 and $350, can treat the entire upper lip area, which is part of the reason that collagen injections are three times more popular than fat injections.

Initially, some doctors will overfill the wrinkle, leaving the patient looking slightly swollen or lumpy, but that dissipates quickly as the collagen is absorbed into the skin. Over a period of three to six months, the body will absorb most of the collagen and the treatment will need to be repeated.

Keep in mind that despite the fact that thousands of women seem to be sprouting this look, collagen is not FDA approved for injection into the meat of the lips. Don't be alarmed by this, though. Collagen's lack of FDA approval for that one purpose is a similar situation to the one Retin-A was in not too long ago. (Retin-A was only approved for acne, even though many doctors prescribed it for wrinkles.)

GOOD NEWS FOR CONSUMERS Because collagen therapy must be repeated, the Collagen Corporation, the company that is the primary maker of collagen, has introduced its own kind of frequent flyer program. For every four vials a patient uses, the fifth should be free; for every six vials, the seventh and eighth should be free. In addition, the company recently introduced a 2 cc vial that is only 30 percent more expensive than the 1 cc vial. New patients should also be offered a free patch test. The company, of course, sells to the doctors and encourages them to pass the savings on to patients, so be sure to ask about pricing.

HOMEMADE COLLAGEN If you're planning a tummy tuck or other form of surgery that will involve cutting away fat and skin, you may want to consider having the excess skin sent away to Collagenesis, a company that will process it into your very own collagen for injecting into wrinkles. Because Collagenesis is a very new company that is trying to gain ground on the well-established Collagen Corporation, they will process your own collagen for about the same price as the bovine product.

You will, however, have to pay your doctor to do the injections and pay Collagenesis to store the excess unprocessed tissue for future use. Although your own collagen will be more expensive, autologous collagen is not a foreign substance like bovine collagen, fibrel, or Gore-tex, so adverse reactions are virtually eliminated.

In fact, Dr. Dale T. DeVore, who patented the process, says that there have been no adverse reactions among the four hundred patients who have used the autologous collagen thus far.

FAT INJECTIONS When patients are allergic to collagen, the doctor may recommend using autologous fat injections. This is a two-step process, involving harvesting the patient's own fat from the thighs or buttocks, and then injecting the fat in the wrinkle as with collagen. Because it is a double procedure, fat injections cost much more than collagen—between $500 and $800 for facial wrinkles—and the injections must be repeated every three to six months.

Harvesting fat for soft tissue augmentation should not be done through common liposuctioning, according to Dr. Romo, who is also the academic director for two New York hospitals, because the high pressure extraction kills the fat cells. Gently removing cells with a needle will keep them alive and when they are transferred into the wrinkle, after being washed and decanted, 20 to 30 percent of the cells will "take" and become a permanent part of the wrinkle correction. The other 70 to 80 percent of the cells will be reabsorbed by the body, just as collagen is reabsorbed.

Doctors who harvest fat and refrigerate it for use in a few weeks will be injecting dead fat cells that have no chance of permanently filling the wrinkle, says Dr. Romo.

FIBREL Fibrel is a pig protein that is mixed with the patient's own blood plasma and used, although not nearly as often as fat, when collagen is contraindicated.

Interestingly enough, fibrel can last considerably longer than collagen or fat (one to two years) and less than 1 percent of patients are allergic to it. (A patch test is also required with fibrel.) To top it off, fibrel injections cost less than collagen—between $150 and $400.

So, you might ask, why isn't fibrel used more often?

Because of the fear of HIV, some doctors are reluctant to work with blood when they don't have to and fibrel treatments involve drawing blood, separating the plasma, then mixing the fibrel with the plasma.

In addition, fibrel stings like a novocaine injection and can leave the treated area inflamed for several days. However, according to Dr. Gary Monheit, an assistant professor of dermatology at the University of Alabama who works extensively with fibrel, most patients are back to normal in less than three days. Fibrel is also somewhat technique-dependent. (For best results, it should be injected in the uppermost layers of the dermis.)

Still, a correction that lasts longer and is less expensive sounds like a good option.

Germ Warfare: Botox

Just when you were beginning to think you had picked up a science fiction book masquerading as a women's lifestyle book, along comes the section on botox to convince you.

Botox is the nerve toxin found in botulism, minus the bacteria. When a person eats contaminated food, the bacteria multiply quickly and the toxin paralyzes the body's respiratory system, causing the patient to stop breathing and die. The paralyzing effect is what doctors have put to work on wrinkles.

When the facial muscles are paralyzed, it's impossible to make the faces that cause the wrinkles to appear. While botox does not remove wrinkles, it does, in effect, reduce the look of the wrinkles. Let's be clear about this. Botox is not a fill. It renders the muscles in the forehead unable to flex. By not being able to wrinkle your brow, you can prevent future wrinkles and avoid drawing attention to the ones that are already there. It is particularly good for people who seem to have a permanent scowl. You know them—they're the ones you think are always angry or unhappy.

For those individuals, says Dr. Alastair Carruthers, the Vancouver plastic surgeon who first presented botox to the American Academy of Dermatological Surgery in 1991, botox is an important discovery because they have more than just a cosmetic issue. "They're giving off the wrong body language all of the time," said Dr. Carruthers. "That kind of a permanent scowl affects the way they are understood by others."

Botox injections also take away the ability to raise a questioning eyebrow or knit your brow in disapproval, which makes botox somewhat inhibiting for those who rely on facial expressions to communicate. The paralysis, however, does not extend below the eyebrows (when done properly), so you can still smile, frown, and let your eyes twinkle away.

The paralysis lasts three to six months and while there are no known side effects and no recovery time, it's still important to select an experienced doctor so that you avoid the complications resulting from too much injected toxin. An overdose of toxin can invade surrounding muscles and cause droopy eyelids.

The botox takes effect in twenty-four to forty-eight hours and begins to wear off after four or five months, at which time the muscles will be weak, but not paralyzed. After six months the paralysis wears off completely.

Dr. Steven Bloch is a Chicago plastic surgeon and past president of the Chicago Society of Plastic Surgery who has been injecting thirty patients a month for the last two years and is himself a botox user. Dr. Bloch is incorporating botox injections with laser resurfacing for a more complete correction. Even though botox prevents the muscle from making the wrinkle, a lifetime of muscle flexing may have implanted a wrinkle on the skin. Once Dr. Bloch disables the muscle, he applies a laser to finish off any wrinkles that still appear when the face is relaxed.

Before seeking out one of the hundreds of doctors working with botox, be sure your forehead wrinkles are not the result of keeping your eyebrows out of your line of vision. If you are wrinkled from holding up your eyebrows, botox will paralyze the muscle that enables you to do that, causing your eyebrows to interfere with your sight.

If you find the idea of injecting a deadly toxin into your face a little frightening, you're not alone. This is why, according to Dr. Carruthers, it has been slow to catch on. But, in fact, the amount of toxin injected is only a fraction of a percent of what would be needed to produce the deadly symptoms of botulism. To be precise, 100 million molecules are all that are injected. To understand just how miniscule that is, consider this: Doctors everywhere are still using the same 150 mg batch of botox made in 1979; that batch, equivalent in size to half an aspirin, has been enough to perform all of the trials as well as the millions of injections in North America.

The cost of botox injections is between $250 and $500, but because the effects wear off, they must be repeated two or three times each year.

GORE-TEX THREADING Interestingly enough, Gore-tex, the product that's used to make ski jackets, has been used successfully in vascular surgery for the last fifteen years, but it's only been the last year or so that surgeons have been using it for soft-tissue augmentation.

Just as you'd thread elastic through a waistband casing, doctors fish Gore-tex threads into the nasolabial folds to fill up the void created between the edge of the nose and the corner of the mouth. The fiber fills up the crease just as other injectables do, but Gore-tex is not absorbed by the body, so the results are permanent. To keep the skin from pushing out the thread like a splinter, the material should be placed in the fat below the skin, says Dr. Skouge of Johns Hopkins, who works extensively with Gore-tex.

According to Dr. Skouge, infection is rare and he's seen no allergic reactions to the material. Considering that the fix is permanent (unlike collagen, fat, or fibrel), the cost is a minimal $600 to $1,000, and the recovery time is only a day or two, I expect you'll see doctors offering Gore-tex more and more.

Dr. Skouge, who believes that uses for Gore-tex will explode in the next five years, is also using Gore-tex to enhance the lip line that can sometimes flatten out with age. Again, he threads the fiber right along the vermilion border, the line where the lip meets the skin, to enhance the definition.

FACIAL SURGERIES

Lois, fifty-eight, celebrated her son's wedding only six weeks after having a face-lift. She's also had her stomach and thighs liposuctioned. "You reach a point that you are so unhappy with the way you look that you forget about the dangers and just do it. I'm so pleased with the results that I wouldn't hesitate to repeat any procedure if I needed it."

At fifty-five, Gail was looking forward to her daughter's wedding and wanted to look better for it. "I went to a very qualified plastic surgeon, but developed a hematoma underneath the skin that needed to be drained. I was taken back into surgery where all of my stitches had to be removed to allow the blood to drain. All told, I was in surgery for seven hours and I still have lumps and bruises under my skin. If I had known this, I never would have had a face-lift."

Rhytidectomy: Face-lift

A face-lift is the most effective and most drastic way to restore youthful looks. Depending on the patient's needs and desires, a face-lift can tighten jowls, remove furrows from between the brows, smooth out lateral wrinkles across the brow, decrease the nasolabial folds, and eliminate the general sag that is the result of time and gravity. Doctors say a face-lift is most effective for women between the ages of forty and fifty, when the skin is still elastic enough to respond well and there is still enough to be gained from going through the surgery.

Although a face-lift can be performed under local anesthesia with enough sedation, many surgeons prefer general anesthesia. If you are going to one of the many cosmetic surgery centers that have cropped up around the country, make sure that there will be an anesthesiologist or nurse anesthetist attending to your surgery.

The placement of the incisions will depend on the patient's particular needs and goals for the surgery. To lift sagginess, an incision would start behind the ears, travel in front of the ears and up into the hairline above the temples. If the surgeon is correcting a furrowed brow, he or she might use the small incision technique mentioned in the brow lift section (see later in this chapter), or make an ear-to-ear incision above the hairline.

During a face-lift, the surgeon separates the skin and subcutaneous fat from the muscles, pulling it back and up and cutting away the excess. Because there is so much cutting involved, the surgeon must be careful not to cut any facial nerves or paralysis could result.

The most common complication is a hematoma, a swelling that contains blood, which is why many surgeons choose to insert drains under the skin. This can also reduce bruising. Hematomas are most common to those with untreated high blood pressure, uncorrected blood clotting factors, and those who smoke or take aspirin. Following surgery, patients may experience a lack of skin sensitivity, or crawly sensations as the nerves regenerate. Swelling can cause a limitation of muscle movement too. Most of these symptoms, however, dissipate with healing. Skin pigmentation can change, particularly in the neck, and you can expect to have a higher hairline as a result of a face-lift.

Other procedures, like laser resurfacing, a phenol peel around the mouth, or blepharoplasty (surgery around the eyes) are often done at the same time as a face-lift so that the patient can recover from everything at once.

Recovery takes two to three weeks. Bruising will subside within two weeks, but puffiness may linger. It will be six months before you'll be able to see the maximum improvement in your appearance, but the results will last from five to ten years. The cost for a face-lift can range from $4,000 to $10,000, but tack on additional charges if you are also having other procedures such as a blepharoplasty, laser resurfacing, or other services.

Face-lift of the Future
Dr. Thomas Loeb, a Manhattan plastic surgeon, is employing a combination of techniques for a new kind of face-lift that eliminates the possibility of the overpulled mummy look that frightens so many patients. He does a facial laser resurfacing, liposuctions the jowls, and then performs a neck-lift. The neck-lift will take away the crinkly turkey-neck look for fifteen years and the laser resurfacing will wipe off wrinkles, while the liposuction in the jowls will give you a tighter jawline. If needed, Dr. Loeb will use fat injections to fill in the nasolabial folds.

Rhinoplasty
Reshaping the nose, or rhinoplasty, is one of the most common cosmetic surgeries performed. It is most often and most effectively performed on young women, under age thirty-five, while the skin is still elastic enough to adapt to a new shape and so that the nose can age with the face. However, with extra finesse on the part of the doctor, the surgery can be performed on older women.

Still, some older women undergo rhinoplasty to touch up a nose that may be drooping, or to have the new look they've always wanted.

To get the best results, it is important to work closely with your doctor to determine your exact desires from the surgery and what is possible for him or her to accomplish for you. (Take a realistic look at yourself before seeing the surgeon. You probably won't be happy with the results if you ask the doctor to give you the pert little nose of a twenty year old when you're sixty.) Together you'll work with photographs or computer-imaging to design the nose of your dreams. Keep in mind, though, that computer-imaging is a sales tool to help you see possibilities. The computer, however, will not be operating on your nose and your surgery may not come out exactly as the computer predicted.

Most rhinoplasties involve incisions in the nostril and then a reshaping of the bone and cartilage that make up the nose. With a saw and chisel, the surgeon can remove a bump on the nose, or rearrange the cartilage to turn up the tip of a droopy nose. Crooked noses can be broken and set straight. Sometimes a nose seems out of proportion to the rest of the face because the chin is too small. A doctor can remove some of the cartilage from the septum and move it to the chin, to create a more balanced look.

When you wake up from surgery, your nostrils will be packed, and possibly splinted. You'll probably soon have black eyes and your nose will feel numb. Most of the swelling will be gone in about two weeks, but give your new nose a full six months to take its final form.

As with any surgery, complications and bad results are always possible. Be sure to discuss those possibilities with your doctor, as well as what can be done to correct the problems if they occur.

Dr. Henry Kowamoto, a third generation Japanese American and clinical professor of plastic surgery at UCLA in Santa Monica, cautions ethnic women to be particularly careful about selecting a surgeon for a rhinoplasty. "The nose landmarks are different for an Asian nose than a Caucasian nose. Black and Hispanic landmarks are also different. If you shape a Caucasian nose on a Mexican person whose heritage is Spanish, they'll look fine, but if their heritage is American Indian, they'll look ridiculous," he said. Some patients, however, want the "Western ideal" and are striving for a Caucasian nose.

Patients who want to retain the look of their heritage while improving upon an imperfection should ask their doctor specific questions about his or her experience doing that particular kind of nose.

Surgeon's fees for a rhinoplasty range from $2,100 to $4,300.

Cheek and Chin Implants

Using bone, cartilage, silicone forms, or a new product called Medipore, doctors can enhance recessed chins and cheekbones.

A chin implant can restore balance to a face or make a slightly large nose seem more in proportion to the rest of the face. The chin can also recede because of premature loss of the lower teeth. Because osteoporosis tends to shrink facial bones and alter the face's shape entirely, implants are becoming more common among older women, not to get Sharon Stone cheekbones but to restore the good looks of youth.

Dr. Romo is using Medipore extensively for cheeks and chins when he performs a face-lift because the lifted skin drapes more naturally when the face's architecture is restored. The body treats Medipore like part of the family and within months of implantation, this custom-carved bioframework will bleed just like regular tissue. The body treats silicone like the foreign object that it is and encapsulates it. Should the area ever require additional surgery or experience a trauma, the implant would slip out of position because it never becomes a permanently integrated part of the face.

Unless the doctor will be taking bone or cartilage from somewhere else—usually in conjunction with a rhinoplasty—a chin implant is performed under local anesthesia and the incision is usually made inside the mouth or beneath the chin.

Following mandibuloplasty (chin surgery), the patient will be restricted to a soft diet. Complications from this surgery are rare, although the implant can slip and numbness is a possibility.

Malarplasty (cheek surgery) uses materials similar to chin implants, typically made from bone, silicone, and Medipore, although some doctors are working with Gore-tex, too. The incision is made either in the mouth, through the lower eyelid, or behind the hairline. Cheek implants will cause the facial skin to drape a little differently and in the very thin, the implants may be apparent on close inspection.

As with chin implants, cheek implants can drift and infection is always a possibility. That drift is why doctors are working with "new" substitutes for cheek and chin implants including biocompatible bone and injectable coral.

Biocompatible bone is harvested from cadavers, sterilized, treated to remove minerals, and then reconstituted with water prior to surgery. Rejection is virtually nil and because it is malleable, doctors can get a much more natural look with the material. Coral is chemically similar to bone and when it is ground and mixed with a patient's blood and collagen, it forms a paste that can be injected and shaped during surgery. With both materials, the body develops a blood supply to the implant, further limiting the risk of infection.

Chin augmentation can cost between $1,000 and $2,500, while cheeks run from $1,500 to $2,500. Recovery time takes one to two weeks for both procedures and the improvements are permanent unless the implant drifts.

Blepharoplasty

The eyes are one of the first areas to show the signs of aging and I'm not talking crow's-feet or smile lines. Thanks to gravity and a lifetime of sun exposure, top eyelids begin to droop and become hooded and lower lids get wrinkly and baggy. Fat pockets also develop around the undereyes, causing permanent puffiness. Eyelid surgery can be done as an outpatient under local anesthesia, although because many people have trouble letting anything near their eyes, much less knives or lasers, an additional anesthesia is often advisable.

On the upper lid, the surgeon will make an incision following the natural creases in the eyelid and cut away the excess fat and skin. For the lower lid, the doctor will make an incision below the lash line or inside the lid.

Doctors are now using lasers for blepharoplasty because there is less bleeding and less swelling afterward. However, Dr. Rohrer, who specializes in laser work, says that incisions made by scalpels heal faster than incisions made by lasers. "There are pros and cons to each method," he said. "A laser is just a sexy way of cutting, but for simple excision, it's not necessarily better than a scalpel."

Dr. Loeb uses a combination of techniques for his blepharoplasty. He uses a scalpel to cut away excess fat and tissue and then performs a laser resurfacing to erase the wrinkles and fine lines.

You'll never see the scars of a successful eyelid surgery. Recovery generally takes one to two weeks, for results that last from five to ten years. Some complications include temporarily blurred or double vision, the lower eyelid turned out due to excess swelling (this usually disappears over time), or drooping eyelids from excess scarring. Naturally, infection is a concern as it is with any surgery, and a patient may require eyedrops to soothe dryness for the long term. If you wear contact lenses, plan to be without them for up to a week following eyelid surgery. Naturally, your doctor will advise you to steer clear of eye makeup for several days. Most of the painful swelling and bruising will dissipate in forty-eight hours and the rest of the swelling will usually subside in a week.

Dr. Kowamoto points out that the Asian ideal of beauty is somewhat different from the Caucasian ideal and that too often Asian women end up with Caucasian-looking eyes that can be perceived as offensive in the Asian community. Asian women who want to retain the shape of their eyes should seek out a surgeon who is sensitive to those desires.

"I was not made aware of this when I was in training to be a plastic surgeon. It wasn't until I began lecturing in China and Japan that it was brought to my attention," said Dr. Kowamoto, who pointed out that the Westernization of Asian eyes is more common in Japan, Hong Kong, and Bangkok than it is in the United States.

The surgeon's fees for eyelid surgery will run between $2,500 and $3,500 for top and bottom lids, and between $1,500 and $2,000 for top or bottom lids only.

Brow or Forehead Lift

While botox can provide temporary relief from lateral wrinkles on the forehead, if you want to raise droopy eyebrows, remove wrinkles, and forestall a face-lift, you may want to consider a brow lift (also known as a forehead lift). The improvements will last from five to ten years. Like most cosmetic surgeries, brow lifts are done on an outpatient basis under local anesthesia and a sedative.

For a brow lift, incisions are made in the scalp or above the hairline and the skin is pulled up and cut away, smoothing out wrinkles and raising the eyebrows to relieve that angry, sad, or tired look that comes from hooded brows. A brow lift can also correct crow's-feet and if needed, can remove deep creases between the eyebrows.

Not long ago, a brow lift involved an ear to ear incision, but a new surgical technique called small-incision brow lifts have almost entirely replaced the old methods. This small incision procedure is particularly good for women with thinning hair because the small incisions remain well hidden. According to Philadelphia's Dr. Shapiro, the only time the older method would be used is when a patient has an unusually high hairline to start with or if there is a lot of skin to remove.

The risks for this surgery include infection, the spreading of the scar, blood beneath the skin, patches of numbness, short-term hair loss, and an inability to raise your brows. Following surgery, the patient is advised not to use hair color as the chemicals can irritate the scar.

A good brow lift will leave the patient looking refreshed and well rested, but you'll know someone had an overzealous surgeon if she looks perpetually wide-eyed or surprised. Brow lifts are done alone or as part of a total face-lift. When only a brow lift is performed, you can expect to pay the surgeon between $2,000 and $3,200 for this procedure.

Neck Sculpting or Neck Lift

Smoothing away the loose skin I call turkey neck or trimming up a double chin can take years off your appearance and is a popular alternative for patients who want the youthful boost of a face-lift without the recovery time.

A small-incision neck lift will do the job well if your problems are a loose neck or double chin, but if you're looking to firm up the jowls or improve the nasolabial folds (the crease between the nose and the mouth) a full face-lift may be in order. The incisions for a neck lift are made behind the ears so the surgeon can't get the pull needed to tighten jowls or remove nasal/labial creases.

Depending on the patient's needs, neck sculpting may be as simple as liposuctioning excess surface fat, or may include removing excess skin and tightening the platysmal muscle, which acts as a corset but can become slack over time.

Recovery time from liposuction on the neck is about twenty-four hours but more extensive neck work will require about a week's recovery. Swelling and bruising are the most common side effects, and occasionally there can be some excessive bleeding.

If a neck lift is the right procedure for you, the costs can be as little as $1,000 to $2,000 for liposuction alone and up to $4,000 if skin and muscle are tightened, but you can expect the results to last as long as twenty years!

BODY PROCEDURES

Breast Surgery

Breasts can be enlarged, reduced, lifted, and totally reconstructed, thanks to the wonders of plastic surgery. While most of the procedures are considered cosmetic, most insurance plans recognize breast reconstruction following mastectomy as rehabilitative and will pay for the procedure.

Breast Augmentation

Breast implants are the topic of great controversy and interest for the millions of women who have already had them or are contemplating them. Until the early nineties, breast implants were the most common cosmetic surgery performed; however, a 1992 FDA ruling changed all that. Now, according to the Society of Plastic and Reconstructive Surgeons' figures, close to forty thousand women had implant surgery in

1994 and nearly thirty thousand had old silicone implants removed. (Those figures do not include surgeries performed by doctors who are not members of the SPRS, so the real statistics are considerably higher, though probably proportionally similar.)

In 1992, the FDA became concerned about implants after reports of leakage, inflammation, and the possible relation to immune and connective tissue disorders, like arthritis and lupus, but by then two million women already had the implants. At that time the FDA determined that the safety of silicone gel implants was not established and that future implants should be limited to patients involved in clinical trials.

The FDA further advised that women who were not experiencing problems with their implants should not have them removed. The clinical trials that are currently underway seek to determine how often the implants break or leak, how long they last, the instance of adverse effects, how and to what extent the implants interfere with mammography, and whether there is a relationship between implants and the risk of cancer, immune-related diseases, and connective tissue disorders.

In February of 1996, Dr. Charles Hennekens of the Brigham and Women's Hospital in Boston released an analysis of reports on more than four-hundred thousand women. The study concluded that of three thousand women with implants, one was likely to develop a connective tissue disease, a risk that researchers characterized as small but significant. Attorneys on both sides of the implant litigation pointed to the study to prove their point. (Tens of thousands of women have sued implant manufacturers and approximately ninety thousand joined a class action suit reporting illnesses from their implants.)

Studies on the safety of silicone implants are ongoing. Only women who are undergoing restoration or those who currently have silicone implants but need to replace them can participate in the clinical trials. Women who simply want implants for augmentation must receive implants filled with saline.

Clinical trials are also underway for soybean oil–filled implants. According to Dr. Neal Handel, a Los Angeles plastic surgeon who is one of the primary investigators, the body will metabolize the oil if the implant ruptures, the oil does not interfere with mammography the way silicone or saline can, and the feel is somewhere between silicone and saline. The next phase of trials will involve only fifty women and it will be two or three years before they are on the market.

For most people, breast augmentation is usually accomplished by inserting an inflatable silicone sac containing saline. The patient's measurements and the amount of skin available to cover the implant are taken into consideration in determining the size of the implant. Incisions are made either below the breast, at the armpit, or now, thanks to the inflatable prosthesis, around the areola with a far smaller incision.

Implants will cost between $1,800 and $3,500. The risks are many, including loss of nipple sensation, interference with cancer detection, infection, uneven appearance, tightening of the scar tissue causing unusual firmness, and the formation of calcium deposits in surrounding tissue. The FDA says that implants should not be considered lifetime devices and that patients should anticipate the need for future surgeries to replace ruptured or leaking implants.

Signs of Implant Problems
1. joint pain, redness, or swelling
2. fatigue
3. hardening of implants
4. change in shape or size

Breast Reduction

Over time large breasts can become pendulous, altering posture and causing neck and back pain in extreme cases. For those reasons and many others, including shoulder dents from bra straps and a constant rash under the breasts, many women choose breast reduction surgery.

This procedure is normally performed under general anesthesia in a hospital. Most often with a breast reduction, a T-shaped incision is made, with the top of the T situated under the breast. Tissue is removed from under the breast and then the skin is restitched. Depending on how much is removed, the nipple may be simply lifted but in other cases, depending on how the nipple is situated, the nipple and areola may be removed and then regrafted into position.

Prior to undergoing breast reduction surgery, be sure your doctor knows if you plan to nurse a baby in the future because if the nipple is regrafted on to the breast, the necessary ducts will be cut, making nursing impossible.

Breast reduction surgery normally involves an overnight stay in the hospital with drains removing blood, serum, and liquefied fat, although this procedure is sometimes done as same-day surgery.

Recovery takes two to three weeks and athletic activity can be resumed after a month's time. Risks include infection, loss of nipple sensitivity, and excessive scarring. Eventually the breasts will sag again from their postoperative position, although the relief from back pain is tremendous. The cost for this procedure will run between $4,500 and $5,500.

Breast Reconstruction

Following a radical mastectomy, when the spread of cancer is unlikely, or in cases of severe injury or congenital deformity, patients may seek to have their breasts reconstructed through surgery.

Breast reconstruction can be complicated as it will likely involve skin grafting as well as implants and may involve more than one surgery before completion. These operations are performed under general anesthesia and typically require a longer hospitalization than other breast surgeries.

While perfect reconstruction is not possible, the patient can expect a good simulation that will make her look better in clothes.

In addition to the scarring associated with the mastectomy, breast reconstruction will inevitably result in additional scars at the location from which the skin and tissue are taken (usually the abdomen, buttocks, or thighs).

Many doctors find that it is easier on the patient to undertake the mastectomy and the reconstruction simultaneously, while others prefer a period of healing and observation for recurrence of the cancer between operations.

Because of the great variety of reconstruction techniques and the individual needs of the patient, the surgical costs of breast reconstruction vary widely from $2,500 for simple implants to $8,000 for microsurgery.

Liposuction

Just before the FDA limited the use of silicone implants, liposuction supplanted breast augmentation surgery as the most common aesthetic surgical procedure. Liposuction is the surgical removal of body fat through suctioning. Lipectomy is a less common form of fat removal that involves cutting away the fat. Both procedures are most successful when the skin is still able to redrape without becoming bunched or wrinkled, so it is best done on those under forty or on patients who are unconcerned about the appearance of the skin.

Because the procedure is relatively easy, many physicians are performing the surgery who are not necessarily qualified to do so. Liposuction is essentially a blind procedure and overzealous or untrained physicians have been known to leave hills and valleys by failing to sculpt evenly. This is another case for credential-checking. Patients are cautioned to choose a physician carefully even though this seems like a common and uncomplicated procedure.

While liposuction is an effective means of body-contouring, it is no substitute for diet and exercise and ideally would be used only to take care of isolated trouble spots once diet and exercise had accomplished the patient's other body-shaping objectives.

Liposuction is performed under general anesthesia by inserting suction tubes called cannulae below the skin's surface into fatty areas and suctioning away the fat. Fluid and blood are extracted along with the fat, which is why most doctors will only remove 2,000 ccs at one time. (If more were removed, the patient could go into shock.) The tiny incisions are placed inconspicuously near the naval or in the bikini area for the most common liposuction areas: the abdomen, hips, and thighs. Knees, ankles, upper arms, and under chins are also commonly treated with liposuction.

Following the surgery, the liposuctioned areas are strapped in elastic pressure dressings or surgical girdles, if appropriate, to prevent excessive scarring. The elastic dressing should be worn for approximately three weeks following the surgery.

Liposuction is major surgery and patients should prepare for it accordingly by quitting smoking and ensuring current good health. Complications can include blood clots, excessive bleeding, scarring, etc. Liposuctioning any single area will cost between $1,500 and $2,000.

Abdominal Lipectomy

Severe weight loss and pregnancy are two of the most common reasons women seek out a tummy tuck. After so much stretching, the abdomen can become slack or even pendulous, and the skin and fat may have separated from the muscle walls making it impossible to exercise the abdomen into submission.

In these cases, a surgeon will make an incision—usually along the pubic line from hip bone to hip bone, but sometimes laterally between the belly button and the pubic line—and the excess skin and fat are cut away. Sometimes the loosened muscles are pulled together and sutured to tighten up the area, and often the naval is relocated.

For the surgery, the patient's knees and upper body are both raised so that the most tissue can be removed.

Following surgery, the patient will wear a surgical girdle to help compress the scars and prevent keloids from forming. Usually the girdle is worn for six weeks following surgery.

Complications can include infection, excessive bleeding, and tissue loss.

A tummy tuck will firm up the abdominal area, and the look of any stretch marks will be improved, but will not be eliminated completely.

Because this is major surgery, performed under general anesthesia, patients should be in excellent health before undergoing a tummy tuck. Even then, full recovery can take several months. Expect to spend between $3,000 and $7,000 for this procedure.

NONMEDICAL OPTIONS
Beauty Lifts
Hollywood makeup artists used to rig up a rubber band, glue, and thread contraption to smooth out the trouble spots of actresses who didn't want, or hadn't yet undergone, cosmetic surgery.

Today, we have Years Away Beauty Lifts, surgical tape and elastic bands that instantly give the effect of a face-lift. Because the tape is transparent, it blends in with the skin, and hair hides the bands. Your skin can breathe through the tapes (called lifts, by the company) and the adhesive is hypoallergenic.

I use Years Away and think that for $29.95 per kit (plus postage and handling) they are a great alternative to a face-lift and they work so well that people have asked me if I've had a real face-lift. The kit includes thirty-eight lifts, four bands for a neck lift, four bands for face and eye lifts, complete instructions, and a videotape, in addition to Years Away toner to help gently remove the lifts and an eye cream. For $24.90 ($19.95 plus shipping and handling) you can get an additional set of lifts and bands. Although the package doesn't recommend it, you can use the lifts for more than one wearing. Just pull the ends of the bands out, leaving the lifts in place. The next day, you can reinsert the bands. If your skin tends to be sensitive, I wouldn't recommend this little cost-cutting trick.

I find Years Away Beauty Lifts to be especially useful for special occasions and television appearances when looking my best is an absolute must. You can, however, wear them every day and I often do.

You can purchase Years Away Beauty Lifts by calling 800-207-4411.

Facial Exercise

There are varied opinions about whether or not facial exercise can tighten facial skin and improve wrinkling or sagging.

On one hand, experts remind us that it's repeated motion, like smiling, laughing, chewing, smoking, etc., that help cause wrinkles in the first place and that facial muscles get more exercise than any other muscles in the body.

On the other hand, facial exercises are generally intended to improve sagging, not superficial wrinkles, so if a crinkly neck or limp jawline are your problem, facial exercise may be a good alternative to cosmetic surgery, especially when there are so many other ways to tackle wrinkles.

After conducting studies on Facial Flex, Dr. Gary Grove of the Skin Study Center in Broomall, Pennsylvania, is a firm believer in resistance exercise for the face. Unlike the many books and videos that teach people strange contortions to exercise the face, by incorporating resistance, Facial Flex (a small device that is inserted horizontally between the lips) provides an efficient way to exercise the face, giving the appearance of a face-lift.

Linda Hellings, vice president of marketing for Facial Flex, explains that the face, neck, and chin muscles respond to resistance training just like the other muscles in the body. Unlike other muscles that become bulky with exercise, tiny facial muscles become flat and compact as they grow stronger.

If you are beginning to see the signs of gravity on your face, Facial Flex, priced at only $79.95, may save you the time, trouble, and expense of a face- or neck lift.

It's interesting to note that Facial Flex is patented, design-protected, and FDA-registered, making it the only product of its kind. Also, it only requires two or three minutes twice a day to see results.

If you've had a face-lift already, ask your doctor about Facial Flex as a way to preserve your investment.

Facial Flex is available in fine salons, through health and fitness catalogs and the Home Shopping Network—which sells the device for $10 less—or by calling 800-469-FLEX.

ONLY YOU CAN DECIDE

Plastic surgery, lasers, peels, and injections are not for everybody, even though close to half a million people had some kind of procedure last year and 21 percent of them were repeat customers.

I've been considering a face-lift for the last two years to correct some of the sagging that I just can't resolve with skin care. Frankly, as appealing as a tight jawline may be, I was frightened by the prospect of someone taking a knife to my face and neck. Thanks to the Beauty Lifts, I've been able to procrastinate, but I think eventually I'll just shore up my courage and do it, especially now that I've met Dr. Loeb and some of his patients. When I visited Dr. Loeb's office, he introduced me to several patients (with their permission, of course) who had come for follow-up visits. Each woman looked fabulous and the comparisons with their "before" pictures were amazing.

This pointed out to me the value of referrals and meeting a doctor's patients prior to surgery. I can't overemphasize how important it is to feel comfortable with your doctor's work and the best way to do that is to meet former patients. Think of it this way: You buy a certain brand of clothing, cars, or cosmetics based on the manufacturer's reputation for quality and reliability. It only makes sense to take the same approach when selecting a plastic surgeon.

Even if you've found the most skilled surgeon in the world and are the bravest woman ever born, there is a lot to consider when contemplating cosmetic improvements. Remember to first examine your motivation and do it for yourself, not for anyone else. Then consider cost, risks, and recovery time. After you've weighed all of those factors, see a few doctors and get more than one opinion, particularly if you're considering surgery. Be careful not to let yourself be dazzled by the prospects of a smooth face and tight neck and allow the doctor to go crazy with a laser beam. Once you're finished, you'll still have the same hands and chest, and you don't want to look ridiculous with a twenty-year-old face on a fifty-year-old body. Be realistic in your plans and your expectations.

If you decide to take the plunge, give yourself every advantage by practicing faithful skin care a month or two prior to your procedure. Also be sure to follow your doctor's directions carefully immediately following. Some doctors are even employing estheticians to supervise a patient's postoperative skin care. Once you're healed, be sure to do everything you can to preserve your investment. If you begin working with a dermatologist for ongoing skin care following your surgery, you may never want or need to see the surgeon again.

Part 2

MORE THAN JUST A PRETTY FACE

Chapter 6

EATING RIGHT

"To lengthen thy life, lessen thy meals."

— B<small>ENJAMIN</small> F<small>RANKLIN</small>

G ood health is the very foundation of good looks. A healthy, physically fit person with rosy cheeks, clear eyes, shiny hair, and a well-proportioned body will always look good no matter what they use for moisturizer or mascara. If you're healthy and physically fit, everything else is gravy.

Unfortunately, too many of us are not healthy or physically fit. In fact, most of us are overweight. Over the course of this century, as our society has switched from agricultural and manufacturing work to service and technology, we've become less active and increasingly overweight. At the same time we've become obsessed with watching our weight and shedding pounds. While this split personality is certainly good for the economy—causing new businesses like Jenny Craig, Quick Weight Loss Systems, the Richard Simmons empire, and Slimfast to evolve—losing weight and keeping it off is tough and, as anyone who has tried it knows, dieting really doesn't work in the long term.

Staying trim was once solely about looking good but, today, controlling weight and exercising is more about staying healthy. Unless you've been living in a cave for the last ten years you know that carrying around excess pounds will put you on the fast track to heart disease and might increase your risk of cancer.

In its 1995 updated Dietary Guidelines for Americans, the U.S. Government says that women who had no weight problem as young adults should allow themselves to gain no more than fifteen pounds as they get older. Additionally, women who gained more than forty pounds over a fifteen-year period are seven times more likely to die of heart disease and 50 percent more likely to die of cancer than women who gained less than ten pounds.

Medical science seems to be gaining convincing evidence that some obesity is genetic and that it is properly grouped with diabetes and hypertension in a category known as "complex diseases," those ailments that arise from a combination of genetics and environment. Whether or not we are predestined to struggle with our weight, we have clear and convincing evidence that we will live longer and healthier lives if we win the fight early on.

Since the primary goal of most women is to stay healthy and active while they're living longer, this chapter will include some information about the impact of aging on our weight-maintenance efforts. While it's true that metabolism slows with age, it's not hard to make appropriate adjustments to compensate. In fact, Dr. Walter Bortz II of the Palo Alto Medical Center in California says that weight gain with age is not inevitable, it's simply a matter of calories in, calories out. We become inactive and the pounds pile on.

Dr. Bortz is probably correct, scientifically at least, but ask any woman who has been through menopause and she'll tell you it's not that simple. Pounds and inches just seem to appear from out of nowhere.

From age twelve until she was forty-six, Julie weighed between 114 and 116 pounds. Then she started gaining two pounds a month, despite her active lifestyle. No matter what she does, or how little she eats, she just can't seem to shake the extra pounds. "I've exercised more in the last ten years than I have in my whole life. I only drink skim milk, I don't use butter, I have fish and chicken, I don't eat cheese—I'm gaining weight on air. The more I give up, the harder it gets. I'm frustrated, hungry, and feel very fat." Julie seems to be doing everything right to control her weight, but menopause is really throwing her for a loop. And she's not alone. Although doctors can point to no particular reason why menopausal women tend to gain weight, the overwhelming experience of millions of women makes the phenomenon impossible to ignore.

IT'S NOT "ALL IN YOUR HEAD"

There is a lovely dress shop near my home where I often go for special occasion dresses. When I went in for a dress for my daughter's wedding, I headed straight for the dressing room while the saleswoman, who knows my taste, went in search of a few selections. She came back with an armload of size fours and couldn't believe it when

I sent her back for size eights. Menopause had hit in between visits to the dress shop and doubled my dress size.

According to Debra Waterhouse, author of *Outsmarting the Female Fat Cell,* there is a real reason that hormone replacement therapy causes women to gain weight. Furthermore, there is a bona fide reason that men are more successful at losing weight and keeping it off.

Women's fat cells are designed to efficiently store fat, and our hormones boost this self-preservation feature so that our bodies can stay fertile and bear children. In theory, a pregnant woman could survive a famine and still deliver a healthy child by relying on her fat reserves. That's why puberty, pregnancy, oral contraceptives, and hormone replacement therapy are typically associated with weight gain. The hormones are telling our bodies to stockpile extra fat and calories in case a baby comes along.

Understanding this fat-cell phenomenon may help you to be a little less hard on yourself and help you to approach weight loss or weight maintenance more sensibly. You can't starve your thirty billion fat cells into submission, but, according to Waterhouse, you can outsmart them by eating small portions several times a day. Don't let yourself get to the point where your stomach is growling because that will cue your fat cells to switch into conservation mode. Constant fueling keeps your metabolism burning up calories.

Before you make yourself crazy trying to erase extra inches, have a complete physical and ask your doctor to check your thyroid. For unknown reasons, the thyroid can become underactive, causing tiredness, weight gain, dry skin, hair loss, and constipation. The condition is known as hypothyroidism and can be controlled with medication, so before you start eating carrots sticks like Bugs Bunny, have a complete physical if you're suddenly gaining weight. The thyroid can also become overactive, causing dramatic weight loss and while most of us wouldn't mind having that problem, it should be investigated just the same.

Having a regular physical is a good habit to get into anyway, even if you don't have a particular problem to address, and it is especially important before starting any new exercise regimen.

THE MIGHTY METABOLISM

From about age thirty on, we start to burn calories more slowly. That's why we start to pack on extra pounds without having changed what we eat. It's another one of nature's cruel tricks, but it's one we can manage. Consuming fewer calories is probably the most obvious way to steer clear of the midlife weight gain, but you can also give your metabolism a boost by exercising and changing some of your eating habits.

Mother always said that breakfast was the most important meal of the day and she was right. Breakfast — and I don't mean a cup of black coffee — is your body's wake-up call. At rest, your body goes into slow-burn mode. Your metabolism will kick into gear once you get moving and give it some fuel. It's just like stoking a furnace.

Your metabolism is the reason dieting seldom works. Initially when we begin to eat less, our bodies burn reserve fat. That's the good part. A short time later, our bodies kick into preservation mode and adjust to less fuel. The body stops burning fat just in case another famine (diet) comes along. This is why it is so important to fuel the body with foods that are high in fiber and carbohydrates. They're easily burned and eliminated and don't turn to fat so readily.

Exercise is another great metabolism boost because your body burns more calories when it is active. Furthermore, muscles require more fuel than other tissue, so building muscles through weight training, in addition to aerobic exercise, will cause your body to burn more calories when exercising and even at rest.

The bottom line is that unless you want everything you eat to end up on your bottom, get your bottom moving.

DIET WILL ALWAYS BE A FOUR-LETTER WORD

Nobody likes to feel deprived, and for most of us, dieting is just that — depriving ourselves of the not-so-good-for-you "good stuff" in favor of rabbit food. Many people have dieted for years, shedding pounds only to put them back on again.

Our thinking about diet has been changing slowly over the years. We once thought of dieting as a temporary sacrifice of the foods we liked. It was a verb, something we hated to do, like scrubbing floors. And, according to a 1996 Harris Poll that found that three-quarters of American men and women are overweight, it is clearly not something we do very well.

Today we are beginning to think of diet as a noun. Our *diet* is the collection of what we normally eat. Experts tell us to eat a low-fat *diet*. Our *diet* should be loaded with fresh fruits and vegetables. Still, the word "diet" has negative connotations for many of us. In fact, its first three letters sort of sum up the way it makes us feel. That's why I like to substitute the word "menu" for diet. Eat from a low-fat menu. Our menu is full of fresh fruits and vegetables. Doesn't that sound much more appealing?

Now, with that little bit of attitude adjustment concerning the "d" word, let's review the basics of a healthy diet — er. . . menu.

FAT IS THE ENEMY

Officials from the Department of Agriculture to the American Heart Association all recommend that we derive no more than 30 percent of our total calories from fat. Some experts have recently adjusted that recommendation to 20 percent. The Center for Science in the Public Interest and the late Dr. Nathan Pritikin recommend no more than 10 percent, but that's fairly unrealistic for most people.

That "cut back on fat" message seems to have taken hold in the public consciousness. In 1977–78, Americans got 40 percent of their calories from fat, but by 1994 the number had decreased to 33 percent. It's still too high, but at least the trend is going in the right direction.

Eating fat makes you fat — it's that simple. Fat is the leading culprit in heart disease and obesity and it's even been linked to an increased incidence of cataracts. Studies also implicate fat in a variety of cancers, including breast and colon cancer. It's not that fat causes cancer, but some experts believe that fat provides an environment that promotes the growth of cancerous tumors.

Fat is found in almost everything: meat, dairy products, prepared foods, wonderful rich sauces, butter, margarine — everything except most fresh fruits and vegetables. Even a salad can lose its healthful benefits if it is drowned in too much fat-laden dressing. Did you realize that some salad dressings have as many as 130 calories in a tablespoon and that 90 percent of those calories are from fat? That can turn a healthy lunch into a fatfest in a hurry.

To keep your fat intake to 20 percent, remember this simple formula from registered dietitian Marie Ward, who is the cardiac rehab dietitian at the Center for Continuing Health at the Medical College of Pennsylvania. Foods should have no more than 2 grams of fat for every 100 calories consumed in order to stay under 20 percent fat. (Obviously 3 grams for every 100 calories will keep you under 30 percent.)

It can be fairly easy and painless to eliminate a good bit of fat from your diet and still eat the things you like. Each month more than 1,500 new products are introduced to grocer's shelves and the great number of them are reduced-fat products ranging from sour cream and cream cheese to cookies, cakes, and salad dressings. I know that some of these products have no taste and others have a consistency that differs significantly from the "real" stuff, but the products are getting better all of the time and are worth trying again even if you didn't care for them when they first came out. Just as we got used to drinking diet soda and coffee with artificial sweetener instead of sugar, once you get used to low-fat items like skim or 1-percent milk, the full-fat products will start to seem heavy.

Avoiding fat has almost become a national pastime and many manufacturers are lining their pockets thanks to the low-fat craze. Turkey and chicken consumption is up and snack-food manufacturers and commercial bakers are making a killing selling fat-free cookies, cakes, and snack foods. But watch out for those fat-free brownies. While they really are fat-free, the only reason they taste good is because they're loaded with sugar. Read the labels and don't assume that because a bag of cookies is marked "low fat" or "fat-free" you can make a meal out of them. Certainly they're a good substitute for the three regular cookies you allow yourself before bed, but just remember, if it seems too good to be true, it probably is.

One of the best, low-fat products available, believe it or not, is the I Can't Believe It's Not Butter spray. Unlike cooking sprays in aerosol cans, this pump spray has no chemical smell, looks like butter, and actually tastes good. For use with popcorn, toast, and steamed vegetables, etc., it's really a great alternative.

I confess that I have a sweet tooth, and until menopause and hormone therapy, I didn't really struggle with my weight. Now, it's a whole different story. I've tried every variety of Snackwell's cookies, make chocolate pudding with skim milk, and "treat myself" to Edy's low-fat frozen yogurt. Would I love to have a cream doughnut or a hot fudge sundae made with ice cream? You betcha. But if I didn't die from the Jewish guilt after my little binge was over, the workout on the treadmill to burn off the calories would kill me.

Every diet book tells you what to eat for breakfast, lunch, and dinner, and heaven knows I know to eat fresh fruit and vegetables, but nobody ever gives you good recipes to satisfy that after-dinner craving for sweets. (Fruit and Jell-O don't always cut it.) Because I don't know a woman who doesn't like desserts, I've included a few of my favorite low-fat dessert recipes in this chapter.

There are dozens of low-fat cookbooks available to help you on your quest for a low-fat menu. (The American Heart Association puts out several excellent volumes.) I strongly suggest that you visit your local bookstore and spend some time perusing several of them for recipes that you think you'd be likely to make and enjoy. If the recipes are too complicated or exotic, you probably won't make them, so check it out carefully before buying. Your local newspaper's food section is also a good source of low-fat recipes, as are friends and relatives. To make the search a little easier, I've listed a few low-fat cookbooks and magazines that I like because the recipes are easy to follow and the ingredients are not so exotic that you have to spend the whole day shopping.

In addition to seeking out low-fat recipes, here are a few cooking tips that will help you reduce fat in your diet.

1. Many prepared foods call for a tablespoon or two of oil. Usually that oil can be eliminated altogether with no loss of flavor or consistency. This is especially true of prepackaged rice and pasta dishes.
2. Try sautéing foods in chicken broth or other flavorful liquids like fruit juices or wine. If I'm rehydrating sun-dried tomatoes in water, I use the tomato water to sauté chicken, veal, or other vegetables. It's very tasty and adds no fat to the recipe. Nonstick cooking sprays also help eliminate calories.
3. Once you've browned your ground meat and before you proceed to the next step in the recipe, spoon the meat into a colander and rinse with hot water. Wash out the frying pan, too. This can eliminate a good bit of fat from the recipe.
4. Ground turkey and ground chicken are great hamburger substitutes. Try using them in any recipe that calls for ground beef. Make turkey loaf or chicken lasagna, don't tell anyone in your family, and see if they notice.
5. When making soups or stews, always chill the finished product before serving. The fat will rise to the top and solidify, making it easy to spoon off.
6. All poultry is not created equal. Turkey breast has only 20 percent of the fat that chicken breast has. If it's all the same to you, choose turkey.

Elaine's Exclusive

BOOK 'EM

Check the health and diet section of your local bookstore as well as the cookbook section for low-fat cookbooks. The store managers can also tell you which books are best-sellers and the most requested. Aside from a good cookbook, treat yourself to Oprah Winfrey's book *Make the Connection,* which she coauthored with her trainer, Bob Greene. In it, they tell of Oprah's journey from 237 pounds to the cover of *Shape* magazine and provide inspiration and guidance for overweight women everywhere.

DON'T FORGET THE BASICS

Many people work hard at eating a low-fat menu, but still somehow continue to pack on pounds or fail to lose weight. It's hard to say exactly why that happens, but I have a hunch there are still a few things they need to address, like serving size and calorie intake.

All nutritional information is listed by the serving, so if a serving is two cookies and you normally eat six, then you are consuming three times as many fat grams as the label indicates. While the product itself may be low fat, you can still accumulate a day's worth of fat pretty quickly. Often the serving size is ridiculously small, so be sure to read the labels carefully.

Calories still count. You can't ignore calorie intake in favor of counting fat grams and still expect to lose weight. Pasta with marinara sauce may be low in fat, but it still has plenty of calories to burn off.

On average, women consume 1,800 calories per day. With an 1,800-calorie diet, you should have no more than 60 grams of fat, 18 from saturated fat. With a 1,500-calorie menu, you should have no more than 50 grams of fat, 15 from saturated fat. On a low-calorie (1,200) diet, eat no more than 40 grams of fat, 12 from saturated fats.

OLESTRA: A FAT BY ANY OTHER NAME

As I'm writing this, the newspapers are full of the "good news" that Olestra, the first man-made fat to withstand the high temperatures needed for cooking, has received its final FDA approval after twenty-five years of testing and a $200 million investment by Proctor & Gamble. While it may seem like the answer to our dieting prayers, Olestra does have some drawbacks. As it slips through the body without being absorbed and stored as fat, it takes with it some important, fat-soluble vitamins like vitamins A, D, and K. It also can have a mild laxative effect and can cause cramping.

Like anything else, Olestra is probably fine in moderation. That's the problem. One ounce is considered a serving of potato chips, and frankly I don't know anyone who eats such a small portion. If you absolutely have to have potato chips with your tuna sandwich, then choose baked chips or have a few Olestra chips, if you must. Better yet, have some pretzels. They're baked and most are naturally fat-free.

To put Olestra into perspective, remember when we thought sugar-free soft drinks and Sweet 'N Low would solve all of our dieting problems? We're still an overweight nation.

Man-made or otherwise, fat is the enemy.

COMPLICATED CHOLESTEROL

Cholesterol is the topic of confusion among some people. First we learned that cholesterol is bad, that it clogs arteries and contributes to heart disease. Then we learned that some cholesterol is good for your heart and that there are two kinds: LDL, the lousy cholesterol, and HDL, the healthy cholesterol.

Cholesterol is a non-water soluble substance that moves through the blood on the backs of lipoproteins and is used by the liver and tissues to make cell membranes throughout the body. If too much cholesterol is in the blood, some of it begins to collect on the walls of the arteries, an affliction known as atherosclerosis or hardening of the arteries. High density lipoproteins (HDL) do not clog arteries, but low density lipoproteins (LDL) do. HDLs may also help whisk away LDLs.

Why is all of this important? Clogged arteries limit blood flow and consequently oxygen flow to the heart. A heart that is not getting sufficient oxygen can suffer a heart attack. Heart disease is the number one killer of postmenopausal women. Ten percent of women age forty-five to sixty-four and 20 percent of women over age sixty-five have some form of heart disease. Add to those figures the 1.6 million women who have had a stroke and the fact that one in five Americans has high cholesterol (total blood cholesterol over 240 mg/dl), and you can see why watching cholesterol is close to edging out baseball as the national pastime.

Only 10 to 25 percent of your body's blood cholesterol level comes from cholesterol in foods. Only foods that are derived from animals contain cholesterol, so limiting your intake of animal products, including meat, cheese, and other dairy products, will help keep your cholesterol count in check. The rest, approximately 1,000 milligrams a day, is manufactured by the liver in response to dietary intake of saturated fats. In general, solid fats, butter, stick margarine, cheese, and ice cream are high in saturated fats and the National Cholesterol Education Program recommends that everyone over age two keep their saturated fat intake under 10 percent of total calories consumed each day.

Polyunsaturated fats, however, encourage the generation of HDLs, so choose soft or liquid margarines and vegetable oils instead. Monounsaturated fats found in olive oil or canola oil are also good alternatives.

If all of this seems complicated, that's OK. It is. Think of it this way. If the fat is hard and sticky, it will be the same way in your bloodstream and stick to the walls of your arteries. If it is liquid and flowing, it is less likely to clog up the works.

By now everyone knows that eggs are high in cholesterol. In fact one egg yolk contains almost the entire recommended daily allowance of cholesterol — 272 mg out of 300 mg. In cooking, use two egg whites for every whole egg the recipe calls for. I guarantee you'll never notice the difference. If you're making quiche or an omelette, egg substitutes like Egg Beaters are a fabulous alternative. I love to bake and I use Egg Beaters all the time. There's no difference in the way my baked goods turn out.

Remember, even if your weight is under control and you are physically fit, your blood cholesterol level can still be dangerously high, so have it checked periodically.

My cholesterol was over 300 at one time, even though I exercised regularly and had never had a weight problem. If it hadn't been for a routine physical, I never would have known I was having a cholesterol crisis. Even now, my cholesterol count is high (285), but because my ratio of total cholesterol to HDL is 5:1, my doctor says I'm not at risk for a heart attack or stroke. The American Heart Association recommends a ratio below 5:1, with the optimum being 3.5:1. A desirable total cholesterol level is under 200, with 200 to 239 considered borderline-high.

Regular exercise will help lower LDL and raise HDL, and losing even a few pounds can help too. As we all know, smoking is bad for your heart and lungs, but did you know that it lowers HDL? Moderate amounts of alcohol are linked with increasing HDL, but not enough to cause the AHA to recommend drinking for people who do not already do so.

Menopause and its attendant estrogen deficiency is known to contribute to elevated cholesterol levels, making heart disease the number-one killer of postmenopausal women. This is why doctors believe hormone replacement therapy, which increases a woman's estrogen level, reduces the risk of heart disease. The American Heart Association lists premature menopause without hormone replacement therapy in its list of elements increasing heart attack risk.

The National Heart, Lung, and Blood Institute publishes some terrific literature on cholesterol that you may wish to consult for further information on this topic. Their number is 301-251-1222.

LABEL LINGO

Thousands of products enter the market each month aimed at menu-conscious America. They're packaged beautifully with terms like "low fat" screaming from the label. It wasn't long ago that companies could make these claims just by making only the slightest changes in the original recipe, but now the FDA has established guidelines that specifically define the terms that manufacturers use on their labels. Knowing the package label terms can help you make better selections at the grocery store.

LIGHT A product that claims to be light has half the fat or one-third the calories of the original product. In a low-fat, low-calorie product, light means that the sodium content has been cut in half.

LOWER, REDUCED, FEWER, LESS Products labeled "reduced calorie," "lower fat," and "less sodium" have 25 percent less of the undesirable ingredient than the regular product.

LEAN Less than 10 grams of fat, 4.5 grams of saturated fat, and less than 95 mg of cholesterol per serving.

EXTRA LEAN Less than 5 grams of fat, 2 grams of saturated fat, and less than 95 mg of cholesterol per serving.

LOW FAT Less than 3 grams of total fat per serving. For a main dish or meal, low fat means that there are less than 3 grams of fat per 100 grams of food and less than 30 percent of the calories are from fat.

LOW SATURATED FAT Less than 1 gram of saturated fat per serving and 15 percent or less of its calories from saturated fat. For a main dish, 1 gram or less of saturated fat per 100 grams of food and less than 10 percent of calories from saturated fat.

FAT FREE Less than .5 grams of fat per serving.

LOW CHOLESTEROL Less than 20 mg of cholesterol per serving and less than 2 mg of saturated fat per serving. For a meal or main dish, 20 mg of cholesterol per 100 grams of food, with less than 2 mg of saturated fat per 100 grams of food.

CHOLESTEROL FREE Less than 2 mg of cholesterol per serving.

LOW SODIUM Less than 140 mg of sodium per serving, or for a main dish, less than 140 mg of sodium per 100 grams of food.

VERY LOW SODIUM Less than 35 mg of sodium per serving.

SODIUM FREE Less than 5 mg of sodium per serving.

FABULOUS FIBER

As children, we were all admonished to eat our "roughage" because it was good for our system. Our mothers recognized that roughage, or fruits and vegetables, passed through easily and prevented constipation. Little did they know how good their advice really was.

In addition to keeping things moving, so to speak, fiber is now believed to help prevent colon and rectal cancer. In fact, the National Cancer Institute has predicted that cases of colon cancer would fall by 50 percent if Americans ate 20 to 30 grams of fiber a day. Most of us, however, only get about 11 grams of fiber from our menu.

Not only is fiber good for warding off some cancers, but fiber whisks away LDL cholesterol, reduces estrogen levels, and may help control diabetes. Think of fiber as an internal loofah scrubbing out your insides and sloughing off fat, cholesterol, and carcinogens.

High-fiber diets, by their very nature, are usually lower in fat. Most fruits and vegetables, with the notable exceptions of avocados and black olives, are low in fat and high in fiber. Fiber-rich foods also tend to be packed with vitamins and nutrients, too. As long as you don't load up on hollandaise sauce or butter, you can pick up plenty of extra fiber and vitamins by adding extra veggies and whole-grain bread and cereal products to your menu. Bran, rice, oats, whole-wheat breads and pastas, and legumes are great sources of fiber. With bran muffins and high-fiber cereals readily available at the grocery store, it's easy to trade in your morning toast for a bran muffin and be on your way to a higher fiber menu.

A quick jump in your fiber intake can have some rather unpleasant side effects, so take it easy at first and let your system build up the bacteria needed to digest all of this extra fiber. In other words, don't switch from a menu that's full of Wonderbread and white pasta to one that's packed with All-Bran, salad, and brown rice overnight. Gradually increase your fiber intake to avoid the sometimes noisy and uncomfortable side effects.

Drinking plenty of water, eight 8-ounce glasses a day, is important to overall good health and healthy skin, but it becomes especially important as you increase the fiber in your menu. Without adequate amounts of water, fiber can clog up your system and do the exact opposite of what you intended.

COOKBOOK RECOMMENDATIONS

1. *365 Easy Low-Calorie Recipes*, Sylvia Schur and Vivian Schulte, R.D., Ph.D.: HarperPerennial, $17.95 plus $3.50 shipping and handling. Call 800-331-3761.
2. *Everyday Cooking with Dr. Dean Ornish: 150 Easy Low-Fat, High Flavor Recipes*, Dean Ornish, M.D.: Harper-Collins, $25.00.
3. *Better Homes & Gardens Family Favorites Made Lighter,* $14.95; *Better Homes & Gardens Healthy Family Cookbook*, $29.95; *Better Homes & Gardens Cooking For Today: Vegetarian Recipes*, $14.95: Better Homes & Gardens Books, Meredith Corporation.

4. *Sunset Light & Healthy Cookbook,* $14.99; *Sunset Low-Fat Cookbook,* $9.99: Sunset Books and *Sunset* Magazine.

5. *The Twenty Minute Low-Fat Gourmet,* Karen A. Levin: Contemporary Books, $9.99.

6. *American Heart Association Low-Fat, Low-Cholesterol Cookbook,* Scott M. Grundy, M.D., Ph.D., and Mary Winston, Ed.D., R.D., Editors: Random House, $13.00.

7. *Beyond Alfalfa Sprouts & Cheese,* Judy Gilliard and Joy Kirkpatrick, R.D.: Chronimed Publishing, $12.95.

8. *Williams Sonoma Collection—Healthy Desserts*: Time Life Books, $18.95.

9. *Baking Without Fat,* George Matelijan, President of Health Valley Foods: Villard Publishing, $15.00.

10. *Betty Crocker's Easy Low-Fat Cooking*: Macmillan Press, $19.95.

11. *Fat Free Living Desserts,* Jyl Steinback: Fat Free Living, Inc., $15.95.

12. *Weight Watchers Magazine Dessert Classics*: Weight Watchers Publishing Group, $9.95.

13. *Great Taste: Healthy Cooking from Canyon Ranch*: $25 plus $4.75 shipping and handling. Call 800-726-8040.

14. *Cooking Light Annual Recipes*: Oxmoor House, $29.95. Available in bookstores or by calling 800-765-6400.

Note: The Sunset and Better Homes & Gardens books have the best and simplest recipes. From them you can learn how to convert your own favorite recipes into guilt-free creations.

LEADING MAGAZINES
Bon Appetit has a Cooking for Health section that features low-fat recipes; *Cooking Light* is a great magazine with many easy low-fat recipes.

VITALITY THROUGH VITAMINS

As I'm writing this book, vitamins are capturing headlines every day with new findings about the cancer-fighting prospects of antioxidants. In his book *Antioxidant Revolution,* Dr. Ken Cooper, the physician who got everyone doing aerobics, is now pushing antioxidants as the true fountain of youth and the cure for almost all evils, especially cancer and heart disease. In addition, Jean Carper's best-seller *Stop Aging Now* suggests that all diseases are the result of age-damaged cells and, therefore, if we focus all of our attention on fighting aging, then cancer, heart disease, even Alzheimer's, will be drastically delayed or eliminated.

Read on to learn more about vitamins' potential and how you can sift through all of the sometimes confusing information.

Alphabet Soup

If you follow the news, you'll notice that medical science announces some new vitamin finding almost every week. Frankly, it's hard to keep up and hard to know what to do.

Here are some examples:

- The National Cancer Institute says that too much beta-carotene (one of the good-guy antioxidants) could increase a smoker's risk of lung cancer and that it provides no protection against cancer or heart disease.
- Too much vitamin A can cause birth defects.
- Calcium supplements are important in warding off osteoporosis, but there's no sense taking them without adequate amounts of vitamin D to help the body absorb it.
- And as if all of that were not enough alphabet soup to swim in, studies show that those of us living in the northern section of the world may be deficient in vitamin D in the winter months because of sun deprivation. (Our bodies manufacture vitamin D when exposed to the sun.) Of course, we all know we should protect ourselves from the sun to prevent skin cancer and that sunlight creates free radicals that can be neutralized by antioxidant vitamins.

According to Dr. H. James Day, an internationally known hematologist and oncologist who is the chief of hematology at Abington Memorial Hospital in Abington, Pa., a multivitamin tablet along with calcium supplements taken in conjunction with a sensible diet that's heavy on fruits and vegetables is the best course of action for most people. Postmenopausal women will want to be sure that either their multivitamin or their calcium tablets have extra vitamin D. How's that for simplification?

Calcium tablets made from bone meal and dolomite have been known to have lead, mercury, or arsenic in them, so many doctors recommend taking Tums, the chewable antacid tablets. They're flavored and easy to chew, inexpensive, loaded with calcium, and they'll ward off heartburn after a spicy dinner. Who could ask for more?

I've spoken to women who were concerned about developing kidney stones because of taking calcium supplements, but according to the National Institute of Health, people who are not otherwise at risk for kidney stones can safely take up to 2,000 mg of calcium a day. That would be the equivalent of seven 8-ounce glasses of skim milk per day plus a few spears of broccoli. If you are confused about which form of calcium is best, ask your pharmacist for some guidance.

Menstruating women especially should be sure their vitamin pill is fortified with iron. While iron can build up to toxic levels, the human body only absorbs about 10 percent of what it takes in, so according to Dr. Day, you'd have to eat rusty nails to be in any real danger of building up too much iron.

The National Research Council's Food and Nutrition Board has established Recommended Dietary Allowances (RDA) for vitamins and minerals, and according to the RDA guidelines most healthy people get sufficient amounts from their diet. As we age, however, our appetites tend to decrease and the risk of a vitamin deficiency becomes greater, making the need for a supplement more critical.

Although you will probably meet your RDA with a nutritionally complete diet, taking a multivitamin in addition is not going to cause you to overdose on vitamin A or iron. In fact, most people can take as many as two or three multivitamins without running the risk of getting too much of any one vitamin.

Carper and Cooper claim that the RDA is woefully inadequate and arbitrary and recommend significantly higher doses (between 10 and 200 times the RDA) to ensure good health and prevent disease.

I'm impressed by Carper's and Cooper's books. Because of them, and the influence of a friend who is "into vitamins," I've begun taking a multivitamin every day in addition to chewing on a few Tums for extra calcium. I realize that these additional precautions may not help me live long enough to see my great grandchildren graduate from college, but they can't hurt and they just might help, so why not?

Free Radicals and Antioxidants

The biggest news in vitamins these days is the ongoing research into free radicals and antioxidants. Here is a quick review to help you understand what all of the commotion is about.

FREE RADICALS Despite the name, free radicals are not guys like Timothy Leary or Pat Buchanan. Free radicals are highly charged molecules with one spare electron that are created, ironically, by the things we do to stay alive, such as eating and breathing in oxygen. In addition, exposure to ultraviolet rays (sunlight), pollution, and smoke, causes the formation of free radicals. Like humans, electrons like to be part of a pair, so the unstable molecules attack stable molecules in search of a partner for the lonely electron. But in picking up a partner, the molecule breaks up the previously stable molecule. This kind of cellular gang warfare destroys DNA, fat, and protein molecules. Many believe that a lifetime of free-radical damage is the root of all kinds of age-related disorders, including wrinkles and most notably cancer.

ANTIOXIDANTS Think of antioxidants as a your body's back-yard bug zapper, working to neutralize the free radicals. Vitamins A, C, D, and E, and beta-carotene (a vitamin-A derivative) are the most common antioxidants, but with the exception of vitamin C, antioxidants are fat-soluble and can be stored in the body so that they are ready to fight off any free radicals that come along.

Some knowledgeable people, following the lead of vitamin gurus like Dr. Cooper, drink what are called antioxidant cocktails, concoctions that contain megadoses of vitamins, to promote their own good health and prevent cancer. But according to Dr. Day, that won't do you much good. He says that eating your antioxidants is the only way to obtain any real cancer and heart disease-fighting benefits.

However, you'd need to eat anywhere between 45 and 170 oranges a day to get the amount of vitamin C Dr. Linus Pauling said was necessary to extend your life twelve to eighteen years. (Pauling, who lived to be ninety-three before dying of cancer, credited vitamin C with delaying the onset of his cancer by twenty years.)

Clearly it's not possible to eat enough food to get the kind of antioxidant protection that Carper and Cooper describe in their books, so if you find their ideas appealing, supplements are the only viable alternative.

But the fact of the matter is that the jury is still out on whether or not antioxidants provide any real protection against heart disease or cancer. First, the benefits of beta-carotene were dismissed based upon a study funded by the National Cancer Institute. In addition, there's evidence that even though vitamin E produces blood-thinning effects that reduce the risk of heart disease, those same effects may raise the risk of stroke. Every day another medical journal comes out with some new findings.

While a daily multivitamin and calcium supplement are sensible recommendations, I suggest consulting your physician before you become a vitamin-pill junkie.

Money-Saving Tips

Americans spend $3.5 billion a year on vitamin supplements, but that doesn't mean that a little insurance pill has to be a budget buster for you. Buy your vitamins in the grocery store, mass-market retailer, or discount drugstore for the best savings and buy the largest bottle possible. Avoid health-food stores, where the same products will cost five or six times as much. Also look for multivitamin pills. There is no real advantage to taking each vitamin individually.

Natural vitamins are not worth extra money since the body absorbs natural and synthetic vitamins comparably and any difference is not worth a price premium. In fact, you can safely buy the generic, store brand of vitamin to save additional money. Just look for labeling that says USP (United States Pharmacopeia) or "dissolves in sixty minutes" to ensure that the vitamins meet the standards for purity.

The American Association for Retired Persons (AARP) has a mail-order pharmacy that offers great prices on vitamins as well as prescription drugs. They send out a quarterly catalog that's full of special discounts on everything from contact lens solution and adult diapers to heart medication. And the best part is you don't even have to be a retired person to use the service. You can call them at 800-456-2277.

Pharmacists are great resources for vitamin supplements as well as the medicines they dispense, and I've yet to meet a druggist who wasn't happy to share advice and wisdom. The owners and employees of health-food stores also tend to be extremely knowledgeable, but since their prices are high, I would buy vitamins somewhere else and use health-food stores for herbal products and specialty items. When you do shop at health-food stores, ask about discount days and special clubs for frequent shoppers. I know that General Nutrition Centers (GNC) have such a program, offering discounts on Tuesdays, and I'm sure other companies do, too.

To learn more about vitamins and minerals, call Health Media of America at 619-688-0377 and ask for their Nutrition Report. A year's subscription costs $48, but it is full of the latest research compiled from more than six thousand publications.

WATER, WATER, EVERY DAY

For some reason, many people, myself included, find it difficult to drink eight 8-ounce glasses of water every day. We drink plenty of coffee, tea, soda, and juice, but we avoid water and milk, the two beverages our bodies need most. No, all liquids do not benefit your body equally. Even though coffee and tea are made from water, they don't count toward your eight glasses per day.

Prior to "the change," if I drank water at all, it was a fake lemonade concoction with lemon juice and Sweet 'N Low. After menopause, when my hair and skin started to dry up, I complained to my doctor about my throat and mouth being dry, too. That's when I realized how little fluid I was actually taking in every day.

Now that water is a regular part of my life, I see a tremendous difference in my hair, skin, and body functions. It helps keep things flowing, so to speak, and helps control my weight too.

Water is fat- and calorie-free, whisks away impurities, helps keep your skin looking great — it's practically perfect.

To get into the water-drinking habit, I spent $5 for a Weight Watchers bottle that holds 64 ounces. Every day I fill it up and keep drinking until it's empty. Now, if I have a busy day and don't get to it until later in the day, I can really feel it. I feel dried out, even sluggish sometimes. I rarely drink diet soda anymore because there's nothing like the fresh taste and feel of a cool drink of water.

Even though most tap water is just fine, some people prefer to drink flavored waters, seltzer, or spring water. Just watch what you're buying, it's easy to pick up sugary concoctions by mistake.

Elaine's Exclusive

LEARN SOMETHING NEW EVERY DAY

The University of California at Berkeley Wellness Letter is a treasure trove of good, reliable information on the latest in nutrition, exercise, stress management, and much more. It's a bargain at $24 for twelve issues. Call them at 800-829-9170.

ALCOHOL

60 Minutes aired a segment in 1991 called "The French Paradox," which pointed out the lower incidence of heart disease among the French despite their fat-laden diets. Since about that time, research on the health benefits of moderate alcohol consumption has gained a lot of attention in the United States. Wine sales soared by 44 percent in the year following the segment, and researchers undertook more studies to explain the phenomenon.

Initially, the medical community believed that red wine, with its high levels of antioxidants, held the premium on heart protection, but additional research found that women who drank one glass of red or white wine per day decreased their risk of heart disease by 30 percent. In addition, women who had one beer or one drink of hard liquor also greatly reduced their risk of heart disease.

What we know is that alcohol increases HDL, which sweeps the artery-clogging LDL out of the bloodstream, thereby protecting the heart and keeping the blood flowing smoothly. Alcohol also makes platelets less sticky so that they can't cling to fatty deposits and clog arteries. In addition, one or two drinks will reduce tension and boost relaxation, which is also good for the heart.

The key here is one drink, or two, with meals. Not three or four a day.

Studies that have been published since 1991 have ascribed health benefits to heavier (three to five drinks) drinking. A Danish study of thirteen thousand men and women found that those who drank three to five glasses of wine daily had half the risk of dying of any cause. Non-wine drinkers and wine drinkers alike were only one-third as likely to die of cardiovascular disease. Those who drank the equivalent amount of hard liquor boosted their risk of death 36 percent over those who did not drink at all and beer drinkers increased their death rate by 22 percent.

While this study allowed for three to five glasses of wine, most published reports suggest only one or two glasses for healthful benefits. Certainly at five glasses of wine a day, most people might have healthy hearts, but their heads would feel lousy the next day and they'd be consuming a lot of empty calories, too.

Clearly alcohol is another example of the need for moderation — we all know too well the results of excessive alcohol consumption. In addition to the unpleasant side effects of a hangover, heavy drinking causes water retention, which gives you that bloated look and feel the morning after. The swelling and subsequent deflation causes the skin to stretch unnecessarily which, over the years will cause your skin to wrinkle and become loose. Of course, if you drink that much, you probably have bigger problems than baggy skin.

In its Dietary Guidelines for Americans, updated in 1996, the Department of Health and Human Services changed it's long-held antialcohol policy to say the following: "Alcoholic beverages have been used to enhance the enjoyment of meals by many societies throughout human history. Current evidence suggests that moderate drinking is associated with a lower risk for coronary heart disease in some individuals."

The bottom line is, if you drink alcohol, an occasional glass or two of wine with meals seems to have real health benefits. On the other hand, if you don't drink alcohol, the potential health benefits are not enough of a reason to start.

THE LATEST CRAZES

Nearly every week we hear news about some miracle, herb, hormone, pill, or tablet that will help us live longer, happier, healthier lives. Even though we like to think of ourselves as mature, intelligent human beings who couldn't be suckered by a sales pitch, doesn't the fact that so many of us have been buying hope-in-a-jar for the last twenty or thirty years indicate that we're all somewhat inclined to believe in miracles?

Because these products are available in health-food stores, many people assume that their quality is assured and that they are harmless. Good sense, however, suggests otherwise. In addition to the hype that accompanies every promising new study, each year there is some sort of scare associated with health foods.

Not long ago there was the L-tryptophan scare. People were taking the amino acid as a sleep aid, but a contaminated batch killed thirty-eight people and another fifteen hundred got a painful connective tissue disorder. The FDA eventually banned L-tryptophan supplements entirely, but that kind of action doesn't happen often.

In 1994, Congress enacted the Dietary Supplement Health and Education Act, which classified vitamins, minerals, and herbs as food supplements, thereby reducing the FDA's jurisdiction over them. Now, unless the FDA can prove that something is dangerous, it has no standing to regulate it. Of course those who market herbs and vitamins can't make drug claims, but they can promote what the product is known to do and they can name the product whatever they want. With those guidelines a company can market caffeine pills as Nature's Energizers or Rocket Pills and it's all perfectly legal.

All of this should not scare you away from health-food stores or vitamins. After all, many herbal remedies are beneficial, and so much of conventional medicine is rooted in herbs and folk medicine that it should not be dismissed as quackery.

If you decide to seek out diet supplements as a way to improve your health, be sure to buy known brands from reputable stores like GNC or local, independently owned health-food stores. Often the proprietors are very knowledgeable and eager to talk and make recommendations. In addition, if you are taking any serious medication for depression, blood pressure, or a heart condition, for example, you should discuss with your doctor any plans to start taking any medications, vitamins, or health-food products.

Fat Burners

Take a trip to the health-food store and you'll find shelf after shelf of products called "fat burners," products that presumably will help melt away body fat. The fact of the matter is that these products are primarily vitamins, minerals, and amino acids, chemical compounds that are the basic structural units of all proteins, not anything newly discovered or invented.

Some also contain natural stimulants like caffeine or ephedrine, which can raise blood pressure and heart rate. (Ephedrine or pseudoephedrine is the active ingredient in decongestants). Ephedrine is the ingredient used in the "natural drugs" you may have heard about in news reports. Kids are getting high "naturally" with drugs called Herbal Ecstasy and Cloud 9, but the stimulant, which is combined with caffeine, has been known to have deadly effects.

One popular ingredient found in many fat burners is chromium picolinate, a mineral that improves glucose tolerance and reduces blood serum cholesterol. One study involving young athletes indicated that it may help the body shed fat, but other studies have yet to bear it out. In addition, news reports say that the body stores chromium and it can reach dangerous levels if taken for too long.

L-carnitine, an amino acid that is a common ingredient in fat burners, does indeed lower cholesterol levels and help the body metabolize fat and build endurance.

Some of the ingredients in fat burners have some healthful bene-fits that may facilitate weight loss or improve overall fitness. If you purchase well-known ephedra-free products from reputable health-food stores, you probably won't get hurt and you might lose a few pounds and see some improvement in your general health. Keep in mind, however, that every fat-burning product recommends a regi-men of sensible eating and exercise that, if adhered to faithfully, would probably deliver the same results.

Truthfully, if some combination of herbs, vitamins, minerals, and amino acids were proven to burn fat, it would be the biggest news since the end of World War II. If fat burners really worked, don't you think the inventor would have been on the cover of *Time* by now?

If you're considering taking fat burners, be aware that they are not recommended for women who are pregnant or nursing, or for anyone with high blood pressure, a history of cardiovascular disease, thyroid disease, diabetes, prostate problems, or people taking M.A.O. inhibitors. In addition, people who are sensitive to stimulants or aspirin are not good candidates for fat burners for obvious reasons. Be sure to take the products only as directed and to stop taking them immediately if you experience any of the contraindications noted on the package.

Melatonin: Mother Nature's Miracle?

By now you've probably heard or read about melatonin, the sleep-inducing hormone that can control jet lag. It, too, is available in health-food stores and ever since the 1995 publication of several books on the subject, even big health-food chains like GNC are hav-ing a hard time keeping it in stock.

The body produces melatonin in the pineal gland, a pea-sized gland in the center of the brain. This hormone maintains the body's circadian rhythms, the sleep/wake cycle that can be disrupted by changes in daylight and darkness patterns—the same reason it takes a few days to get adjusted to daylight savings time. As youngsters, we produce plenty of melatonin, but blood levels drop sharply around puberty and decline steadily as we grow older.

Jet-setters and people who travel frequently for business have long known about melatonin's ability to help with jet lag, but now insomniacs are snatching up melatonin as a natural sleep aid that has virtually no side effects.

Studies that were documented in the best-seller *The Melatonin Miracle* suggest that melatonin may also be a hormonal youth dew. Removal of the pineal gland seems to accelerate aging in mice, so scientists are hopeful that increased amounts of melatonin could slow the aging process. While researchers are a long way away from proving youth-prolonging benefits in humans, for many people — older people especially — a good night's sleep could go a long way to restoring energy, if not youthful vitality.

I am, however, concerned about the lack of long-term studies on melatonin. If used occasionally for a sleepless night or to control jet lag, it's probably fine. In August of 1996, experts attending a meeting sponsored by the National Institute on Aging to evaluate the available research on melatonin concluded that there was not enough scientific evidence to support the widespread use of melatonin.

Melatonin is moving beyond health-food stores into the mainstream. It's now sold in supermarkets and drugstore chains and I recently saw a newspaper coupon for it. It is available in tablets or lozenges that dissolve under the tongue, and because it works so well at making you sleepy, be sure not to drive a car or operate heavy machinery after taking it.

Longevity magazine reported on Dr. Michael Cohen, a Virginia endocrinologist who developed a pill called M-Oval, a combination of melatonin and low doses of estrogen for menopausal women. Because melatonin extends estrogen's effects, this doctor found he could give women the protective benefits of estrogen while minimizing the risks of estrogen's side effects. He is working on FDA approval for this drug, which should take about four years. He is also developing a birth control pill that suppresses ovulation with a combination of melatonin and progesterone. Because it does not contain estrogen, the risk of breast cancer is reduced or eliminated and the fifteen hundred women who have taken it did not retain water or lose their libido. The birth control pill is expected to take two years to get FDA approval for marketing.

DHEA

If you haven't heard much about DHEA (dehydroepiandrosterone) yet, you probably will soon. It's a hormone that is produced by the adrenal glands, and like melatonin it is plentiful in the young and practically nonexistent by the time you reach age sixty.

Researchers think that low levels of DHEA make people more susceptible to the diseases commonly associated with old age, namely heart disease, cancer, and Alzheimer's. Its proponents say that it reduces the risk of heart disease, breast and other cancers, and Alzheimer's. They also credit it with lowering cholesterol, stimulating weight loss, and giving the memory a boost. Researchers have also found that HIV-positive patients do not develop full-blown AIDS until their DHEA output drops.

Since research into DHEA is relatively new and long-term studies haven't been done yet, no one is sure about long-term use of the supplement. And it may also have side effects. For example, the body converts DHEA into testosterone and estrogen, so it is possible that the risks of hormone replacement could apply to DHEA. On the other hand, doctors might be able to stimulate estrogen production in older women, thereby eliminating the need for estrogen replacement therapy.

Dr. Nicholas Perricone, a Connecticut dermatologist and clinical professor at Yale Medical School, is convinced that DHEA's benefits outweigh its possible drawbacks. He includes DHEA in an aggressive regimen of antioxidants, melatonin, amino acids, and hormone replacement therapy for patients who want to live longer, healthier lives and are willing to experiment a little.

Studies are ongoing with DHEA, but it is now available in health-food stores. Beware of products that claim to cause your body to make DHEA. These are supplements derived from wild yam and are not pure DHEA. They are sold as dioscorea. Scientists have only done their research on the real DHEA, not on the wild yam precursor.

DHEA, like melatonin, has many credible supporters and with the tremendous possibilities for these supplements, it's easy to feel as though you're missing the chance of a lifetime if you're not taking them. My best advice is to speak with your doctor about them, then read on your own to learn as much as possible before taking the plunge.

If you do decide to take DHEA, be aware that even those who heartily endorse the supplement recommend dosages of 25 to 100 mg per day. Also be aware that 90 mg or more per day has had a masculinizing effect on women, namely causing lowered voices and an increase in facial hair.

THINK POSITIVELY AND LET THEM EAT CAKE

At the beginning of this chapter I mentioned that dieting often meant deprivation and I think that's where diets run off course. If your diet is driven by foods you should avoid—chips, hamburgers, cookies, ice cream, etc.—you end up spending a lot of time thinking about what you are trying to avoid. Instead, if you focus on eating healthy foods instead of avoiding unhealthy foods, you're spending your time thinking positively instead of negatively. You will be full from good food and, before you know it, eating well will become a habit.

According to dietitian Marie Ward, emotional cues cause us to consume 75 percent of what we eat. We eat because we're happy, sad, mournful, celebratory, nervous, tense, bored, you name it—which means that we're really only hungry for 25 percent of our food. As Americans we use food as comfort from early on. Have you ever given a crying child a cookie to help them feel better? But have you ever actually healed a scraped knee by rubbing Chips Ahoy on it? You get the idea.

Try to get into the habit of eating only what you need to fuel your body. Then when you've had a truly horrendous day, you can eat the whole pint of Häagen-Dazs and not feel the least bit guilty, because you don't do it all the time.

And finally, there's nothing wrong with a treat now and then. In fact, many dietitians tell their patients not to put anything on the forbidden list, because psychologically if you feel you're being deprived of something you'll want it all the more and your efforts will be derailed quickly. I think that's especially true for special-occasion treats like birthday cake. If you care enough about someone to celebrate their birthday, share their cake—even a small piece.

GUILT-FREE DESSERTS

BLACK MAGIC CAKE

Prepare and allow to cool:
2 cups strong black coffee
$1/2$ cup cholesterol-free margarine (stick, not whipped)

Sift together in large bowl:
$2^1/2$ cups flour
2 cups granulated sugar
1 cup baking cocoa
2 tsp baking soda
2 tsp vanilla extract

1. Blend dry ingredients with coffee, cooled, melted margarine, and vanilla extract. Batter will be runny.
2. Bake in 9 x 13-inch pan at 350 degrees for 35-45 minutes or until toothpick comes out clean. Dust with powdered sugar.

This cake is great warm from the oven.

18 servings • 105 calories per serving • 5.8 gm fat • 0 mg cholesterol

---

PINEAPPLE CHEESE PUDDING

Blend in food processor for 10 seconds:
2 cups fat-free cottage cheese
$1/2$ cup egg substitute or 3 egg whites
1 tbs melted margarine
$1/2$ tsp vanilla extract

Add the following and process 10 seconds more:
$1/3$ cup sugar
2 tbs flour
1 cup crushed pineapple, drained

1. Pour mixture into 10 x 6 x 2-inch pan coated with cooking spray and sprinkle with $1/8$ tsp cinnamon.

2. Place dish in larger pan with one inch of water in bottom and bake 40 minutes at 350 degrees or until knife comes out clean.
3. Serve warm or at room temperature.

10 servings • 98 calories • 3 gm fat • 2 mg cholesterol

SMILING ANGELS ICE CREAM CAKE

1. Slice one angel food cake into three layers.
2. Sprinkle each layer with Amaretto (approximately 3 tbs total).
3. Spread fat-free praline ice cream or frozen yogurt on two layers and assemble layer cake.
4. Ice cake with fat-free Cool Whip.
5. Dust with finely chopped almonds.
6. Freeze until firm.

Variations:

Grand Marnier, orange sherbet, and vanilla ice cream
Godiva liquor and mint chocolate-chip fat-free ice cream

15 servings • 366 calories • 3.9 gm fat • 5 mg cholesterol

CANYON RANCH STRAWBERRY-RHUBARB COBBLER

Contributed by Canyon Ranch Health & Fitness Resort.

FRUIT FILLING
2 cups quartered strawberries
2 cups rhubarb cut into ¹/₂-inch pieces
¹/₄ cup fructose
2 tsp cornstarch

DOUGH
²/₃ cups all-purpose flour
¹/₃ cup whole-wheat pastry flour
1¹/₂ tsp baking powder
1¹/₂ tsp fructose
2 tbs margarine
¹/₂ cup buttermilk
1 tsp ground cinnamon

1. To make fruit filling, combine rhubarb, strawberries, fructose, and cornstarch in a small bowl. Mix well and set aside for 15 to 20 minutes.
2. Preheat oven to 325 degrees.
3. To make dough, combine flours, baking powder, and fructose in another bowl. Using pastry blender or two knives, cut in margarine until mixture is crumbly. Stir in buttermilk and work until mixture is the consistency of biscuit dough.
4. Lightly spray 8 small serving dishes with nonstick vegetable spray. Spoon $1/2$ cup of fruit mixture into each dish and drop a heaping tablespoon of dough over each. Sprinkle with cinnamon.
5. Bake 15 to 20 minutes or until filling is bubbling and the top is golden.

Variation:

Use blueberries, apples, peaches, or other fruits in season.
8 servings • 130 calories • 3 gm fat • trace cholesterol

CANYON RANCH FUDGE BROWNIES

Contributed by Canyon Ranch Health and Fitness Resort.

2 oz semisweet chocolate

3 tbs butter

2 tbs vegetable oil

1 cup sugar, divided into two equal parts

1 cup all-purpose flour

5 tbs cocoa

$1/2$ teaspoon baking powder

pinch salt

2 tbs apricot jam

3 egg whites

$1/4$ cup nonfat fudge sauce

1. Preheat oven to 325 degrees. Lightly spray 8 x 8-inch pan with nonstick vegetable coating and set aside.
2. Melt chocolate, butter, and oil in a small saucepan over low heat. Remove from heat and set aside.
3. In a medium bowl, sift together $1/2$ cup of sugar, flour, cocoa, baking powder, and salt. Add apricot jam and mix well.

4. In a separate bowl, whip egg whites and remaining $1/2$ cup sugar until soft peaks are formed. Gently fold half of chocolate mixture into egg white mixture and mix until incorporated. Fold in remaining chocolate mixture. Fold flour mixture into chocolate mixture.
5. Pour batter into prepared pan and bake for 30 minutes, or until knife comes out clean when inserted in middle.
6. Remove from oven. Drizzle with nonfat fudge sauce when slightly cooled.

16 servings • 145 calories • 5 gm fat • 5 mg cholesterol

CHOCOLATE YOGURT MOUSSE IN PHYLLO CUPS

Contributed by Cheryl Lace, Lace & Co.,
Philadelphia, Pennsylvania.

MOUSSE
8 oz plain nonfat yogurt
1 oz melted chocolate
$1/4$ cup cocoa powder, sifted
8 egg whites
$1/3$ cup powdered sugar, sifted

1. Drain the yogurt overnight in the refrigerator using a cheesecloth-lined strainer.
2. Bring the yogurt to room temperature, then stir in melted chocolate and cocoa.
3. Whip the egg whites to soft peaks with an electric mixer. Slowly sprinkle sugar over egg whites and continue whipping until medium peaks are achieved.
4. Fold the meringue into the yogurt mixture and chill thoroughly.

PHYLLO CUPS
3 sheets of frozen phyllo pastry, thawed
2 tbs low-fat margarine, melted

1. Preheat oven to 350 degrees.
2. Spray a muffin tin with nonstick cooking spray.
3. Cut each phyllo sheet into 6 squares. Using a brush, spread a small amount of melted margarine on one square. Place

another square on top at an angle, brush with margarine, and top with third square at a different angle. Place all three in muffin tin to form a cup. Repeat process five times.

4. Bake cups 10 minutes or until golden.
5. Divide the mousse among the phyllo cups, garnish, and serve.

Garnish ideas:
orange zest
whipped cream
fresh berries
6 servings • 164 calories per serving • 6.5 gm fat • 1 mg cholesterol

---

CHOCOLATE MERINGUE COOKIES

Contributed by Cheryl Lace, Lace & Co.,
Philadelphia, Pennsylvania.
3 egg whites
1 cup sugar
2 tbs cocoa powder, sifted
1 tsp vanilla extract or coffee liqueur (optional)

1. Preheat oven to 200 degrees.
2. Whip egg whites to firm peaks with an electric mixer. Slowly sprinkle the sugar over and continue whipping until stiff peaks are achieved. Fold in the cocoa powder and vanilla extract or coffee liqueur.
3. Line a baking sheet with parchment or wax paper. Drop by tablespoonfuls or pipe with pastry bag into desired shapes on sheet.
4. For a crisp cookie with a chewy center, bake for 30 minutes. For a crisp cookie, bake for 60 minutes.
5. Cool on sheet for 15 minutes before removing. Once cooled, store in airtight container for no more than 2 days.

Tip: These cookies are best made on dry, humidity-free days.

Variation:
Fold 1 tbs of orange zest into the batter.
Sandwich your favorite spreadable fruit between cookies and dust with cocoa.
Yield 4 dozen cookies • 24 servings • 36 calories per serving • 0 gm fat • 0 mg cholesterol

---

LOW-FAT CHOCOLATE CUSTARD

Contributed by Colleen Winston, Pastry Chef,
Passarelle Restaurant, Radnor, Pennsylvania.

7 tbs sugar
¼ cup cocoa powder
2 tbs corn starch
1 tsp powdered gelatin
2 cups low-fat milk
⅔ cup whole milk
2 eggs
2 tbs vanilla

1. Sift sugar, cocoa powder, cornstarch, and gelatin into a pot.
2. Pour in milk, eggs, and vanilla.
3. Whisk all ingredients together.
4. Cook over a medium flame until thickened, stirring constantly to prevent scorching.
5. Remove from stove when mixture begins to boil.
6. Pour into six glasses or small bowls.
7. Chill and serve topped with fresh fruit, dusted with confectioner's sugar.

6 servings • 145 calories • 3.7 gm fat • 6.7 mg cholesterol

BROWNIES WITH FUDGE SWEET

Contributed by Chef Michel Stroot, The Golden Door Spa,
Escondido, California.

BROWNIE
¾ cup unbleached flour, white
½ cup unsweetened cocoa powder
1 tsp baking powder
½ tsp baking soda
3½ oz ripe bananas (1 medium banana)
¾ cup light brown sugar
½ cup unsweetened apple juice
1 tsp vanilla
½ tsp chocolate extract

4 egg whites (room temperature)
$^1/_2$ tsp kosher salt

GARNISH
**$^1/_4$ cup Fudge Sweet chocolate sauce (a product of Wax
Orchards, Vashon, Washington)**
10 oz oranges (2 medium oranges cut into 6 wedges each)
1 cup blueberries

1. Preheat oven to 350 degrees.
2. Spray a nonstick 8 x 8-inch baking pan with vegetable spray. Set aside.
3. In large mixing bowl, sift together flour, cocoa powder, baking powder, and baking soda. Set aside.
4. In blender, combine banana, brown sugar, apple juice, vanilla, and chocolate extracts. Process until smooth and fold into dry ingredients.
5. In bowl of electric mixer fitted with a whip, beat egg whites and salt together until egg whites form soft peaks. Fold half of egg whites into batter, then fold in remaining egg whites.
6. Pour batter into pan and bake for 30-35 minutes or until brownie springs back when touched in center.
7. Cut brownies into 12 squares and drizzle Fudge Sweet over top. Place brownie on each plate and garnish with an orange wedge and a few blueberries.

Brownies are best eaten the day they are baked. Wrap and seal leftovers tightly.

12 servings • 122 calories • 1 gm fat • 0 mg cholesterol

EXOTIC FRUIT SALAD WITH MINT
AND GINGERSNAP CRUMBLE

Contributed by Chef Michel Stroot, The Golden Door Spa, Escondido, California.

SYRUP
1 cup white grape juice concentrate
$^1/_2$ cup water

1 tbs lime peel (zest of two limes)

$^1/_2$ vanilla bean, split

1 whole star anise

1 whole clove

2 sprigs fresh mint

1 tbs fresh lime juice

FRUIT

1 mango, peeled, cored, thinly sliced

2 kiwi, peeled, sliced

2 peaches, peeled, sliced (or 5 oz frozen peaches)

$^1/_4$ fresh pineapple, peeled, cored

2 cups fresh blueberries, blackberries, or raspberries

GINGERSNAP CRUMBLE

2 gingersnap cookies crumbled in food processor

1. In a small saucepan, combine syrup ingredients, except lime juice. Simmer and reduce by one-third. Add lime juice, strain and cool.
2. Place prepared fruit in nonreactive bowl. Pour syrup over fruit and refrigerate overnight.
3. Spoon portions into chilled glass bowls and top with gingersnap crumble.

4 servings • 138 calories • 1 gm fat • 0 mg cholesterol

APPLE PIZZA

Contributed by Chef Michel Stroot, The Golden Door Spa, Escondido, California.

PIZZA DOUGH

1 tbs active dry yeast

$^3/_4$ cup tepid water

$^1/_2$ tsp sugar or honey

1 tsp kosher salt

1 tsp olive oil

$^3/_4$ cup unbleached white flour

$^1/_2$ cup whole wheat flour

1 tbs cornmeal (to sprinkle on baking sheet)

APPLES

**4 Golden Delicious apples, peeled, cored, halved (Granny
Smiths also work well)**
1 tsp ground cinnamon
¼ cup white sugar

APRICOT GLAZE
¼ cup sugar-free apricot preserves
1 tbs orange liqueur

1. In mixing bowl, combine yeast, water, and sugar. Let stand
   for 5 minutes. With a mixer fitted with a dough hook, or by
   hand, mix in salt, olive oil, and the two flours. Knead until
   dough forms a ball and is smooth and elastic. Place in mixing bowl and cover with a towel. Set in warm place and let
   rise approximately 20 minutes.
2. While dough is rising, prepare apples. Place halved apples
   on work surface and thinly slice crosswise. Set aside.
3. Spray pizza pan or baking sheet with vegetable spray and
   sprinkle with cornmeal. Set aside.
4. After dough rises, transfer onto floured board and knead
   well with hands. Divide and shape dough into 2 large balls.
   (You'll only use one for this pizza.) Using lightly floured
   rolling pin, spread and shape on ball of dough into a large
   circle 14 inches in diameter. Transfer to prepared pizza pan
   or baking sheet.
5. Preheat oven to 350 degrees.
6. Fan the thin apple slices on the dough, starting with the
   outside edge, making a large ring. Working toward the center, fan smaller circles of apple slices until all the dough is
   covered. Combine sugar and cinnamon and sprinkle over
   apples.
7. Bake for 20-25 minutes until light golden brown.
8. In small saucepan, combine apricot preserves and orange
   liqueur. Over low heat, stir until dissolved.
9. Brush pizza with glaze and serve immediately!

8 servings • 175 calories • 1 gm fat • 0 mg cholesterol

SONOMA FAT-FREE RICE PUDDING

Contributed by Chef Suzanne Gunther, Main Street Restaurants, Manayunk, Pennsylvania.

5 cups cooked brown rice

8 egg whites

3¾ cups skim milk

1¼ cup honey

½ cup quick oats

1 cinnamon stick

2 Granny Smith apples, cut into ½ inch cubes with peel on

¾ cup golden raisins

1. Preheat oven to 300 degrees.
2. Place rice in casserole dish. Whisk together egg whites, milk, and honey. Toss oats, cinnamon stick, apples and raisins in with rice. Pour in egg white mixture. Stir to mix evenly. Bake in a water bath about 35 minutes or until the liquid is three-quarters gone. Take out and let stand 15 minutes. To serve, sprinkle on cinnamon and add a little extra skim milk if you like.

15 servings • 242 calories • 1.1 gm fat • 1 mg cholesterol

THE BEST OF LOW-FAT SNACKS

Between-meal snacks don't have to be your downfall if you pick the right ones. Below are my favorites. Be sure to watch the serving sizes—some of them can be pretty skimpy.

PRODUCT	SERVING SIZE	CALORIES	FAT (GM)
Baked Tostitos	1 oz	110	1
Baked Lays Low Fat Sour Cream & Onion Potato Chips	1 oz	110	1.5
Orville Redenbachers Smartpop	1 cup	15	2
Herr's Carmelcorn	1¼ cup	160	2.5
SmartFood Popcorn Toffee Crunch	¾ cup	110	1.5
PopSecret Butter Artificial Flavor	1 cup	20	2
Nabisco Wheatthins Aircrisps	24 crackers	130	4.5
Campfire Marshmallow Munchies	1 bar	90	0
Snackwell Fudge-Dipped Granola Bars	1 bar	110	3

PRODUCT	SERVING SIZE	CALORIES	FAT (GM)
Nabisco Fig Newtons	2 cookies	110	2.5
Haägen-Dazs Sorbet 'n' Yogurt Bars	1 bar	90	0
Edy's Carmel Praline Crunch Frozen Yogurt	$\frac{1}{2}$ cup	100	1.5
Ben & Jerry's Sorbet	$\frac{1}{2}$ cup	140	0
Snackwell Creme Sandwich Cookies	2 cookies	110	2.5
Reduced Fat Oreos	3 cookies	130	3.5
Angel Food Cake	$\frac{1}{12}$ cake (1 slice)	140	0
Sugar-Free Jell-O	$\frac{1}{2}$ cup	8	0
Rold Gold Pretzels	1 oz	110	1
Chocolate Pudding (made with lowfat milk)	$\frac{1}{2}$ cup	90	3

Chapter 7

SHAPE UP

"Just do it."
—NIKE ADVERTISING SLOGAN

"If you rest, you rust."
—DENISE AUSTIN

Many Americans don't get enough exercise. Older Americans, in particular, tend to take to their chairs as they age, although exercise may in fact become even more important as the years go by.

A study conducted by the U.S. Army showed that exercise can make an older person's heart and lungs behave like those of a younger person. Furthermore, if you are active throughout your adult life, your cardiovascular system will function more effectively, which means more oxygen for the brain and greater mental acuity for you. Additional benefits of regular exercise include:

- weight control
- increased HDL (healthy cholesterol) levels
- lower blood pressure
- a stronger immune system
- less depression
- less risk of diabetes
- osteoporosis protection
- lessened risk of cancer

By adolescence we have all the muscle cells we'll ever have. The cells simply grow and shrink based upon use, but they always retain the ability to enlarge.

Studies done at Tufts University prove that with regular exercise, we can retain most of our muscle mass and strength well into old age. A few years ago, researchers at Tufts studied ten frail men and women up to age ninety-six. After two months of exercising with free weights, they had increased thigh strength by almost 200 percent and muscle mass by 9 percent. Five volunteers doubled their walking speed and two others were able to throw away their canes.

Dr. Walter Bortz II, the author of *We Live Too Short and Die Too Young,* says that exercise is at the root of all weight control. "Exercise is a sacrament," he says. "If you do the exercise, diet (and consequently better health) will follow." He even places exercise above smoking cessation in order of priority.

"I don't try to get people to stop smoking," he said. "I get people to exercise. Exercisers don't smoke. Exercise is an affirmative step toward good health and gives people a sense of self-efficacy. You need to have a sense of autonomy for things to work. When you say, I choose to exercise, you are taking control."

For many of us, exercise is still a necessary evil that we do only to maintain our weight and stay healthy. There are days when I'd give anything to be able to turn that stationary bike into a clothes rack. But, since I like the way exercising makes me look and feel, I make myself do it.

As I talked to women about this book, time and again they told me their greatest fear was becoming incapacitated and dependent upon others. With that in mind, I propose that we should begin regarding regular exercise as a kind of insurance policy against premature death and helplessness.

I vary my activities to prevent boredom from setting in. I play tennis, ride my bike, and do light weight training. For me, having a variety of exercise activities helps to keep me on track. If I only walked the treadmill or climbed the Stairmaster, I'd be bored in no time. I do enjoy playing tennis. When I can't do that, I ride my stationary bike, which isn't as much fun, but I do feel better after I've pedaled my buns off.

Every health-care professional in the world recommends regular exercise for a lifetime of good health. It helps with weight maintenance, strengthens the heart and lungs, and, especially important for women, it helps prevent osteoporosis.

Furthermore, according to Dr. Bortz, it's never too late. "The renewal capabilities of the human organism are infinite," he says.

THE TOO-BUSY BLUES

More than anything else, women will tell you they're just too busy to exercise. While I appreciate that women's lives are jammed with careers, children, husbands, homes, car pools, churches, grandchildren, and much more, I really believe that once you make exercise a priority, you'll find time.

Most experts recommend twenty to thirty minutes of aerobic exercise at least three times a week, coupled with strength training to firm up muscles and prevent bone loss. That's only one to two hours per week, which isn't a lot for improved health.

Even better for busy women is the fairly recent notion that you can accumulate your thirty minutes of exercise over the course of the day, doing ten minutes here and ten minutes there. You can do ten deep knee bends while you're curling your hair and fifteen leg lifts washing dishes. In her book *Jump Start,* exercise expert Denise Austin suggests several leg and buns exercises you can do while brushing your teeth, drying your hair, even cooking dinner. Leg lifts, squats, and stretches are all easily adapted to everyday chores. As long as you're working your muscles and getting your heart rate going, it doesn't have to be an involved process that requires a change of clothing and another shower.

"When women tell me they're too busy to exercise, I suggest that they schedule it in their appointment book just as they would a business engagement or a doctor's appointment," said Karen Lane, the personal trainer who helped me develop my free-weight routine. "When we want to do something, we generally can make the time for it, even if it takes a little bit of effort."

Karen also suggests finding an exercise partner and making exercise fun. "Having a partner will help keep you motivated," she says. "Listening to music, watching TV, or getting some fresh air will also make exercise a more pleasant experience."

Fitness expert Joyce Vedral, who developed the Pritikin Center's exercise program, says that just as your body craves the nutrition it needs, once you get in the habit of exercising, your body will demand that you do it. You'll feel sluggish or just out of sorts if you skip your workout for too long.

Until exercise becomes a habit, you have to make yourself do it. When you were a child, your parents had to nag you to brush your teeth and take a bath. Would you consider reminding any adult to brush their teeth? Exercise can become as routine as brushing your teeth once you get going.

GETTING STARTED

The first thing anyone should do before starting an exercise program is have a medical checkup. Make sure there are no reasons for you to avoid strenuous exercise. Once your doctor gives you the all clear, it's time to get moving.

Take a careful and honest look at yourself before choosing an exercise plan. Do you need the motivation of a partner? Do you like team sports? Will paying for a club motivate you to use it? How much time do you have to dedicate to your exercise? How are your joints? Consider all of the factors that have impeded you from sticking to an exercise program in the past before deciding on a new program.

Many women tell me they can't exercise because they have a "bad back." This condition is often caused by poor posture, which is directly related to poor abdominal muscle tone, which, of course, won't improve without exercise. It's a vicious little cycle.

If you have a bad back and your doctor gives you the okay to begin exercising, you don't have to start doing sit-ups to strengthen your abdominals. You can start by holding in your stomach, standing as straight and tall as possible, and walking around the block or as far as you can go. Swimming, which works all of the muscles and puts virtually no strain on the joints, is another good alternative for strengthening the back itself.

The mission here is to strengthen the back's supporting structure, which will eventually relieve the pain. Once your back is getting adequate support, then you can start doing modified sit-ups or abdominal crunches to get your tummy flattened. If you suffer from back pain, you may want to work with a physical therapist who can encourage you through the inevitable pain that comes from putting those muscles back in action.

When you're getting started, you may want to consider splurging on a few sessions with a personal trainer to get you on the right track. My husband gave me a few sessions with a trainer as a gift once and it was one of the best gifts I ever received. When we started out, Karen did a full assessment to see how much I could handle and prescribed a routine that would challenge me without making me quit. At first, one push-up would kill me, but now I can do forty without stopping. Karen got me going and now she comes back on occasion to fine-tune the routine, add repetitions, and make sure I'm using my equipment properly. There's no need to hire a trainer to supervise every workout, but it's a great idea to get you started.

Slow and Steady Wins the Race

Model your exercise after the tortoise and the hare to avoid injury and the painful aftershock of overexertion. Warming up and stretching are not the same thing. Because cold muscles can snap when stretched, it is important to always warm up your muscles first, then stretch and proceed with the rest of your workout. I warm up with five minutes or a quarter mile on the treadmill at a medium pace. I stretch after the warm-up, and then I get back on the treadmill or stationary bike and go faster and longer.

Weekend warriors who go out and run ten miles in one day to make up for five days of inactivity will do themselves more harm than good. The same thing goes for starting out in the springtime. If you've been relatively inactive all winter, don't try to walk six miles your first day out in April just because that's how far you went in October before the weather turned cold.

For example, if walking is going to be your exercise of choice, take two or three brisk trips around the block for starters. Don't head out to investigate the Boston Marathon course.

All the Right Stuff

Exercise fashion didn't come into vogue with body-hugging leotards and leg warmers. Long before Jane Fonda slipped into a Danskin, women were selecting perky tennis dresses and golf skirts for their exercise wardrobe. But you don't need to wear anything special for your workout. Any comfortable, loose-fitting clothing will be just fine. Don't let yourself be fooled into thinking that you need a color-coordinated bodysuit and thong in order to have a good workout. Not only can those items be expensive, unless you're in really good shape already, they won't be especially flattering for you either. So why start out feeling self-conscious? You will find that once you start getting into shape, you'll want to wear something wonderful to show off your new physique.

Lycra and spandex fabrics are great because they breathe and perspiration can evaporate easily. However, clothing made from those fibers tends to be more form-fitting than many of us would like. Cotton is another excellent fabric choice, but because it's absorbent, you can end up soaking wet after a rigorous workout.

Whatever you choose, pick something that makes you comfortable so that you won't dread suiting up to exercise.

Feet First

The only thing you really need to start exercising is a good pair of sneakers that are comfortable and support your feet properly. Dr. James McGuire, D.P.M., P.T., the Director of the Department of Physical Therapy at the Foot and Ankle Institute in Philadelphia, says that just about any shoe priced over $50 is probably well constructed, and if it fits your feet, buy it. If it costs more than $75 or $80, look for a lower priced shoe that fits just as well. Once you find a model that fits, stay with it until the model is discontinued. Also, it doesn't matter whether you choose canvas or leather, both materials can support your feet well.

When you go to a store looking for workout shoes you may be surprised or confused by the enormous selection. When I was a kid, sneakers were sneakers — you had Keds, Converse, PF Flyers, and high-tops for basketball. Today there are different shoes for tennis, aerobics, running, walking, basketball, hiking, and cross training, etc. While that may seem like a whole bunch of marketing aimed at getting you to buy different shoes for different activities, there really is some difference between them, so select a shoe that is made for the activity you've chosen.

If you're new to working out and are unsure whether you'll be sticking with aerobics, a walking program, or picking up tennis or racquetball, start out with a pair of cross-training shoes. They offer the best support and the most versatility for a variety of activities.

Light hiking shoes are a fairly new entry in the market. They're basically walking shoes and are generally a good buy. They offer good support for day-to-day walking, shopping, and light hiking, and the best part is you can often find a good pair that offers terrific support, looks nice, and is waterproof for around $30.

Remember, when you're shopping for any shoe, always measure your foot and try on the next half-size larger and smaller than what you normally take. Manufacturer's sizes will vary and your shoe size will also vary with age, so spend the extra few minutes to make sure you get a good fit. Shop for shoes at the end of the day when your feet are as large as they're likely to be.

Feet change with age, just like every other part of your body, which is why Dr. McGuire recommends everyone see a podiatrist around age forty and once every two years thereafter. A podiatrist can identify and help address the changes that aging brings on, such as the loss of fat padding in the soles of the feet and the collapse of bony structure that results in a widening, lengthening, and flattening of the feet.

He also says that staying active and healthy is the best way to stay footloose and fancy-free. Keeping muscles strong and subjecting the feet to the stress of walking, etc., will keep tissues stimulated and viable.

HEALTH AND FITNESS CLUBS

Health and fitness clubs are great if you don't have the room in your own home to set up some exercise equipment. I do, however, have concerns about health clubs.

Memberships. Most of the bigger clubs offer big discounts for "lifetime memberships," knowing full well that you'll probably stop going in six or eight months. The consumer ends up shelling out a lot of money for a lifetime of services that they just don't use. That's why I recommend asking for a free trial workout and using the trial when you would normally go to the club to see how busy it is. Next, take a month's trial membership and see how often you go. If you're going two or three times a week, try to get a six-month membership or take another month. While the per-month cost will be much higher than the per-month cost of a lifetime membership, that lifetime member-ship is very pricey if you stop going after four months.

I would strongly recommend getting into the habit of exercising before you join a club. If you've been exercising faithfully for six months and want to treat yourself to a club membership, go for it. If you're hoping that a club will motivate you to exercise, however, you've probably put the cart before the horse.

When you're checking out a club, make sure the locker rooms are spacious, clean, and have plenty of towels. Ask about the staff's certifi-cation and notice how many pieces of equipment are out of order.

Finally, trust your gut. If you feel uncomfortable being surrounded by spandex Susies, and you're fully dressed, just imagine how you'll feel working out next to them.

If you decide to join a gym, one of the nice benefits is the availability of personal trainers, who will work with you one-on-one for a nominal fee.

Before you spend big money for a health club, look into your local YMCA or high school or college continuing education programs. They often offer programs specifically targeted to the over-fifty set that might be just what you're looking for at a fraction of the price.

WALK AWAY

Not everyone is comfortable joining a club, having someone tell them what to do, or bouncing around a room with other women trying to get into shape. If you fall into that category, there's one activity that almost everyone can do, and since experts are saying we should plan to exercise for the rest of our lives, there's no better habit to get into than walking. It's the one form of exercise most people can keep doing no matter how many years go by.

Walking is perhaps the best workout of all because it's so versatile and it's free. You can do it alone or with a partner. You only need comfortable walking shoes, and it's something you can do regardless of the weather. Walking outside is certainly more pleasant and gives you the chance to create some vitamin D by taking in a little sunshine, but there's nothing wrong with taking a few laps around the mall during lousy days. Check with your local mall to see if they sponsor a walking club.

If you're not an exerciser yet, start out slowly — ten or fifteen minutes will be just fine — and remember to stretch first so you don't hurt yourself. (Yes, you can get hurt just walking.)

Get going at a comfortable pace that gets your heart pumping, but still allows you to speak. Build up your speed and your distance over time, increasing both gradually. If you become so fit that walking alone won't get your heart going fast enough, add hand weights or hills to boost the aerobic effect and burn more calories. Speed walking or racewalking are also popular alternatives to jogging because they get the heart pumping without jogging's joint-jolting effects.

Contrary to popular opinion, physically fit older women can safely take up jogging by slowly adding a few minutes of jogging into a walking regimen. Most, however, steer clear of jogging because the pounding of feet against the ground can exacerbate any tendencies toward arthritis. If you're just starting to exercise, stick with walking.

Call the American Running and Fitness Association at 800-776-2732 for free information about starting a walking or exercise program. If you send a self-addressed, stamped ($.55) envelope, they will send you information and a handy chart to help you record your progress. AARP also has a free fitness book for midlife and older persons that was prepared in cooperation with the President's Council on Physical Fitness. Write to AARP at 601 E. St. NW, Washington, DC 20049, and request publication D549. The President's Council has also published Nolan Ryan's Fitness Guide, which is available free of charge by writing to: Nolan Ryan Fitness Guide, P.O. Box 22091, Albany, NY 12201-2091.

AEROBICS TAPES AND CLASSES

If you prefer to work out in the privacy of your own home, then aerobics tapes can be a great alternative for you. There are currently any number of tapes on the market for every fitness level.

Be sure to read the cover material before spending money on any tape. If it concentrates on floor exercise and you have a hard time getting up and down, you probably should choose something else. Many tapes are available from your local library or video store, so you can try one out before purchasing it.

Abington Memorial Hospital in Pennsylvania even has a workout tape that is aimed toward people who can't walk well. It provides a good aerobic workout and you never have to leave your chair. Check with your local hospital's cardiac rehab department for this kind of program if you're having trouble getting around.

Before spending $20 or $25 for an exercise video, rent a few from you local library or video store and see which one you like best. Also, video stores often sell used tapes for as little as $5 or $10, so be sure to ask if the one you like is available for purchase.

Here are a few things to consider when selecting an aerobics tape or class:

1. Be sure you can follow the instructor's cues easily.
2. Pick a class or tape that is a little challenging. If you can do the entire class or tape without breaking a sweat, you need the next level.
3. Choose classes or tapes that allow sufficient time for warming up and cooling down.

4. Listen to your body. If you've had enough for the day, quit or slow down until you catch your breath. But don't quit altogether.

Elaine's Exclusive

FOUR THINGS TO CONSIDER WHEN CHOOSING A WORKOUT VIDEO

1. Type of workout: What do you want to achieve? Weight loss, strength, toning, cardiovascular benefits?

2. Fitness level: How fit are you? Have you ever exercised before? If you're new to exercising, choose tapes that are labeled for beginners. Don't choose the Killer Abs tape right off the bat.

3. Length of workout: How much time can you dedicate to the workout? Do you have half an hour, an hour, or just fifteen minutes? Choose accordingly.

4. The style: Do you like seeing a group presentation or do you prefer the one-on-one feel of a single leader? Do you like and feel comfortable with the person leading the exercise? If you're sixty and flabby, will you feel intimidated by or resentful of a twenty-year-old beauty?

Denise Austin strongly suggests that you only use tapes that are prepared by someone with a background in exercise physiology. Super models and actresses certainly have plenty of experience keeping themselves in shape, but that doesn't mean they are qualified to help anyone else do it safely.

Jill Ross is the Director of Customer Relations for Collage Videos, a consulting company that evaluates every workout video by actually doing each workout. They help consumers select appropriate videos for their individual levels, so the tapes don't end up in the back of the closet. They'll send you a catalog of recommended tapes, plus regular updates, or help you make a selection over the phone. You can buy directly from them. For more information, call Collage at 800-433-6769.

I've listed some of their top recommendations:

AEROBICS

TITLE	LEVEL	LENGTH (MINS)	PEOPLE	PRICE ($)
Leslie Sansone Weight Loss Walk	beg	60	5	19.95
Jamaica Me S'wet Low Impact Aerobics (filmed on beach in Jamaica)	beg	40	5	19.95
Donna Richardson's Donna Mite (Motown music)	int	50	8–10	14.95
Kathy Smith's March to Fitness	beg	30	3	14.95
Victoria's Cardio Soul (low-impact dance)	int	45	5	14.95
Low Impact & Stretch (by Jay Blahnik & Linda McHugh—IDA exercise Instructor of the Year)	adv	53	2	24.95

WEIGHT WATCHERS SERIES

Low Impact Aerobics	beg/int	41	5	14.95
Step & Sculpt	beg/int	41	5	14.95
Tone & Stretch	beg/int	33	5	14.95
Kari Anderson Great Moves (complete choreography— dancier workout)	int	38	1	16.95

STRETCH VIDEOS

Karen Voight's Pure & Simple Stretch	beg	38	1	14.95
The Firm: 5-day Stretch (do 7–10 minutes per day)	beg	43	10	14.95

YOGA STRETCH

TITLE	LEVEL	LENGTH (MINS)	PEOPLE	PRICE ($)
Kathy Smith's New Yoga Basics	beg	54	1	19.95
Ali McGraw's Yoga Mind & Body	int	45	5	14.95

TONING WITH FREE WEIGHTS

Donna Richard's 4-Day Rotation (four 15-minute workouts)	beg	58	10	14.95
Kari Anderson's Tone It Up (includes free Dynaband)	int	38	5	14.95
Karen Voight's Great Weighted Workout (very precise instructions)	adv	83	5	19.95

WALKING (CASSETTES FOR HEADPHONES)

TITLE	LEVEL	TIME	PRICE
Kathy Smith's WalkFitt	beg–adv	varies	14.95
The '60s Power Walking	adv	60	12.95

HOME FITNESS CENTERS

I find that working out at home is the best option for many people, especially those on a tight schedule. If you have to schlep out to aerobics class or the gym, you're more likely to skip class on rainy days, or busy days, or sunny days—you get the idea. If your workout equipment is accessible and in a pleasant place, you'll be more apt to use it.

Once all of my kids moved out, I set up a separate room for my fitness center. I have a television and a stereo in there, as well as mirrors, a barre, and my equipment. Although using a section of the basement was an option, a personal trainer recommended choosing a more inviting location—and boy was she right. I just know that the basement would have been a turnoff and I would not be as faithful to the routine.

I do a combination of aerobic training on the bike and treadmill along with some weight training. While the free weights increased my overall weight, because muscle weighs more than fat, I am firmer than ever before. My butt is tight, my legs are less flabby, and my breasts are a little more perky. Yes, I guess I'm bragging a little, but believe me, I've worked hard to get this body and I'm proud of it. I'm only unhappy with one area right now—the flabby parts under my arms—and I don't think that any amount of exercise is going to fix them.

Whether you walk, run, bike, do aerobics, lift weights, play sports, whatever, the only rule is to be faithful. Just do it—three or more times a week.

EXERCISE BURNS CALORIES

ACTIVITY	CALORIES BURNED/30 MINUTES
Aerobics (low impact)	300
Bicycling	210
Cross-country skiing	350
Dancing	180
Free weights (like Bottom's Up workout)	395
Housework	100
Jogging (easy pace)	215
Nordic Track	245
Rowing	225
Shoveling snow	200
Stair-stepping	300
Swimming	305
Tennis (singles)	200
Walking 2 m.p.h.	120
Walking 3 m.p.h.	160
Yardwork	100–150

EXERCISE AND ARTHRITIS

Grace is seventy-seven and has lived with both osteo- and rheumatoid arthritis for at least thirty years now. She's been through every treatment imaginable, including gold shots, steroids, and methotrexate, a cancer drug. While the arthritis in her back has slowed her down somewhat, she still makes a good effort at walking every day to keep her body from stiffening up.

Because arthritis comes in a hundred different varieties, having arthritis is like saying you don't feel well. It's almost true that if you live long enough, you'll one day suffer from some form of joint stiffness—the one common link between all one hundred forms of the disease. The most common forms of arthritis, osteo- and rheumatoid, affect approximately forty million people. With the baby boomers moving into their fifties, that number is expected to grow tremendously in the coming years.

Osteoarthritis is a degenerative disease that follows excessive wear and tear or insult to a particular joint. The cartilage that cushions the knees, hips, spine, etc., just wears away. This is why it is most common among older people—and why walking has supplanted jogging as the aerobic exercise of choice. While estimates say that one hundred and twenty-one people out of a thousand have mild forms of the disease—the aches and pains of old age—nearly sixteen million people suffer enough to seek medical help, which can range from pain and anti-inflammatory medication to surgeries such as hip, knee, and shoulder replacements, and spinal fusions.

Rheumatoid arthritis is a crippling disease that affects the entire body. Unlike osteoarthritis, which effects only one or more joints, rheumatoid arthritis is related to a malfunction of the immune system, not to the degeneration of particular body sites. This is the most severe and painful form of arthritis and the second most common, affecting nine people in one thousand, mostly women. Rheumatoid arthritis can, however, go into remission for months or years at a time, whereas osteoarthritis doesn't go away unless the afflicted joint is replaced surgically.

Surprisingly, the medical community does not know a whole lot about arthritis or what causes it. What we do know is that osteoarthritis of the hands can be hereditary, and that obesity can aggravate it, particularly in the back and knees. A lifetime of excessive stress has also been attributed to rheumatoid arthritis.

Exercise strengthens muscles around the afflicted joints, which helps them maintain their mobility. While taking to the couch may seem like an attractive idea when you're in the middle of an arthritis flare-up, it will eventually lead to even greater joint and muscle stiffness. It is especially important for arthritis sufferers to emphasize range of motion and extensions in their exercise routines.

As the codirector of the arthritis units for West Jersey Hospital Systems, Dr. Sheldon Solomon strongly recommends swimming and water aerobics for his arthritis patients. These activities give people the benefits of working their muscles without placing added stress on the joints.

Although arthritis can be painful and crippling it is, for the most part, not life-threatening and therefore, researchers have focused their attention on other, more pressing problems. Although a good deal of the research on osteo- and rheumatoid arthritis is as much as thirty years old, I believe that once the baby boomers start really feeling the effects of arthritis, medical science will heed their demands for more research and relief. Until then, if you have arthritis, or are experiencing excessive joint and muscle stiffness, redness or swelling around the joints, or hot spots on the joints, see a rheumatologist, a doctor who specializes in arthritis. In addition to medication and other treatments, including heat and rest, your doctor can also suggest appropriate exercises to help maintain your mobility.

THE INCREDIBLE SHRINKING WOMAN

> I went to the doctor recently to have my thyroid checked because I can't stop gaining weight. While I was there, I mentioned that even though I was heavier, my slacks were dragging on the floor. When he measured me, I was shocked to learn that I had shrunk an inch. Now I'm scheduled for a bone scan to see if I have osteoporosis. In the meantime, I'm taking calcium faithfully and exercising more than usual.
>
> *Carol, age fifty-six*

Twenty-five million Americans suffer from osteoporosis, the disease of thinning bones, which strikes one in four women. Osteoporosis is to blame for 250,000 hip fractures each year and 50,000 deaths. In fact, 20 percent of the patients who break a hip will die from complications such as pneumonia or a blood clot within one year. While this is certainly sad and terrifying news, the tragic part is that osteoporosis is a largely preventable disease.

With age, many women literally shrink before your very eyes because their bones are losing mass. (Tiny fractures in the spine are usually responsible for the loss of height.) While most women lose 1 to 2 percent of their bone mass each year starting at age thirty-five, the onset of menopause causes many women to lose bone mass much more quickly.

Bone mass is much like a bank account in that the more calcium you take in, the more bone mass you accumulate, up until age thirty-five. After thirty-five, women who have successfully stockpiled bone mass through exercise and calcium intake are in a much better position when their bodies start to shed bone.

With a calcium-rich diet, calcium supplements, and proper exercise, women who are beyond age thirty can still minimize the risks of osteoporosis and maintain a solid structure that will safely carry their bodies through life. Hormone replacement therapy is also a good stopgap for many menopausal women, but regular weight-bearing exercise can lay the foundation for strong bones long before menopause sets in and help maintain those strong bones well into old age.

Just as resistance causes muscles to develop, we now know that bones create more cells when they are faced with weights or other forms of resistance. Brisk walking, aerobics, dancing, jogging, and tennis are all aerobic exercises. They also qualify as weight-bearing exercises for the purpose of bone-building because they increase the weight of gravity on your bones and they work the legs and hips, areas that are particularly vulnerable to osteoporosis.

Diagnosing and Monitoring Osteoporosis

Today, the DEXA scan is considered to be the gold standard in the diagnosis and treatment of osteoporosis. Using one-fiftieth of the amount of radiation used for a chest X ray, this scan measures bone density.

Until the DEXA, the only way doctors could predict a patient's risk of osteoporosis was to look at factors such as heredity, gender, race (Caucasians are much more likely to suffer from osteoporosis than Hispanics or Blacks), smoking, and calcium and alcohol intake. Unfortunately, once risk factors could be compared against the results of the scan, doctors realized how unreliable those predictors actually are. In fact, a full 30 percent of women with several risk factors did not have osteoporosis when checked with the scan. Conversely, the scan pointed out osteoporosis in 30 percent of women thought to be at low risk for the disease.

The DEXA scan is a good test to have in your forties, as a checkup to see how well your bones are holding up. If, at the onset of menopause, you are considering forsaking hormone replacement therapy, Dr. Solomon strongly recommends a scan before making the final decision. Women who are shedding bone rapidly may want to reconsider hormones based on the results.

A new urine test called the NTx measures the rate at which the body is shedding bone and is helpful in diagnosing osteoporosis. Don't be confused by these two tests. The DEXA scan tells the doctor your current bone density; and the NTx determines the rate of bone loss, which can tell your doctor how well hormones, calcium, exercise, and any other treatments are working to help you prevent additional bone loss. The cost of an NTx test is around $50 and is now reimbursed by Medicare and many insurance plans.

By the turn of the century, one and a half million osteoporosis-related fractures will cost the government and insurance companies $10 billion per year. With that staggering bill coming due in just a few years, research is racing forward to find new and better ways to prevent osteoporosis and build up bone mass in women who already suffer from it. It may not be long before a baseline DEXA will be as routine as a baseline mammogram. For now, though, even if your insurance company won't pay for the scan until you are perimenopausal, if you can afford it, it may be worth the $100 to $200 to have a baseline scan in your early thirties, when you have achieved peak bone mass.

Science has also recently introduced three new drugs to combat osteoporosis. Two of them received FDA approval in 1996. Fosamax is the first nonhormonal treatment for osteoporosis. It must be taken half an hour before eating, because it can cause stomach irritation. Fosamax thickens bones twice as fast as Miacalcin, a nasal spray, which is easier to take. A third drug, slow-release sodium fluoride, which was recommended for FDA approval, is not yet on the market. Unfortunately, these drugs must be taken for life if the benefits are to last. By the year 2020, one in every six Americans will be over age sixty-five, so you can be certain that treatments for osteoporosis will be released at an astonishing clip over the next several years.

With or without the benefits of scientific advances, we can just about eliminate our risks of osteoporosis if we get plenty of calcium and exercise before we're thirty. If you're already beyond that age, the same prescription will help you maintain and even improve upon your current bone-density levels. The bottom line here is that you have control. You don't have to rely on medical science to keep your body strong and healthy.

Just remember that the smoothest skin and the most expensive makeup won't make you any more beautiful if you're bent like a question mark and no one can see your face. So get moving.

WEIGHT TRAINING

Many women balk at the idea of weight training for fear of looking like Arnold Schwarzenegger with a manicure, but the fact of the matter is that sufficient exercise, and weight training in particular, plays an important role in maintaining shapeliness and preventing osteoporosis. Aerobic exercise helps strengthen the cardiovascular system and is important for weight loss and weight maintenance. Weight training, on the other hand, not only increases muscle density and definition, but increases bone density as well.

Certainly you can gain some of the muscle-defining benefits of weight training through aerobic exercises. Running or walking, for example, helps build leg muscles, but they don't do much for your arms. Rowing may be great for the heart and the arms and shoulders, but your legs lose out. See what I mean?

If you don't know much about weight training, don't be surprised. It wasn't until a few years ago that the American College of Sports Medicine updated its official guidelines to include weight training. But if you think weight training is just for muscle heads, you're woefully mistaken and could be cruising for a lifetime of helplessness. In addition to holding your body together, you need muscles—the stronger the better—to do just about everything.

Muscles begin to atrophy a little at a time, starting around age thirty, which is why it is especially important for older women to do some weight training. To my mind, the best reason to get into some kind of weight training has less to do with looking good and more to do with long-term health and fitness. We all know older women who have trouble walking, or going up and down even a few steps. I don't want to spend my final years like that—do you?

When I grow up, I want to be a spry old lady, the one everyone admires on the dance floor or the tennis court. I don't want to be bent over because my muscles have atrophied and they can no longer hold me up. I don't want a flight of stairs to be my undoing, and I certainly don't want to spend ten years sitting in a chair reading and playing bridge because I just don't have the strength to do anything else.

The body has infinite regenerative capabilities. You can begin rebuilding lost muscle immediately and keep yourself from becoming a helpless little old lady.

I've been working with a Muscleman machine for a few years now. It has enabled me to develop a tight, well-toned body that I never had, even when I was in my thirties. While I've always been slim, I look better now than ever before, even though I weigh more than I ever have. That's because even though muscle takes up less space than fat, it also weighs more. Therefore, a well-toned person will look slimmer than a nonmuscular person even though they may weigh exactly the same.

When it comes to weight training, the best advice I can give you is to trust the mirror instead of the scale, because you might put on a few pounds while you're molding your muscles.

Weight training is also inexpensive and something you can do at home with minimal coaching. And since you're not going to be working with heavy weights, you're not likely to get hurt unless you drop a five-pounder on your toes.

Joyce Vedral has two great books, *Bottoms Up!* and *Definition,* that provide complete and easy-to-follow weight-training regimens that will build strong, well-defined muscles quickly. I like her books because they give clear instructions, explain why weight training is important, and tell readers what kinds of results they can expect by making a realistic commitment to weight training. Her routines don't require spending your life at the gym and you can do the entire workout at home with a minimal investment in free weights.

The best part about her book, though, is that she provides therapeutic alternatives for exercises that strain the back or knees, something that is particularly beneficial as we grow older.

Dr. Vedral credits exercise with the fact that, at fifty-three, she has the bone density of a woman half her age. She also cites other women who started out with bone densities below the 50th percentile for women their age, who, through exercise, have risen into the 70th percentile in less than two years.

"Ninety-nine percent of women my age are unhappy with the

way they look," said Vedral. "They complain that things are sagging, flabby, etc. I tell them that I can change that, guaranteed. They start exercising to look better. They continue exercising because they feel better and want to be strong and healthy into old age."

EXERCISE AND INJURY

Everyone has heard of people who have fatal heart attacks mowing the lawn, jogging, or shoveling snow. Some of us use those stories as excuses not to exercise. Certainly there is some risk of injury from exercise, which is why everyone should consult their physician before beginning a new routine. According to Vedral, however, older women are less likely to hurt themselves exercising because they are more cautious and willing to start out slowly, working up to fast paces, longer distances, and heavier weights. Yes, you could pull a muscle or strain a ligament if you don't warm up properly, but that can happen to anyone.

Don't let your age or other people's horror stories keep you from doing what's good for you. Just approach it sensibly.

BEYOND EXERCISE: OTHER BODY BOOSTERS
Up in Smoke
According to the Centers for Disease Control, 22.5 percent of American women smoke cigarettes. While that 1993 statistic is an improvement over the 1991 figure of 24.8 percent, I'm still shocked by how many women are damaging their health this way.

The best thing you can do to prolong your life and good health is to quit smoking.

In addition to cancer, emphysema, and heart and lung disease, smoking is a contributing factor in osteoporosis, it depresses the immune system, and *it does not keep weight in check*. In fact, most women only gain five pounds when they quit smoking and the benefits of quitting far exceed any risk from a five-pound weight gain. You'd have to gain 75 pounds to offset the health benefits of quitting smoking.

The health issues associated with smoking are so well documented that you certainly don't need me to remind you about them, but what you may not realize is that smoking will cause your skin to wrinkle, too. So, even if you can fool yourself into thinking that you smoke to stay thin, what's the point if you'll be thin and prune-faced?

In a study done at Wake Forest University in North Carolina, researchers found that on average, smokers looked five to ten years older than their actual ages. By robbing your body of oxygen, smoking loosens up the elastic tissues in the skin, causing it to wrinkle.

Twenty-five years ago I joined Smokenders on a bet and I'm proud to say it's the best money I ever spent. Smokenders classes focus specifically on behavior modification while weaning participants from the nicotine. In addition to the group meeting format, they also have at-home study programs available. For more information about Smokenders, please call 800-828-4357.

There are also other smoking-cessation programs and aids to help you come out from under the cloud. Hypnosis, psychotherapy, and nicotine gum and patches, which were recently approved for over-the-counter sale, have helped millions of people get on the road to a more healthful life.

Even though there is help and support aplenty, quitting smoking is still very difficult, so be kind to yourself and understand that it may take a few tries before you finally kick the habit for good. Yes, it's difficult, and yes, you may feel lousy for a few weeks, but when you consider the alternatives, it's clearly worth the trouble.

Because the body has infinite regenerative resources, you can undo years of smoking damage by quitting now. Your lungs will immediately begin to heal themselves and after five years of not smoking, they can be as healthy as if you never smoked at all.

Stress

Like smoking, stress is linked to almost every disease and ailment, except maybe cancer. Stress is associated with weight loss, weight gain, depression, reduction in the immune system, sleeplessness, heart attack, stroke, high blood pressure — you name it and stress is likely to be a contributing factor. Unlike smoking, which you can avoid, stress is a part of life. There are deadlines, demands, and pressures that we all must face, unless we're prepared to trade in our lives for a few solitary years at Walden Pond. Since that's not likely to happen, the best we can do is learn how to cope with stress when it does come our way.

Stress is a natural physical reaction to some mental or physical threat to our well-being. When we sense any kind of danger, our bodies release adrenaline and other chemicals that, among other things, raise our blood pressure and essentially put our entire systems into overdrive. In order to bring the adrenaline level back to normal, our bodies need to do something physical. That's why you'll sometimes get that "jumping out of your skin" feeling when you're under pressure. Your body really wants to jump around and burn off those chemicals.

The body's instinctual reaction to stress is what allows women to pick up cars to free their trapped children and avoid being run over by a train. It's the adrenaline rush that comes from recognizing danger. And in those kinds of instances, stress is a good thing.

Unfortunately, our instincts don't recognize the difference between physical danger and mental danger, so the reaction is the same. Your mind says, yikes, the report is due in half an hour and I just started, and your body whips up some adrenaline in response. It's sort of like pumping the gas pedal too often and flooding your car. Sooner or later, your car is overwhelmed with fuel and it won't start. With too much stress, your body can just quit on you.

Many people choose some pretty unhealthy ways of dealing with stress. They overeat, smoke, drink to excess, and some become physically or verbally abusive to those around them. While no one would recommend any of those methods of stress reduction, there are plenty of techniques for coping with and alleviating stress before it becomes a health hazard.

Get a grip. In more ways than one, getting a grip on your stress will make you feel better. First, squeeze a rubber ball or one of those hand exercisers to release a little tension. Second, get a grip on your responsibilities by getting organized. If you don't feel overwhelmed by all that you need to do, you'll be less stressed.

Run away from it. Exercise — especially aerobic exercise — is one of the best ways to relieve stress. In addition to all of the other health benefits mentioned earlier in this chapter, exercising helps your body use up the extra adrenaline and other stress-related chemicals.

Make it go away. Yoga and meditation are great stress relievers if you put in the time and effort to learn to do them properly. Until you find a yoga class or a book on meditation, simple relaxation will do the trick — and you don't have to sit cross-legged on the floor. Just turn off the television, close your eyes, tune out the world, and listen to quiet for a few minutes.

Shrug it off. If you're like many people, stress collects in your neck and shoulders. Tilt your chin to your chest and then roll your head in a complete circle to loosen up those muscles. Shoulder shrugs help too. Others collect stress in their chests. Take a few deep breaths and let them out slowly to reduce that tightness.

The best medicine. There's nothing like a good laugh to reduce stress. Turn on the Comedy Channel, call a friend and ask her to tell you a joke, or better yet, buy yourself a joke-of-the-day calendar to ensure you have a ready source of laughs.

Reach for the sky. Do a few stretching exercises, touch your toes, swing your arms around, and do a few side bends.

Elaine's Exclusive

RECIPE FOR A HEALTHY LIFESTYLE

- If you smoke, quit. The sooner the better.
- Eat a low-fat menu that is full of fresh fruits and vegetables.
- Drink eight 8-ounce glasses of water each day.
- Exercise regularly.
- Take a multivitamin every day along with calcium supplements.
- Enjoy a glass of wine with meals.
- Get some fresh air and sunshine.
- Laugh out loud.
- Never say no to birthday cake.

KEEPING IT SIMPLE

You could spend the rest of your life reading books about staying fit, living longer, losing weight, and getting exercise. Certainly those books are useful and I've consulted many of them preparing this chapter. Most of them, however, take one view to an extreme and don't allow for the many demands in all of our lives.

If you're raising a family, working, tending to your home, and volunteering, you have plenty of other things to do without having to worry about developing buns of steel.

I do, however, believe that a fit and healthy body is the very foundation for a lifetime of good looks and that's why I've dedicated this entire chapter to the basics of exercise. Just keep in mind the importance of balance in your life. If you're heavy, you didn't get that way overnight and you're not going to get fit overnight either.

Take your time to make health and fitness a part of your everyday life. That way, your commitment and your good health will last longer than the latest hemline.

HEALTH CHECK

It's something of a cliche to say that if you have your health, you have everything, but now that I'm getting older, I realize how very true that moldy oldie really is. You can be wealthy, have every possession imaginable and everything else life has to offer, but if you can't take a walk around the block on a warm summer night, bend over to pick a few spring flowers, or climb the steps to kiss visiting grandchildren good night, what difference does it make?

There is a lot you can do to keep yourself healthy and safe, including eating a well-balanced menu, taking vitamins, and getting plenty of exercise. In addition, take these extra precautions:

- Perform a monthly breast examination.
- Carefully examine your skin for new spots or bumps. (Because it's hard to see behind yourself, this health check can be fun if you have a partner.)
- Keep tabs on your blood pressure. (In between doctor's appointments, take advantage of the free screenings that are always being offered somewhere.)
- Keep tabs on your cholesterol with home test kits like Johnson & Johnson's Advanced Care cholesterol test available in drugstores. It only gives a total cholesterol reading and does not break out HDL from LDL, but it's a reliable measure of your progress in between doctor's visits.
- Always wear your seat belt.

To prevent bone-breaking falls:
- Wear sturdy, low heeled shoes.
- Secure carpeting.

- Use handrails.
- Equip your bathtub with nonskid tape or decals.
- Keep hallways and stairs well lit.

I hound my friends to have annual physicals and urge them to insist on the following tests:

- Baseline cardiogram: Heart disease is the number-one killer of women over fifty, so a baseline cardiogram will give your doctor a point of reference should you develop problems in the future.
- Annual pap smear: Pap smears are essential in the early detection of cervical cancer, which will kills close to five thousand women each year. The test is slightly uncomfortable, but early detection and treatment of dysplasia (abnormal cells) can prevent most women from becoming one of the 15,700 annual cases of cervical cancer. The American Cancer Society (ACS) says that cervical cancer is twice as common among Black women as Caucasians, due largely to lack of regular screening.
- Annual colon cancer test: A digital rectal exam is about as unpleasant a thought as you can imagine, but when you consider that colorectal cancer kills fifty-five thousand people every year, and half of them are women, it's important to grin and bear it. (Well you don't have to grin.) The ACS's 1996 estimates predict that more men will contract this disease than women, but the mortality rate is greater for women. ACS recommends a digital rectal exam every year starting at age forty, followed by annual occult fecal blood tests starting at age fifty. The flexible sigmoidoscope is suggested at age fifty and fifty-one and then only every three to five years if the patient is symptom-free.
- Mammogram: Baseline at age thirty-five, every other year from age forty to fifty, annually after age fifty. Breast cancer strikes one in nine women and we all know someone who has not survived this dreaded disease. Early detection greatly increases your chances for survival, so don't neglect this important test.

- **Complete cholesterol check:** The home test will give you a total cholesterol count, but for a complete analysis of HDL and LDL, you need to see your doctor. Cholesterol clogs arteries, causing heart disease and stroke, but since it can be controlled with diet, exercise, and medication, there's no reason to avoid this test.
- **Thorough visual examination for skin cancer:** Those of us who slathered on iodine and baby oil in search of the perfect tan are now having to contend with more than just wrinkled, leathery skin. Although skin cancer is more likely to turn up on areas that are exposed to the sun, it can appear anywhere, so be sure to have a thorough checkup.
- **Baseline DEXA scan followed by annual NTx test for the rate of bone loss:** For more on these tests, please see the section on osteoporosis.

Chapter 8

BODY BEAUTIFUL

"I have everything I had 20 years ago—except it's all lower."
—GYPSY ROSE LEE

Having a physically fit body, good skin, makeup that enhances your features, and an attractive, face-flattering hairstyle are what most of us think of when we think about a lifetime of good looks, but there are plenty of other ways that your body can betray your age. Hands and nails, legs and feet all show off our age whether we like it or not and there's nothing like menopause to provide you with a little reality check.

These signs of aging are like billboards on the road of life reminding us that we're not as young as we might think. But just because those signs are reminding us about undeniable facts, that doesn't mean that we have to wear their warnings for all the world to see. Read on to learn more about mapping your own course through some of these awkward turns.

LEAVE THE CROCODILES TO DUNDEE

Even if you don't have dryness problems with your facial skin, you may find that your arms and legs become dry, flaky, and scaly, and that elbows and heels, because they are subjected to a lot of pressure, become particularly parched.

Taking warm or tepid showers is one of the best ways to keep from dehydrating your skin. Hot baths and showers may be soothing to tired muscles, but you'll have to decide if the benefit to your muscles is worth the dryness to your skin. If you do go for a hot bath, adding some bath oil to the water will diminish the drying effects somewhat.

Choose a moisturizing body wash or beauty bar for daily bathing and treat yourself to a loofah sponge or one of those antibacterial net sponges. The loofah will whisk away dry, flaky skin, and the moisturizing washes will leave your skin feeling silky smooth.

Antibacterial soaps have gotten a lot of press lately for preventing cross-contamination in the kitchen and for that reason I keep Jergens antibacterial hand soap along with my dish detergent near my kitchen sink. Although they contain ingredients to soften hands, I still keep hand cream right next to them for extra moisture.

Some dermatologists recommend bathing once or twice a week with an antibacterial soap, but when you consider that Americans are the only people in the world who bathe one or more times per day, it's safe to limit the use of antibacterial soap in favor of products that are kinder to your skin.

Apply a body cream or lotion, depending on how dry your skin is, over damp skin to help seal in some extra moisture. It really makes a difference.

As with facial products, you needn't spend a lot to clean and moisturize your skin. There are excellent products available in supermarkets and drugstores for only a few dollars. If you like the pampered feeling, however, there are luxurious bath and body products available in many department store lines as well. I've recommended my favorite cleansing and moisturizing products here.

HAND AND BODY LOTIONS

I was amazed by the fact that so few hand and body products actually contain sunscreen. I think that adding sunscreen would be a big opportunity for some of the popular brands such as Jergens or Vaseline to gain significant market share. In the meantime, don't forget to apply sunscreen over your moisturizer. Price Key: $ under $10; $$ $11–$20; $$$ $21–$30; $$$$ over $30

THE GOLDEN OLDIES

They may not absorb as quickly as the newer products, but these brands have been around for years and are still very effective, very popular, and a good value.

PRODUCT	SIZE (OZ)	PRICE
Eucerin Dry Skin Therapy Original Moisturizing Cream (very dry skin)	2	$
Eucerin Plus Alpha Hydroxy Acid Moisturizing Creme	4	$
Eucerin Plus Alpha Hydroxy Acid Moisturizing Lotion	4	$
Jergens Advanced Therapy Lotion	10	$

PRODUCT	SIZE (OZ)	PRICE
Keri Original Formula	20	$
Keri Silky Smooth Lotion Regular & Sensitive Skin Formulas	6.5/11	$
Lubriderm Bath & Shower Gel	8	$
Lubriderm Dry Skin Care Lotion Original & Fragrance Free	6	$
Moisturel Cream	4	$
Moisturel Lotion	8	$
Nivea Cream	4	$
Vaseline Instensive Care Lotion	10	$

DRUGSTORE BRANDS

PRODUCT	SIZE (OZ)	PRICE
Alpha Keri Moisture Rich Oil	8	$
Cetaphil Moisturizing Cream	16	$$
Cetaphil Moisturizing Lotion	16	$$
Ethocyn Skin Treatment Hand & Body Moisturizer	6.7	$$$
European Touch Skin Normalizing Lotion	8	$
Keri Anti-Bacterial Hand Lotion	11	$
Keri Cream (very dry skin)	8	$
Lac-Hydrin Five (5 percent lactic acid)	8	$$
Lubriderm Seriously Sensitive Lotion	6	$
Neutrogena Body Lotion Sesame Formula	8.5	$
Neutrogena Daily Moisture Supply	12	$
Neutrogena Hand Cream (dry, chapped hands) Norwegian formula	2	$
Nivea Skin Therapy Light Cream	4	$
Physicians Formula Vital Defense Hand & Body Lotion (SPF 15)	6	$
St. Ives Extra Relief Collagen-Elastin Dry Skin Lotion	20	$

DEPARTMENT STORE BRANDS

PRODUCT	SIZE (OZ)	PRICE
Clinique Aloe Body Balm	7	$$
Clinique Hand Repair (SPF 6)	2.5	$$
Donna Karan Cashmere Body Lotion	6.7	$$$$
Elizabeth Arden Visible Difference Moisture Formula Body Care	10	$$$
Lancôme Hydra-Balance Essential Hydrating Body Lotion	6.8	$$$

SPECIALTY BRANDS/PHYSICIAN DISPENSED

PRODUCT	SIZE (OZ)	PRICE
Avon Anew Perfecting Complex for Hand & Body (10 percent glycolic acid)	3.4	$$
Citrix Hand & Body Creme	2	$$$
Kiehls Creme de Corps	8	$$$
Mary Kay Body Care Moisturizing Lotion	7	$
NuSkin MHA Revitalizing Body Lotion	5	$$$

MOISTURIZING BODY SHAMPOOS

These products are a nice addition to the shower and can be found in the grocery store or drugstore for less than $5. Once you have tried a body shampoo, you may never use soap again.

PRODUCT	SIZE (OZ)
Alpha Hydrox Body Wash (formulated for all skin types)	12
Caress Moisturizing Body Wash	10
Dial Moisturizing & Anti-Bacterial Body Wash	10
Dove Ultra Moisturizing Body Wash	10
Jergens Body Shampoo	8
Oil of Olay 2 in 1 Moisturizing Body Wash	7, 12
Soft Soap Anti-Bacterial Body Wash with Moisture Beads	12
Vaseline Intensive Care Moisturizing Body Wash deodorant	9
Vaseline Intensive Care Moisturizing Body Wash Essential Care	9

GIVE YOURSELF A HAND

It's true that nothing shows a woman's age like her hands, which are exposed to the sun's damaging rays as much as her face and withstand years of hard work, harsh detergents, digging in the garden, and much more. And just like our faces, our hands do a great deal of communicating for us. When we meet and greet people our hands do the talking. We use our hands to tell people that things are okay, or that things are just so-so. They say hello and good-bye for us, and we use them to point out an item on a high shelf.

Despite how well our hands serve us, we don't pamper them as much as we could — a weekly manicure is the best that most hands get — and then we're upset when they start to betray our age.

Just as we take care of our skin on a daily basis, we should also take care of our hands daily, too, by applying hand cream throughout the day. Hand cream will help moisturize and strengthen nails. In the skin-care section, I mentioned that the fewer products you use, the less likely you are to have problems with irritation and allergic reaction. The same goes for hand and nail care. Overmanicuring and applying too many chemicals too often can leave your nails weak and irritated, just as too many cosmetics can irritate your skin.

You can also give your hands a hand by protecting them from detergents, hot water, and trauma. Wear rubber gloves for washing dishes or doing housework, and wear sturdy gardening gloves for yard work. Don't bite your nails or cuticles, or tap your nails against hard surfaces. Don't use your nails in place of a screwdriver for light chores and by all means, find a penny to use for scratch-and-win promotions. You get the idea.

Because the skin tends to be thin on the backs of hands anyway, the loss of elasticity becomes immediately apparent before it is noticeable almost anywhere else. The pinch test mentioned in Chapter 2 illustrates this point well. The result is that thinner skin shows off veins and bony knuckles that can already be more prominent anyway thanks to arthritis. Diminishing fat and muscle also make hands look bony and frankly there's not much you can do about that. Products with heavy doses of vitamin C, like Cellex-C or C-ESTA products, may help thicken the skin to reduce the bony appearance. Ethocyn, which increases elastin, may be good, too. For more on those products, see Chapter 4.

Getting into the habit of applying hand cream frequently will help a little because it will act as a temporary barrier against the elements while moisturizing your skin and nails. It won't hide gnarly knuckles, but at least your hands won't look dried out or feel rough.

Elaine's Exclusive

TOOLS OF THE TRADE

If you have a professional manicure or pedicure on a regular basis, invest in your own tools to avoid infection. Clean them with soap and water and wipe them down with alcohol after each use.

Elaine's Exclusive

NEXT TO GODLINESS

If you have an occasional manicure, observe the manicurist's station for cleanliness. Check to see if her tools are kept in a sanitizing solution and if a clean towel is used for each client. Tools and supplies should be neatly organized and clean.

Spotting the Signs of Age

Age spots are the most common complaint of older women. Someone with a fair complexion is likely to see her first age spots in her forties, and they will increase in number from then on. The spots can be lightened with hydroquinone cream or even old-fashioned Porcelana, but for more permanent remedies try laser treatment, Retin-A, or Renova. Vitamin C products are also a good bet.

You are, however, bound to get more age spots unless you keep your hands protected from the sun, so be sure to apply sunscreen to your hands as well as your face each day—and reapply it every time you wash your hands. Cosmetics companies could really cash in by developing more hand creams with sunscreen in them for just this reason. Yves Rocher, the French botanical cosmetics manufacturer, does indeed sell a hand cream, Age Defense for Hands with an SPF of 6, as does Clinique. Yves Rocher products are sold on the Home Shopping Network and through their own mail-order catalogs.

Elaine's Exclusive

NO MORE WITCHY WOMAN

If your hands are beginning to show your age, don't draw unwanted attention their way with long red nails. Trim them to a shorter length and choose a more neutral shade of polish so that your hands will have a refined look that isn't too flashy.

Peels and Paraffins

Some spas and dermatologists will offer AHA peels for the hands and arms for about $100, but according to Betsy Rubenstone, an esthetician with the Center for Human Appearance at the University of Pennsylvania Hospital, the peels don't accomplish anything that good skin care can't do. An AHA peel of the hands will help eliminate age spots, but aging hands don't tend to have the fine wrinkles that respond well to a peel and bulging knuckles, veins, and boniness can't be corrected with a peel.

Instead, Rubenstone recommends using hand cream with hydroquinone to fade the age spots and an AHA to keep up the exfoliation. That should give you the same results as a peel for far less money.

Some doctors are removing age spots with lasers, too, but Dr. Thomas Loeb, a New York plastic surgeon, says that the brown spots are often replaced with white spots that can be even less attractive and the lasered spots take a while to heal.

Many beauty salons offer paraffin treatments for the hands to soften and exfoliate the skin. The treatments soothe and moisturize the skin and for less than $10 it's a nice treat, especially for arthritic hands. The warm paraffin may also provide a temporary respite from the achiness.

Elaine's Exclusives

SISKEL & EBERT SAY. . .

You'll get two thumbs up from your hands if you choose products that *do not* contain these ingredients, which can be drying and irritating to nails and cuticles:
- Formaldehyde and toluene in polishes and hardeners.
- Acetone in polish removers.

NAILING DOWN NAIL PROBLEMS

PROBLEM: Vertical Ridges

Vertical ridges can be a sign of age, just like wrinkles, or they can be the result of overmanicuring or a past injury to the nail. Ridges can also be a sign of illness including arthritis, carpal tunnel syndrome, pneumonia, or psoriasis, so let a dermatologist see any prominent ridges.

SOLUTION

To get a smooth manicure, use a ridge-filling base coat and allow it to dry for a few minutes before applying color.

PROBLEM: Discoloration

Dark polishes can leave behind a yellow residue, as can other nail products and contact with other chemicals, including hair dyes and skin lighteners. Discoloration can also be a sign of illness.

SOLUTION

You can gently buff away stains or leave nails unpolished for a while to allow them to breathe and regain their natural color. Also, be sure to always wear a base coat underneath nail color and wear rubber gloves to apply hair color or work with harsh chemicals.

PROBLEM: Brittle Nails

Brittle nails are the equivalent of dry skin and if you have dry skin, chances are your nails are, or will become, brittle.

SOLUTION

Soak clean, polish-free nails in water and then massage hand cream into your hands and nails. This kind of moisturizing works just the way moisturizing skin works. Also, be sure to wear rubber gloves when doing housework to avoid contact with harsh chemicals.

PROBLEM: Hangnails

Hangnails are caused by excessive dryness, picking at the nails, paper cuts, aggressive cuticle clipping, or biting nails.

SOLUTION

Again, moisturizing and wearing rubber gloves will help prevent the problem. When a hangnail occurs, snip it off with manicure scissors and moisturize the area.

PROBLEM: Horizontal Ridges

Horizontal ridges can indicate a vitamin deficiency or other illness. They can also be the result of an overzealous manicure.

SOLUTION

Always push cuticles gently with an orange stick and take a multivitamin to rule out the possibility of deficiency. You can also gently buff away ridges and use a ridge-filler to smooth out the nail.

PROBLEM: Soft Nails
Crash diets can cause nails to soften, but it is often an inherited trait.
SOLUTION
Protect nails with a hardener, avoid extreme diets, and leave polish on the nails when filing to prevent additional splitting and peeling.

Problem: White Spots
A vitamin deficiency is the leading reason for white spots on the nails, but trauma and illness can also cause this problem.
SOLUTION
Take a multivitamin every day and use a creamy white base coat underneath polish to even up the nail color.

Problem: Separation of Nail from the Nail Bed
If a nail separates from the nail bed, this is an instant tip-off that you have a medical problem such as a fungus, diabetes, or psoriasis.
SOLUTION
See a dermatologist immediately and keep your hands out of the water as much as possible.

TERRIFIC TIDBITS FOR TIP-TOP TIPS
- *To avoid splitting, always file nails in one direction, not back and forth. Keep nails rounded or squared for maximum strength. Pointy nails will break more easily.*
- *Always wear gloves for housework or gardening.*
- *Let your nails go naked for a few days every month so they can breathe.*
- *Acrylic nails can do more harm than good by trapping water under the nail and preventing air from reaching them.*
- *Moisturize your hands and nails every day and apply a sunscreen to the back of your hands.*

MANICURE MUSTS
- *Remove all polish with acetone-free polish remover.*
- *Apply cuticle softener and soak in warm soapy water.*
- *Scrub under nails and push back softened cuticles with an orange stick wrapped in cotton.*
- *Apply a base coat or ridge-filler to dry clean nails, followed by two coats of color and a top coat.*

- *Allow each coat to dry for three to five minutes before applying next coat.*
- *Choose a quick-drying top coat to get you out the door in a hurry. I really like Markron products. Nails are dry to the touch in five minutes and thoroughly dry soon after.*

NAIL CARE PRODUCTS

Everyone has their favorite brand of nail polish, but there are a few products that really leave nails shiny, prevent chipping, and dry nail polish quickly. I'm confident that you will be satisfied with these products, which all cost less than $5.

FAST-DRYING TOPCOATS

Creative Nail Dry & Shine

Cutex Flash Finish

Markron Five Minute Miracle Manicure Quick-Dry Topcoat*

Seche Vite

NAIL HARDENER

Markron Five Minute Miracle Manicure 40 Plus Nail Treatment*

Markron Hydra-Gel Advanced Recovery Therapy (for nails damaged by acrylics)*

Markron Five Minute Miracle Manicure Strengthener & Conditioner*

Nail Magic

Nail Tek

*Toluene & Formaldehyde free

Elaine's Exclusive

HORSE SENSE

Just like your skin, nails and horses' hooves are made from essential proteins, mostly keratin. Horse groomers discovered that the heavy collagen and vitamin E creams they applied to horses' hooves also strengthened their own nails. This caused the spin-off of some horse products for human use. By the way, gelatin and calcium have no proven nail-strengthening benefit.

FOOTLOOSE

Our hands may be underappreciated, but when it comes to unsung heroes, our feet are, without question, the body's own Rodney Dangerfield—they get no respect. From our first baby steps through the end of our lives, our feet carry us an average of 110,000 miles. But for most of us, a pedicure is an occasional treat and some of us don't even get around to trimming our toenails until they come popping through our stockings. We'll complain about calluses or cracked heels but often do very little about them.

Because our feet serve us so well, I suggest that we treat them a little better by giving them an annual or biannual check-up with a podiatrist, who can spot trouble—such as falling arches—take care of corns or heavy calluses, and recommend treatment for other problems like hammer toes and bunions.

In our daily lives, however, we can do a lot to keep our feet feeling fancy-free.

Dr. Charles Gudas, a podiatrist and consultant to Dr. Scholls, recommends the following to keep your tootsies feeling tip-top:

- A fifteen-minute, cool water Epsom-salt soak followed by elevating the feet and a massage of the arches, toes, and calf muscles will restore tired feet in half an hour.
- Because the feet perspire, use foot lotion instead of cream to combat drying and cracking. Creams can be too heavy and trap in perspiration. Peppermint lotions are soothing and help manage foot odor.
- For the same reason, wear wool or cotton socks that absorb moisture.
- Powder and lotion will help combat excessive moisture.
- Keep toenails trimmed straight across to prevent them from becoming ingrown.
- Dampness does not cause fungal infections but it will exacerbate them, so dry feet carefully before dressing. Be particularly diligent around locker rooms and other shared facilities.
- At the first signs of athlete's foot, try an over-the-counter spray or powder. If the problem persists, see a podiatrist for prescription

medication. Be considerate of your family and don't go barefoot until you have the problem kicked.

- Fungal infections can be spread by the foot bathtub used by pedicurists, so be sure the technician uses an antifungal soap and spray in between clients. If you have regular pedicures, invest in your own tools, as you should for regular manicures, to help prevent the likelihood of infection.
- After soaking feet, use a pumice stone on your calluses.
- If you have diabetes, rheumatoid arthritis, or poor circulation, avoid acid-based corn removers. These products can damage surrounding tissue, something you can ill afford if you suffer from other problems.
- Insoles can often help alleviate back pain. If over-the-counter insoles don't help, a podiatrist can fit you with orthotics — custom made insoles designed exactly for the shape of your feet and the way you stand.

With age, many people experience a lack of sensation in their feet due to poor circulation and diminishing nerve endings in the feet. Diabetes often leads to this problem. This lack of sensation impairs balance and makes it difficult to perceive the ground, which is why many older people shuffle their feet and walk slowly, according to Dr. James McGuire of Philadelphia's Foot and Ankle Institute. Staying active, he says, will help keep foot muscles and ligaments in condition and help prevent the loss of nerve endings.

Although not exactly fashionable, both doctors recommend low-heeled, rubber-soled shoes for the best stability and to minimize stress on the feet. In fact, many experts list sturdy shoes as one of the first things a person can do to prevent accidents.

If your feet hurt, everything seems to hurt, and for reasons I can't explain, I always feel more polished when my toes are looking good. A friend of mine balked at having her first pedicure because she said the idea of it made her feel like a poodle and she was uncomfortable with having someone kneeling at her feet. But now that she's tried it, she's hooked.

Depending on how active you are, your feet absorb between five and ten thousand steps each day. Don't you think they deserve a little TLC?

FOOT LOTIONS, SCRUBS, AND DEODORIZERS

Price Code: $ under $5; $$ $6–$10; $$$ $11–$15

PRODUCT	SIZE (OZ)	PRICE
Alpha Hydrox Peppermint Deep Therapy Foot Creme (10 percent glycolic acid—good for knees and elbows, too!)	2	$$
Avon Fancy Feet Double Action Deodorizer	3.5	$
Avon Fancy Feet Double Action Foot Soak	3	$
Avon Foot Massage Lotion with Peppermint	4.2	$
Dr. Scholl's Revitalizing Footbath	4 tablets	$
Dr. Scholl's Super Absorbent Powder	2	$
Dr. Scholl's Super Deodorant Powder	2.75	$
Freeman Barefoot Fresh Herbal Foot Soak	5.3	$
Freeman Barefoot Liquid Foot Powder	5.3	$
Freeman Barefoot Plum & Pumice Foot Scrub	5.3	$

MIRACLE THIGH CREAMS

When thigh creams first came on the market they claimed that if you just rubbed the cream on your thighs, excess fat would melt away in a matter of days or weeks. After the initial hoopla died down, though, products stopped advertising "melting fat" and "decreased inches" and began advertising more realistic claims like "contoured look" and "smoother looking skin."

The active ingredient in most thigh creams is an asthma drug called aminophylline, a bronchial dilator, which one study showed decreased the size and number of fat cells. Aminophylline, along with caffeine and cocoa extract, two other ingredients in thigh creams, are what's known as methylxanthines, which reduce the fat content of cells by blocking the enzyme that slows down the process of breaking down fat. Caffeine also speeds up the metabolism when ingested, but it may or may not have the same result when applied topically. Most of the products also contain alpha hydroxy acids, which exfoliate the skin and stimulate collagen production.

Despite the fact that aminophylline is a prescription drug, the FDA has not chosen to restrict its use in cosmetic creams for several reasons. First, when aminophylline is used as a drug, it is taken orally or injected at certain dosages that are known to be effective. Those who put it in thigh creams, for topical application, use much less of the drug, so the patient's exposure to the drug is considerably less. Second, thigh-cream makers avoid druglike claims for their products by sticking with the "contoured look" language on their labels. Third, consumers approach the products with a healthy degree of skepticism anyway, and so far, there have been no medical problems with the products.

The FDA's John Bailey is a little concerned that asthma patients who already take the drug for their asthma might get too much of the drug if they use an aminophylline cream. He advises asthma patients to consult with their physicians before using thigh creams.

Regulations aside, the only thing most people care about is whether or not the products actually work. And the answer is maybe a little, but most people find that the effect, if any, is minimal and for $40 for a 2-ounce tube, the price just isn't worth it for what amounts to a nice moisturizer. Those who have seen results only retain those results with continued use of the product.

Study participants who have used these creams report varying results. In a study supplied with the press kit for Body Sculpture (a product that does not contain aminophylline) participants lost more than two inches on their thighs in sixty days and more than three inches on their stomachs in the same period, but the report neglects to say whether or not the participants were dieting and exercising while they were using the product.

Remember, the best and most effective way to take the thunder out of your thighs' forecast is exercise. If someone claims that a product will give miraculous results, they've probably spent too much time with the blarney stone.

VARICOSE VEINS

Reports say that half of all Americans over age fifty, or eighty million people, have some problem with their legs. Fortunately, most of the problems don't require medical attention, even though more than one hundred thousand people died from varicose vein complications in 1994. For most people, though, unsightly varicose veins present a cosmetic rather than a medical problem.

A varicose vein is a vein in which the valves don't work properly to regulate the blood flow. The veins become dilated and stretched, which causes the bulging most of us associate with the disorder. But visibility isn't the only sign of varicose veins. Other symptoms that could indicate the presence of a varicosity include swollen legs or ankles, aching, weakness or tiredness, burning or itching legs, and discoloration.

Varicose veins tend to appear more in women than in men, and then they tend to be passed through a family. Low-fiber diets also seem to play a role (another good reason to eat a high-fiber menu). Long periods of sitting in a chair and standing tend to increase the likelihood of developing the problem if you are already predisposed to it, although exercise, which strengthens the walls of the veins, can help prevent the problem.

Varicose veins and their sister disorder, spider veins, can be treated several ways. They can be removed in a procedure called ambulatory phlebectomy, in which small incisions are made near the vein and the vein is removed with the use of a kind of hook. The more common treatment is sclerotherapy, in which the veins are injected with a chemical that causes a clot to adhere to the wall of the vein, blocking off blood flow and causing blood to find another way back to the heart. Lasers can also be used to treat spider veins, but not bulging varicose veins.

If you have a family history of varicose veins, or if you had problems with them during pregnancy, you may find that they crop up again during or after menopause. If that's the case be sure to put your feet up whenever possible. Avoid prolonged periods of sitting or standing and be sure to get plenty of exercise. Keep your weight stable because obesity can aggravate varicose veins, and be sure to get plenty of fiber in your diet.

Finally, if you're experiencing any symptoms of varicosity, alert your doctor so that he can help you keep them from becoming a real health hazard.

Camouflage
Several companies make leg makeup designed to conceal spider veins. While I certainly wouldn't go to the trouble of using these products every day, for special occasions when you'll be wearing sheer hosiery or in the summertime when shorts and swimsuits leave little to the imagination, they are a good option to have. Both Covermark's Leg Magic and Dermablend's Leg and Body Cover do a great job of hiding imperfections without being thick and they have sunscreen built in. These products won't wash off in the pool or in the

ocean. In fact, you'll need an oil-based cleanser or baby oil to remove them.

When applying these products, check the results in a mirror because it will give you the same vantage point that others have when they look at you. The flaws are much less noticeable when you're not right on top of them and you'll drive yourself nuts trying to perfect the coverage from your own point of view.

HAIR REMOVAL

It seems we're never happy with hair. It's either having a bad day, falling out on top, or we're trying to get rid of it from other places.

Most of us begged our mothers for permission to shave our legs and once the novelty wore off, we've regretted it ever since. Underarm shaving is not difficult or time consuming, it's just something else we have to do. Then there are eyebrows that need to be plucked or waxed, mustaches that must go, and bikini lines that need some attention each summer. Once we get all of that under control, menopause hits and with it, hirsuteness that leaves us with never-before-seen hairs on our chinny chin chins. What's a woman to do?

Shaving

Shaving is best reserved for legs and underarms, although I've known women to take care of bikini areas with a razor, too. When women's shave creams were first introduced on the market, I thought they were an unnecessary invention developed to separate women from their money, but some of them really do make legs softer. You can get just as close a shave using any shaving cream and spend a lot less. Remember, just as you are less likely to cut yourself in the kitchen using a sharp knife, a dull razor will hack up your legs more often than a new one. And remember, always shave with the hair, not against it, to avoid folliculitis, inflammation of the hair follicle.

Waxing

Because wax pulls hairs out by its roots, the smooth afterglow of a waxing lasts much longer than shaving, if you can stand the temporary sting of someone yanking out your body hairs. Waxing is especially good for eyebrows and bikini lines. It doesn't hurt as much on the legs, but can be costly for such a large area.

Theories differ about how to make waxing painless. Some estheticians ice the area or use an anesthetic, others swear that the hairs come out more easily if the pores are opened up with steam. I find that the French waxing technique is the least painful. Unlike ordinary waxing, where muslin strips are applied over the wax, with a French wax, the esthetician just zips off the hardened wax, without applying the cloth. Whichever you prefer, if you try it yourself at home, remember to pull in the opposite direction from the way the hair is growing.

Electrolysis

This expensive and time-consuming procedure is sure to be supplanted by the newer laser technologies that require far fewer visits for permanent results. But, since the laser technology is just getting started, electrolysis may be the only permanent hair removal option currently (pardon the pun) available in your area. Electrolysis involves sticking a needle into individual hair follicles and zapping them with an electric current.

I'd recommend restricting electrolysis to pesky facial hairs because of the cost and frequency of treatments to cover a large area. There is always the risk of scarring with electrolysis, so be sure to choose an experienced technician.

Depilatories

Products like Nair simply dissolve unwanted hair, leaving smooth skin behind. Unfortunately they take twenty minutes to half an hour to work and they can be drippy, so I don't recommend them for use on the face, underarms (unless you can hold your arms in the air for half an hour), or on the bikini line. For legs, they work great. Keep in mind, though, that they can be irritating, but the use of an over-the-counter steroid cream can solve that little problem.

Bleaches

Bleaching products are good for facial hair, which can increase when menopause strikes and we have more male hormones vying for the attention of our bodies. I recommend them for mustaches, especially if you're not into waxing them away. I've recommended a few gentle bleaches.

FACIAL HAIR BLEACHES

The following products are available in your drugstore for less than $5. They do not remove hair, but rather, lighten it.

Andrea Gentle Creme Bleach for the Face
Nudit Cream Bleach (Face & Body)
Nudit Cream Bleach for the Face
Zip Creme Bleach

Tweezing

There's nothing like a good pair of tweezers to remove those unwanted stray hairs. Just select and pull quickly. Icing the area will help if you've got a big job to do. I like slant-edge tweezers instead of the pointy-nosed kind.

SMILE AND THE WORLD SMILES WITH YOU

Nine out of ten Americans agree that a smile is an important social asset, yet only half of the people surveyed by the American Academy of Cosmetic Dentistry are happy with theirs.

If you're part of the unhappy half, a cosmetic dentist may be able to help you. New techniques in dentistry make it possible to whiten teeth and repair cracked or worn teeth. Many of these services can put the sizzle back in your smile in just one office visit.

Whitening can be done in the office or at home under the dentist's supervision. Whitening toothpastes help some, but for dramatic results, see a dentist. Obviously, replacing missing teeth through implants or bridgework makes a big difference in your smile and your self-confidence.

Chapter 9

MENOPAUSE

No Longer A Midlife Minefield

It wasn't very long ago that menopause was rarely discussed, and when it was mentioned, discreetly of course, we whispered about "the change of life." Much of that has changed over the last five or ten years with books like Gail Sheehy's *The Silent Passage*, Letty Cottin Pogrebin's *Getting Over Getting Older,* and many others. We now talk more freely among our friends and with our mothers, grandmothers, and aunts in an effort to understand what is happening to our bodies and what we can do about it. Today, we even talk about menopause and its symptoms in mixed company! In fact, my going through menopause has been one of my husband's favorite topics.

Menopause, as everyone knows by now, is the cessation of menses, the menstrual cycle. Usually between ages forty-five and fifty-five, the ovaries stop producing eggs and slow down the production of estrogen, which causes many of the symptoms associated with menopause. A hysterectomy, during which the ovaries are also removed, is a kind of surgical menopause, because the loss of ovaries stops the flow of estrogen through the body.

Medically, a woman is not considered to have gone through menopause until periods have stopped completely for one year, which is why doctors have developed the term "perimenopause" to describe the months and sometimes years from the first hot flash to the final menstrual cycle.

A full 70 percent of menopausal women spend from two to five years experiencing hot flashes and other symptoms, which can vary in intensity and frequency. Additionally, some 20 percent report vaginal dryness as secretions diminish and the vaginal skin thins, shrinks, and loses elasticity. These changes combine to make sex uncomfortable and to make many women more susceptible to bladder and urinary tract infections. And they call these the golden years?

Over the next twenty years, forty million American women will go through menopause with greater understanding of this natural cycle and greater resources to ease the discomfort. We have information galore, medical alternatives, support groups, herbal and nutritional remedies, and, perhaps best of all, a public realization that it's not "all in our heads" and not something embarrassing that needs to be hidden shamefully.

MIDLIFE MIRACLE: HORMONE REPLACEMENT THERAPY

I should probably drop out of the beauty business and market myself as the menopause poster lady, because when the first signs of menopause hit me at age fifty, they all hit at once. It was like being hit by a tidal wave, only drier. I was moody, couldn't sleep, you could fry an egg on my forehead at least five times a day, I had no interest in sex, and everything dried up. I knew I couldn't spend several years feeling that lousy and I wasn't sure I could convince Norman to wear enough sweaters to enable me to keep the house at a balmy 40 degrees all winter.

Once I accepted the fact that I was, indeed fifty—gasp!—and that it was menopause that was making me feel this way, I began reading up on hormone replacement therapy. Then I went to see my doctor, who agreed with my assessment that I would be a good candidate for it.

After starting on the estrogen patch, I noticed the changes immediately. I can honestly say I've never felt better in my life. The hot flashes have stopped and Norman only wears one sweater at a time now. I have energy and a new zest for life, my skin looks and feels good again, and my sex drive has returned with gusto. I now understand why hormone replacement was the most popular prescription drug in the United States in both 1994 and 1995, with ten million women taking it either via the patch or in pill or cream form.

Hormone replacement is not especially new. Doctors and menopausal women have been working with it for thirty years now. What is new, though, is the tremendous number of women who are turning to this kind of treatment for its ability to eliminate the nasty side effects of menopause and prevent other diseases like osteoporosis. In addition, doctors and researchers also understand more about who is likely to benefit most from hormone replacement and who is at risk for side effects. Additionally, doctors are now better equipped to help women decide if the benefits outweigh the risks.

While HRT will eliminate menopause's uncomfortable symptoms, HRT can have minor side effects of its own such as nausea, breast tenderness, fluid retention, and leg cramps and abnormal clotting in women who are heavy smokers or have had a stroke or severe hypertension.

There is enough published information about menopause and hormone replacement to fill a small library, so if you're at a time in your life when HRT may be appropriate for you, I encourage you to read up on the subject before seeing your physician, because there are many factors to consider in deciding whether or not it is right for you. If you are under age fifty and facing a hysterectomy along with the removal of your ovaries, you should discuss HRT with your doctor, too.

The Benefits

No one disputes the many benefits of hormone replacement therapy. Hormone replacement therapy — augmenting declining estrogen levels, and, in the case of women who still have their uterus, progesterone levels — is known to eliminate hot flashes, restore energy and sex drive, alleviate vaginal dryness as well as skin and hair dryness, and help with other lesser-known symptoms such as insomnia, memory loss, and incontinence.

Aside from the symptoms of menopause, hormone replacement is also known to lessen the risk of colon cancer, osteoporosis, and heart disease, the leading killer of elderly women. Research has shown that HRT can reduce the risk of breaking a hip or wrist by as much as 60 percent.

The Postmenopausal Estrogen/Progestin Interventions Trial, commonly known as the PEPI study, was started in 1987 by the National Heart, Lung and Blood Institute (NHLBI) and other branches of the National Institutes of Health. The study followed 875 women at seven clinical sites across the United States. Because of the size of the study, NHLBI has been releasing information as it becomes available and so far, this much is known:

- HRT raises the level of good cholesterol (HDL) and lowers the level of lousy cholesterol (LDL). Estrogen therapy alone raises HDL more than the combined estrogen/progestin therapy.

- Combined estrogen/progestin therapy reduced the risk of over-growth of the lining of the uterus that was associated with estrogen-only therapy.
- HRT did not increase blood pressure.
- Fibrinogen—which allows blood clots to form more readily, thereby increasing the risk of heart disease and stroke—decreased, which is considered to be desirable.
- HRT did not cause weight gain.
- Triglyceride levels increased with HRT. Triglycerides are fatty substances carried through the blood to the tissues where they are stored for use as energy. Their link to heart disease is unclear.
- Insulin levels were not significantly affected, but the reduction in fasting glucose levels and an elevation of glucose levels two hours after eating indicate that more study is needed to determine if this is important in relation to carbohydrate metabolism and diabetes, which could affect the risk of heart disease.

In addition to the PEPI trials, other studies have reported promising news, too.

- Researchers at Columbia University are now more convinced than ever that estrogen, taken long after menopause, reduces a woman's likelihood of developing Alzheimer's disease by as much as one-third. For people who fear debilitation more than anything else about growing older, this is significant news.
- A study conducted by Brigham and Women's Hospital in Boston and published in the *New England Journal of Medicine* found that the combination of estrogen and progestin was highly effective against heart disease, just as estrogen alone is effective.

The Risks

Breast cancer, the killer disease that strikes one woman out of nine, is the number-one reason women choose not to take hormone replacement therapy. Women who have a familial or personal history of breast cancer are usually not considered to be candidates for hormone replacement, but other doctors think that the slight increase in risk is far outweighed by the benefits.

An increased risk of uterine cancer, which was associated with estrogen therapy, was eliminated when researchers added the synthetic version of progesterone, called progestin, to estrogen treatment. Now women who still have their uterus can take the combination of hormones and have no greater risk of uterine cancer than anyone else. Women who have undergone hysterectomy can safely take estrogen alone.

In addition, doctors are still uncertain what effect, if any, hormones play in the development of varicose veins, but until more research is conducted, a woman who is susceptible to blood clots should factor that into her decision to take hormones.

Factors to Consider

> *Risk of heart disease:* Each year, 360,000 women die from heart disease, making it the number-one killer of elderly women in America. Women who are heavy smokers or who have a family history of heart disease may want the protective benefits of HRT. Obesity, lack of exercise, and elevated cholesterol levels also indicate an increased risk of heart disease that might be offset by taking hormones.

> *Risk of osteoporosis:* Fair-skinned, small-boned women, as well as those who are or were heavy smokers or drinkers and those who drink a lot of coffee, are at the greatest risk of osteoporosis. Also, those with a family history of the disease and those who are physically inactive are at greater risk. A DEXA scan can tell you your current bone density and a simple urine test can help you and your doctor determine your risk for developing osteoporosis. You can factor this information into your decision to take or not take hormones.

> *Periods at age seventy?:* One of the few benefits of menopause is the cessation of monthly periods, but one-third of the women who take the estrogen/progestin combination therapy find that their periods return, although flow can vary.

MORE THAN ONE WAY TO SKIN A CAT

For other reasons that don't include breast cancer, many women still prefer to "let nature take its course." After all, menopause is not a disease and as one woman said, "God created menopause for a reason."

For those women, a healthy, active lifestyle and a low-fat, high-calcium diet may provide them with the reduced risk of heart disease and osteoporosis that comes with HRT, but without the drawbacks of hormones. In addition, Fosamax, the first hormone-free bone-builder, is now available to help combat osteoporosis. Certainly, with or without hormones, the diet and exercise advice is worth heeding.

But what about the hot flashes, night sweats, vaginal dryness, and fatigue? First of all, keep in mind that not everyone has severe symptoms in menopause. Some women sail right through with nary a flash and others have moderate symptoms that they don't feel compelled to treat. In fact, the Japanese language has no word for hot flash because so few women experience them. Some scientists attribute that medical tidbit to the high amount of soy in the Japanese diet.

Researchers in the United States are seeing promising results from two studies involving soy products and women experiencing hot flashes that are currently underway. Until the data is in, you could safely add tofu, which also happens to be fat-free, or other soy products to your diet, and perhaps enjoy a residual benefit of diminished flashes.

Cool splashes of water and taking vitamin E supplements can help with hot flashes. (So can putting your head in the freezer, but it's uncomfortable and murder on the electric bill.)

For those women seeking relief from menopause's symptoms, "natural" remedies such as herbal preparations and vitamins may be an alternative. Many of the herbs prescribed for menopause's symptoms contain chemicals called phytoestrogens or literally "plant estrogen." Although these plants, such as licorice root, wild yam, motherwort, ginseng, spirulina, sage, and dong quai, have been used in the Orient for hundreds of years, they have not undergone extensive study. And even though the effective chemicals are plant estrogens, they're still estrogen, and taken in large doses over a long period of time, could increase the risk of uterine cancer just as taking estrogen pills without progesterone.

Health-food stores sell capsules containing a mixture of herbs that are believed to help alleviate menopause's symptoms and the women I know who have taken them do report diminished hot flashes and less dryness, but not the dramatic relief that is common with HRT. Despite the fact that herbs are "natural," they can produce side effects like hypertension from licorice root or intestinal cramping from wild yam, so if you try an herbal remedy and experience those symptoms, or anything unusual for that matter, be sure to discontinue use.

Vaginal dryness can be addressed with a lubricant like Astroglide or estrogen cream; and regular sex, at least once or twice a week, will help too.

Hair and skin dryness can be addressed with moisturizing shampoo and body creams as well as keeping the air in your home moist with a humidifier. Overheating your home will also cause excessive dryness, but if you're having hot flashes, you're probably not keeping the house very hot anyway.

Finally, a patient family and a good sense of humor are the best natural remedies I know of to help you through the irritability and mood swings and, of course, avoiding caffeine late in the day will help with the insomnia, as might warm milk or herbal teas.

HYSTERECTOMY

When a woman develops uterine cancer, fibroids, or excessive bleeding that does not respond to other treatment, the most common form of treatment is a hysterectomy, an operation that involves removing the uterus, surrounding tissue, and sometimes the cervix. Under some circumstances, doctors elect to remove the ovaries, too, especially if the woman is near menopause anyway or if the ovaries are also diseased. Ovarian cancer is very difficult to detect and strikes one woman in one hundred.

When only the uterus is removed, menopause will happen naturally, but when the ovaries are also removed, thereby cutting off the body's supply of estrogen, the woman will be thrown into immediate menopause complete with all of the symptoms she would have normally faced.

For these women, especially, HRT can be helpful in easing the symptoms, but when the patient has already undergone treatment for uterine or ovarian cancer, the risk of breast cancer associated with HRT may be more than she is willing to accept.

In the last few years there have been volumes written about menopause and hormone replacement therapy and as I struggled to deal with the change, I spent a good deal of time reading up on the subject. If you are approaching this time in your life, I urge you to do the same.

We are the fortunate beneficiaries of menopause having come out of the closet and there is no longer any reason to be in the dark as you go through this important and sometimes uncomfortable change.

Part 3

FINISHING TOUCHES

Chapter 10

ABOUT FACE

Making Up Isn't Hard to Do

"The less makeup you wear, the younger you look."
—Bobbi Brown, CEO and Creator,
Bobbi Brown Essentials Cosmetics

"I live by a man's code designed to fit a man's world, yet at
the same time, I never forget that a woman's first job is to
choose the right shade of lipstick."
—Carole Lombard

Many years ago, I worked as an independent cosmetics consultant in a well-known Philadelphia boutique called Nan Duskin. One day a woman in her late fifties came in all made up with her green eye shadow, black eyeliner, and false eyelashes—a look she had obviously perfected years ago that simply didn't work for her now that she was more mature.

By the time I was finished with her makeup, she looked ten years younger. She told me she was thrilled with her new look and everyone in the store told her how fabulous she looked. She obviously loved her new face because she spent close to $300 buying every product I taught her to use.

Two weeks later she was back in the store wearing the same green eye shadow and black eyeliner. I was crushed. But then I realized that she just wasn't ready to look different, even if different meant younger.

There are a lot of women out there like my green-eyed customer. We get used to seeing the same face looking back at us in the mirror and it can be very disconcerting to change styles dramatically. To some, I suspect, needing a change is like admitting that something was wrong in the first place, or worse yet, admitting that time has crept up while we weren't watching.

But, just as you changed clothing styles to coincide with different times in your life, so too do you need to change your makeup. You remember telling your twelve-year-old daughter that lipstick wasn't appropriate for her age, don't you? Different things are appropriate for different times in your life, whether you are twelve, twenty-two, or fifty-two.

More recently, while I was working on this book, I was having lunch with a group of women who were asking how it was coming along. As I was telling them about *Ageless*, one woman proclaimed proudly for all to hear, "Well, I'm not a candidate for your book. I don't even wear lipstick!" I asked why she didn't wear any makeup and she told me that she was comfortable with her years showing and didn't feel she had anything to hide.

That's when it dawned on me that this woman, and many like her, I'm sure, consider makeup to be camouflage, or war paint. She viewed makeup as something that covered up perceived imperfections, not something that enhanced her good looks. Given that line of thinking, it was only natural that someone who was comfortable and confident with themselves would not be interested in such vanity.

Then I looked around the room and noticed that many of the older women in the restaurant were in need of a makeover. It's an easy trap to fall into. You perfected your makeup routine as a young woman and have been sticking with what works. Since most of us have better things to do than fuss in front of a makeup mirror every day, we do the same routine year in and year out and don't really give ourselves a critical looking-over very often. The next thing you know, twenty or thirty years have gone by, your coloring has changed, and your once-beautiful makeup is less than flattering. All of a sudden, your lipstick's too red, your blush is too bright.

No wonder the naked-faced lady was proud that she had decided not to wear makeup. She is a distinct minority, though. Most women over age forty appreciate the value of makeup. However, I see a great many older women who fail to adapt their makeup to the realities of an aging face.

Before you get started changing your look, take an honest look in the mirror. Are you still wearing the same color and coverage that you wore fifteen years ago? Is your eye shadow so frosty that it shows every crease in your lids? If you have bags under your eyes, does your concealer make them more pronounced? Is your foundation caking in your wrinkles and does it adequately hide any imperfections? Does your lipstick develop a mind of its own and start heading for your nose soon after its applied? When was the last time you tried a new shade? Be honest with yourself; no one will know.

Once you've taken a long hard look at yourself, seek out someone to help you make new selections. It might be someone at the cosmetics counter, but since many of those women are too young to really understand what you need, you may be better off seeking out the advice of a friend or acquaintance whose makeup always looks great — chances are she'll be flattered that you asked. And don't forget to take this book with you to the store!

After you've made some new purchases, stay with your new look for a week or two until you get used to it. Don't abandon the new style in the first few days because you feel self-conscious or think you look different. You probably do look different, but in this case, different is better.

Enjoy your new face the same way you'd enjoy a new dress and be sure to go through this exercise every few years, just to stay current. You'll be glad you did.

MAKING UP ISN'T HARD

Just as we need to change our skin-care products and routines to accommodate the changes that age brings, so too does it become necessary to adapt our colors and makeup products to keep up with the times. If you put on your makeup and it just doesn't look right all of a sudden, it's probably not your eyes or the lighting. Your skin has probably grown sallow or less vibrant over time and you're just seeing it. Add a few age spots, spider veins, enlarged pores, and sun damage and all of a sudden, you hardly recognize the woman in the mirror. It happened to me — and even though I've been in the beauty business for close to thirty years and know what happens as women age, I couldn't have been more shocked when it was my turn.

Despite the fact that many women have trouble with it, making up doesn't have to be hard to do. Correcting bad habits is usually a matter of buying a few new products.

"Less makeup, more color," proclaims a makeup artist, who points out that older women's skin tends to become less pink, necessitating a little extra color to brighten the face.

Choosing the right products and the right colors can make all the difference for older women. And applying the right products to skin that is moisturized and exfoliated will help your makeup look its best, too. If you apply foundation or powder to flaky, dead cells, your makeup will eventually crease or look flaky too.

I think that many women get the impression that makeup is difficult because beauty magazines are always full of makeup tips that sound complicated. The truth is that, except for special occasions, most of us want a simple routine that will enhance our best features with a minimum of fuss.

Elaine's Exclusive

BRUSH UP ON YOUR BEAUTY KNOW-HOW

A good set of makeup brushes is as essential to putting your best face forward as a good set of sharp knives is to gourmet cooking. So, when you buy new blush or eye shadow, throw away the worthless applicators that come with the package and use your own sable brushes. Revlon makes Tips and Tools for eyes and lips for only $6.95. (They're great for travel.) You'll also need a few good sable brushes. Astarte's Mari Aldin says to select a brush by running your thumb across the brushes and then shake them before buying. If hairs fall out, don't buy the brush. The only brushes you'll need are:

for loose powder: one dome-shaped brush
for blush: one moon brush $1/4$–$1/2$ inch by $1$$1/2$ inch)
for eye shadow: two $1/4$ inch
for eyebrows: a toothbrush
for lips: a retractable lip brush

FOUNDATION OF GOOD LOOKS

The right foundation is the very basis for a well-made-up face. Just as an artist starts with a clean, fresh canvas, your blush and eye makeup will look their best if you apply them on top of an evenly colored face.

If you've never worn foundation because you were afraid it would clog your pores or give you a made-up look, give foundations another try. Today's technology has enabled cosmetics companies to produce some amazingly lightweight and sheer foundations, and there is truly little difference in quality between the expensive and inexpensive products. The only problem is in finding the right color, which may take some trial and error, especially if you're shopping in a nonservice environment such as a drugstore or supermarket.

Foundation also helps protect the skin from pollutants, which is why some estheticians and dermatologists think that women who wear foundation regularly tend to have better skin. What's more, many foundations today have sunscreen built in, so you can add to the protection you've already applied with your sunscreen and moisturizer.

If you have sensitive skin, watch out for foundations with fragrance, lanolin, or almond oil as these ingredients are known irritants and very common in foundations. Women with oily skin should avoid isopropyl myristate and myristyl myristate, as they are comedogenic.

The Three Cs of Foundation

When choosing a foundation, consider these three Cs: color, coverage, and cost.

COLOR Choose a color that most closely matches your own skin tone. That may seem like simple, obvious advice, but carrying it out can be a little tricky. What's more, we tend to find a foundation we like and stick with it, sometimes longer than we should.

Check to see if your neck is a distinctly different color from your face once you've applied your makeup. If there is a clear line of demarcation where your makeup stops and your neck begins, it's probably time for a new foundation.

Remember that the objective in a foundation is to even out skin tones and hide minor imperfections. You'll use a concealer to cover up major flaws, so choose a foundation that most closely matches your own skin tone.

Essentially, foundations are either yellow-based or rose-based, and you can narrow down your choices by knowing your own coloring. Bobbi Brown says that most women are best suited for yellow-based makeup.

- If your own skin tone is warm, with lots of yellow and gold undertones, then you want to select from the yellow-based foundations.
- If your skin tones are cool, with lots of pink and blue undertones, you'll choose from the rose-based foundations.
- Asian women have a lot of yellow undertones, and should select a yellow-based foundation that matches their skin color.
- Black skin comes in so many shades that finding a compatible foundation is often difficult, but most Black women can safely begin their selection process in the yellow-based foundations.
- Oily-skinned women need to know that rose-based foundation has a tendency to turn orange on women who have oily skin. Also, any foundation applied to oily skin can darken, so be sure to sample a new foundation for several hours before buying it.

According to Helen Lee, a Ford fashion model and makeup artist who operates her own day spa in Manhattan, many Asian women make the mistake of trying to brighten up their faces with rose-based foundations, which leave them looking as if they are wearing a mask. Her recommendation, which applies to all women, is to add color to your face with blush and eye makeup, not foundation. Helen Lee's Day Spa sells a line of products for Asian women and can be reached at 800-288-1077.

Astarte Cosmetics in New York has a line of cosmetics for Black and Hispanic women that are particularly good, too. You can obtain samples and a catalog by calling 212-206-8095.

Contrary to the guidelines above, I find that even though I have warm undertones and am theoretically best suited for yellow-based foundation, I look healthier with a little pink in my foundation. I realize that this goes against every rule, tip, and suggestion ever given to me by a makeup artist, but it's true, at least for me. So, if you've gone through all of the "right" colors for your skin tones and still don't come up with foundation that's really right for you, go ahead and dabble in the opposite end of the foundation color spectrum.

Of course it goes without saying that if you insist on tanning your face in the summertime, you'll need a separate winter and summer foundation to accommodate the color change.

Elaine's Exclusive

FACE FIRST

When choosing a foundation, select three colors that appear to match your skin tone and apply a stripe of each to your jawline. (Obviously you should not be wearing makeup when you do this.) The color that seems to disappear is the color that's best for you.

COVERAGE Foundations come in liquid, cream, cream-to-powders, and sticks, and offer a range of coverage options from sheer to heavy, depending on how uneven the skin tones are. Women with varying pigmentation will want to opt for the light to medium coverage, while women who are fairly evenly complected can choose lighter coverage. Only women who have birthmarks or severe scarring should choose the heaviest makeup, sometimes called "pancake" because it covers like pancake batter.

The type of foundation you choose depends primarily on skin type. However, I feel that creams can end up looking artificial or pasty and that the cream-to-powder foundations can be too matte for mature skin. If you have minimal lines, the cream-to-powder foundations are okay, but they don't give the dewy look that is flattering for older women.

I find that older women get the best results from liquid makeup. Women with mature dry skin should choose an oil-based liquid foundation because it does not settle in wrinkles, creating the cakey look that older women are somewhat notorious for. Generally speaking, mature normal/combination skin still requires an oil-based foundation or some oil-free products made with silicone derivatives. Despite the fact that they are oil-free, they still glide on easily and give the skin a dewy appearance. Oily-skinned women should choose a water-based or oil-free liquid foundation.

According to Julio Ross, the vice president of research and development worldwide color for Revlon, great advances in technology have enabled cosmetics companies to develop foundations that are lighter and silkier than ever before. These lighter products, made with oils and silicones, stay on the top of the skin without clogging pores. What's more, silica and other ingredients, including hydrolyzed whole-wheat protein, mimosa oil, amino acids, lecithin, sodium hyaluronate, and avocado oil all help diffuse light so that fine lines are diminished rather than enhanced by the makeup. That's what cosmetics companies mean when they talk about "age-defying" or "light-diffusing" makeup.

Finally, makeup finishes come in matte, semimatte, and dewy. Since most of us are looking to restore the glow of youth, I recommend that everyone choose the dewy finishes, which include those age-defying or light-diffusing ingredients.

Elaine's Exclusive

UP CLOSE AND PERSONAL

The right foundation is the single most important ingredient in a perfectly made-up face, so don't even bother buying products in frosted bottles or packages that are wrapped in cellophane. If you can't touch the product to feel its consistency and check the color on your own face, don't bother with it.

COST The cost of foundation varies widely from less than $10 for the Revlon or L'Oréal products you find in a drugstore to department store cosmetics that can cost five times as much.

Good quality products are available in mass market, but finding the right color can be a problem if you can't test the products. Revlon and L'Oréal make fabulous foundations, but the packaging makes it difficult to see the shades. When you're shopping in a nonservice environment, keep in mind that twice a year many companies, including Revlon, Max Factor, and Maybelline, sell trial sizes for about $1 so that consumers can try out new products. Although testers for drugstore brands are not readily available, some of your local beauty supply stores and others like Sally Beauty Supply and Cosmetics Plus offer testers for the most popular brands.

While I firmly believe in saving money with inexpensive quality products, because the right foundation is the single most important ingredient in a well-made-up face, it may be worth it to spend extra money to ensure that you get the right shade and texture for your skin.

Elaine's Exclusive

SHOPPING IN A NONSERVICE ENVIRONMENT

If you can find the right color from the many choices offered by popular cosmetics lines like Max Factor, Revlon, and L'Oréal, you can save a lot of money. The trouble is in finding the right color when the bottles are frosted, covered in plastic, or only displayed in one-inch cardboard splotches. Keep these tips in mind when shopping without testers and you'll have a much better chance of finding the best color for you.

1. If you have normal, combination, or dry skin, look for something that appears one shade darker in the bottle.
2. If you have oily skin, buy something that is a shade lighter than your skin. Your own oils will darken the color once it's applied.
3. Be on the lookout for sample sizes that are usually offered every six months.

Custom-Blending

Hardware stores have been mixing up custom colors for the home for years, but it wasn't until Prescriptives came along that custom-blending cosmetics began to take hold. Prescriptives was probably the first large company to offer the service they call "colorprinting," which identifies your skin's undertones and then custom-blends a foundation from a selection of thirty-four different shades. Many beauty salons have been custom-blending makeup for some time now, but the service is becoming more and more mainstream, with Nordstrom's getting into the action in September of 1996 with its C2O—Color To Order line. Vidal Sassoon recently introduced Luminique Custom Blended Cosmetics to its salons in major cities worldwide. Call 212-535-9200 for a salon near you.

Elaine's Exclusive

APPLY YOURSELF

Use a barely damp sponge to apply today's new foundations and you'll get a fabulous, sheer look. If you want a little more coverage, use a dry sponge. Apply a dab of makeup to the sponge and then use the sponge on your face for complete control and perfect, even coverage.

While the cost for a bottle of foundation will be significantly more than what you would pay at the drugstore, if you're having trouble finding the right color, it's worth it to splurge on this one luxury. A bottle of Prescriptives custom-blend foundation will cost $50, at Nordstrom's C2O foundation will run about $35, and you'll pay $40 for Luminique. (You can always make up for the extra expense by choosing less costly blush and mascara.)

Because makeup for Black and Asian women is still somewhat limited — despite great strides by Iman, Flori Roberts, Revlon, and Maybelline — and difficult to choose because of the kaleidoscope of skin shades, I think custom-blending is an especially viable option for women of color.

I had colorprinting done at a department store near my home and was really impressed with the service. Once we established my coloring category, the technician presented me with compatible lipsticks and blushes that complemented my natural coloring. With this kind of a system, it's almost impossible to make a bad selection, but just to be sure, I always recommend leaving the store and checking the makeup in daylight.

Beauty salons are another, often overlooked source for makeup. Many sell great private label products made by reliable manufacturers and offer custom-blending that is not as expensive as custom-blended products from department stores. The only drawback I've noticed buying cosmetics from salons is that the testers can be dirty if the salon does a lot of makeovers.

Nordstrom's custom-blending service offers more than just foundation, too. They can match a discontinued lipstick from the scrapings of your last tube and whip up a blush to match, or take a lip color you like and make it glossier. They can even match a lipstick to a new blouse.

RECOMMENDED FOUNDATIONS

Skin Type Key: N normal; O oily; D dry; VD very dry; C combination; S sensitive; R Renova, Retin-A

Price Key: $ under $10; $$ $11–$21; $$$ $21–$30; $$$$ $31–$40; $$$$$ over $40

DEPARTMENT STORE BRANDS

PRODUCT	SIZE(OZ)	SPF	SKIN TYPE	COVERAGE	PRICE
Adrien Arpel Total Sunblock Creme Makeup	1.25	15	D/VD	med	$$$$
Bobbi Brown Essentials Moisturizing Foundation	1		N/D	vs/sheer	$$$$$
Chanel Pure Perfection	1	8	D/VD	med	$$$$$$
Chanel Teint Natural	1	8	N/D	sheer/med	$$$$$$
Clarins Le Teint Satin	1.2		N/VD	sheer	$$$
Christian Dior Tient Satin	1.2		N/VD	sheer	$$$$$$
Elizabeth Arden Flawless Finish Hydro Light Foundation	1	10	D/VD	sheer/med	$$$
Elizabeth Arden Flawless Finish Sponge-On cream Makeup	.8		VD	med	$$$
Estee Lauder Impeccable Finish Makeup	.42	20	N/D	sheer/med	$$$
Estee Lauder Lucidity Light Diffusing Makeup	1	8	N/D	vs/sheer	$$$
Estee Lauder Enlighten Skin Enhancing Makeup —oil free	1	10	N/C/O/S	sheer	$$$
Lancôme Maqui-Libre Skin Liberating Makeup	1	15	N/D	vs/sheer	$$$
Lancôme Maquivelours Hydrating Foundation	1		N/D	vs/sheer	$$$
Lancôme Maquilumine Creme Powder	.3		N/C	sheer/med	$$$$
M.A.C. Satin Foundation	1		N/D	sheer	$$
Origins Original Skin Some Coverage—More Coverage	1		N/C	sheer/med	$$

PRODUCT	SIZE(OZ)	SPF	SKINTYPE	COVERAGE	PRICE
Prescriptives All Skins Basic	1		N/D	sheer	$$$
Prescriptives Virtual Skin	1		N/D	sheer	$$$
Prescriptives Custom Blend	1		N/D	sheer	$$$$$
Princess Marcella Borghese Natural Finish Makeup	1.8		N/C/O/S	vs/sheer	$$$
Princess Marcella Borghese Cura Naturale Time Defying Makeup	1	8	N/D	sheer/ med	$$$
Shiseido Fluid Foundation	1.1		N/D	sheer	$$$
Shiseido Compact Foundation	.45		N/C	med	$$$
Yves St. Laurent Powder Foundation & Highlighter (2 in 1)	.3		N/D	sheer/ med	$$$$$

DRUGSTORE BRANDS

PRODUCT	SIZE(OZ)	SPF	SKINTYPE	COVERAGE	PRICE
Almay Moisture Renew Makeup	1.25		N/D/S/C	med	$
Almay Time-off Age-Smoothing Makeup	1.25		N/D/S/C	sheer	$
L'Oréal Feel Perfecte	1.12	25	N/D	sheer/ med	$
L'Oréal Luminair	.3		N/C	sheer/ med	$
L'Oréal Mattique	1.12		O	sheer/ med	$
L'Oréal Hydra Perfecte	1.2	12	N/C	med	$
Maybelline Revitalizing Alpha Hydroxy Makeup (oil free)	1.2		C/O	sheer/ med	$
Maybelline Shades of You Oil Free Liquid Makeup	1.25		N/C	med	$
Max Factor Rain Natural Moisturizing Makeup (oil-free)	1.2		N/C	sheer	$
Max Factor Balancing Act Makeup	1.2		N/C	sheer	$
Revlon New Complexion Oil-Free makeup	1.25	4	C/S/O	sheer	$
Revlon Age Defying Makeup	1.25	8	N/D	vs/sheer	$

HOME SALES/ALTERNATIVE OUTLETS

PRODUCT	SIZE(OZ)	SPF	SKIN TYPE	COVERAGE	PRICE
Avon Face Lifting Moisture Firm Foundation	1		N/VD	med	$

ETHNIC PRODUCTS

PRODUCT	SIZE(OZ)	SPF	SKIN TYPE	COVERAGE	PRICE
Astarte Liquid Makeup	1		all	sheer/ med	$$
Iman Second to None Oil Free Makeup	1	8	O	med	$$
Iman Second to None Cream to Powder	.3		D	medium	$$
Flori Roberts Gold Oil-Free Hydrophilic Foundation	1.2		N/D	med/sheer	$$
Maybelline Shades of You	1.25		N/C	medium	$$
Prescriptives All Skins Basic	1		N/D	sheer	$$$
Prescriptives Custom Blend	1		N/D	sheer	$$$$$
Revlon Age Defying Makeup	1.25	8	N/D	vs/sheer	$

BRONZERS AND FACE TINTS

There is no reason to ruin your skin by basking in the sun when you can give yourself that "healthy" glow with any of these products. They all provide a sheer finish, but add that sun-kissed look to your face.

PRODUCT	SIZE(OZ)	PRICE
Clarins Bronzing Powder Duo	1.7	$$$
Clarins Moisturizing Tint (SPF 6)	1.7	$$$
La Prairie Bronzing Powder	1.7	$$$$
Estee Lauder Instant Sun All-Over Bronzer Duo	.51	$$$
Prescriptives Bronze Liquid Lightning	1	$$$
Prescriptives Transparent Face Color (All over tint)(sunscreen)	.5	$$
Revlon Tinted Face Cream Pure Radiance (SPF 8)	.2	$
Ultima II Bronzing	.32	$$

TONERS: TONE DOWN STRONG COMPLEXIONS

You may have read an item or two in a beauty magazine about products called toners that are worn under foundations and act as a color neutralizer. These are products for the most difficult complexions that, because of their strength, tend to change the color of the foundation a few hours after application. Ilana Harkavi of Il Makiage in New York points out that olive-complected women, and those with extremely sallow complexions or inflamed redness from rosacea, often have this problem. If you're one of those women, you need a toner that is the opposite of your skin tone on the color wheel.

If your skin is excessively red, for example, you'll need a green toner to counterbalance the redness. If you are especially sallow, try a violet toner. I know it sounds crazy to apply green or purple makeup to your skin, but it really does work.

The biggest problem with toners is that women who are inexperienced in applying toners can be heavy-handed with the product, so be sure to have it demonstrated to you before taking it home.

CONCEALER: IMPERFECTIONS GO UNDER COVER

Concealers come in tubes, pots, or wands and work wonders for hiding dark, under-eye circles, ruddiness on the cheeks, age spots, spider veins, and any other imperfection that may be too noticeable for your foundation to neutralize.

Always choose a concealer that is just one shade lighter than your foundation and your normal skin tone to get perfect coverage. Dab the concealer on to the trouble spots and blend it in. Apply foundation over the concealer.

Once your makeup is complete, you can also use your concealer, because it is a shade lighter than your foundation, to highlight a brow bone, diminish the tip of your nose, or accent a cheekbone.

A concealer that is a shade darker than your foundation is also a good choice for contouring a sagging jawline, slimming a broad nose, or creating a hollow in cheeks. For extremely dark circles or spider veins, choose an amber- or yellow-based concealer. Dermablend, Covermark, and Matrix's Smartstick are the very best concealers to hide discoloration. Because they tend to be a little thick, apply the product with a sponge so that it doesn't look too cakey.

Remember that light gives emphasis and darkness makes things recede, so apply concealer appropriately. For example, never put light concealer on puffy eyes, they'll only look puffier, and conversely, don't apply dark concealer to a weak chin or cheekbones; it will make them less noticeable than they already are.

Women's magazines are full of makeup tips that promise an instant face-lift, and although we know that's really impossible, we read the section anyway. Many of the recommendations are too complicated for anyone to follow, let alone remember, but here are a few tips that I've gathered over the years that work at least a little magic.

1. Use a concealer that is one shade darker than your foundation to contour your jawline and "erase" any sagging. Apply lightly along the jaw and under the chin and blend well. Dot a little light concealer on your chin for emphasis.
2. Dot a little bit of light concealer between the brows to de-emphasize any lines there.
3. As facial skin thins and fat padding diminishes, noses can look thinner and longer than ever before. To widen your nose, apply a wide band of light concealer down the center. To shorten the look, contour the tip with a darker shade concealer.
4. Use a lighter concealer to hide dark circles.
5. A little highlighter along the cheekbone can widen a thinning, bony face; the same technique can de-emphasize a bony chin.

CONCEALERS

Since most concealers are thick in order to do their job, application is particularly important. If you apply concealer with a small wedge sponge, it will be less likely to cake and will look more natural. Prescriptives concealers are particularly noteworthy because they are sold by skin tone rather than simply light, medium, and dark shades. The following products were recommended for their ability to cover and their creamy texture.

Price Key: $ under $10; $$ $11–$21, $$$ $21–$30, $$$$ $31–$40, $$$$$ over $40

DEPARTMENT STORE BRANDS

PRODUCT	SIZE (OZ)	PRICE
Elizabeth Arden Perfect Covering Concealer*	.35	$$
Christian Dior Hydrating Concealer	.58	$$

PRODUCT	SIZE (OZ)	PRICE
Clinique Soft Conceal Corrector*	.30	$$
Lancôme Maqui Complet Concealer	.25	$$
M.A.C. Concealer	.24	$
Prescriptives Camouflage Cream*	.50	$$
Shiseido Concealer	.22	$$
Ultima The Concealer	.50	$$

* indicates that ethnic colors are available.

DRUGSTORE BRANDS

PRODUCT	SIZE (OZ)	PRICE
L'Oréal Hydra Perfecte Concealer (SPF 12)	.05	$
L'Oréal Mattique Conceal Oil-Free Cover Up	.15	$
Max Factor Erace Colour Precise	.4	$
Revlon Age Defying Concealer (SPF 12)*	.16	$

* indicates that ethnic colors are available.

SPECIALTY CONCEALERS

I've listed the following products separately because they deserve special notice. The Dermablend and Covermark products were developed to cover the most pronounced blemishes including port-wine stains and other birthmarks. As such, they are a little thicker and take some practice to apply perfectly, but they cover beautifully. The Mary Kay products are noteworthy because they come in mint green and lavender, which make them good toners. The Yves St. Laurent Radiant Touch is significantly more expensive than other concealers ($32.50), but worth the extra money because it does such a nice job reflecting light and diminishing dark circles.

PRODUCT	SIZE (OZ)	SPF	PRICE
Adrien Arpel Porcelain Coverbase (violet color corrector)	.7		$$$
Covermark Face Magic (All Skin Tones)	.88	20	$$
Dermablend Quick Fix with sunscreen (all skin tones)	.2		$$
Mary Kay Full Correcting Concealer Neutralizing (mint or lavender)	.5		$
Matrix Colors Smart Stick Treatment Neutralizer for Redness	.2		$$
Yves St. Laurent Radiant Touch	.1		$$$$

BLUSH: BRUSH ON A HEALTHY GLOW

Once you've created a smooth canvas using the right foundation, you can begin to brighten your face and add a youthful glow by applying blush. Unfortunately, one of the most common mistakes older women make is choosing the wrong blush.

When we were younger and our skin color was pinker and our hair color more vibrant, we could wear a brighter blush and look healthy and luminous. But once our hair color tones down a little, and especially if we choose to wear our hair gray or white, bright blush just looks clownish. There's no nice way to put it.

"Too much blush makes you look old," says Bobbi Brown. "The right blush can take years off your face. You want a soft color that makes you look healthy and gives you a glow."

Your skin's undertones will help guide your blush selection. In general, the darker your skin, the brighter the blush you need to add color to your face. Caucasian women with yellow undertones, or sallow skin, and Asian women can brighten their look with cool colors like roses, pinks, or lavenders. Women with cool complexions, those who look pink or ruddy, look best in yellow-based blushes. Select peaches, corals, ambers, and browns. Astarte's President Mari Aldin says that the darkest Black women, those whose skin is ebony or blue/black, should choose a blush with purple or orchid shades, while lighter skinned Black or Hispanic women can wear rosy earth, salmon, or brown tones.

Elaine's Exclusive

BUFF AND PUFF

- Lightly apply concealer with a barely damp makeup sponge. (Squeeze out excess water between paper towels before using sponge.)
- Apply foundation with same sponge.
- Apply loose powder with dry sponge.
- Apply blush with brush.
- Buff and blend everything with the slightly damp sponge.
- Apply more blush and concealer if needed and blend again.

Blush comes in powder, gel, or cream, but unless you're a real pro at makeup application, stick with powder blushes, which are easiest to control. What's more, if you make a mistake, powder blushes are easier to remove or cover over. If you like cream blush, Estee Lauder makes a great product that is easy to control and apply. Use a sponge, dab it on, and blend. The sponge will give you the control that you normally get from a brush.

Treat yourself to a nice, fluffy sable brush for applying blush to your cheeks. Keep in mind that you are looking to add color to your face in a way that looks natural, so don't make the mistake of applying streaks of color from the apple of your cheeks to your temples. Apply a gentle touch of color to your cheeks, being careful not to encroach on your eyes by going too high on your cheekbone.

If age has taken away some of the fat padding in your cheeks, apply your blusher to the area that was once padded, and then highlight the top of your cheekbone with just a smidge of concealer. If you are extremely wrinkled, stay away from frosted blushes because they enhance wrinkles.

BLUSH

The following products are recommended based on the amount of slip (the product's ability to glide on easily without pulling or stretching).
Price Key: $ under $10; $$ $11–$21; $$$ $21–$30; $$$$ $31–$40, $$$$$ over $40

DEPARTMENT STORE PRODUCTS

PRODUCT	SIZE (OZ)	PRICE
Clarins Powder Blush	.18	$$$
Elizabeth Arden Cheek Color Naturals	.18	$$
Estee Lauder Blushing Natural Cheek Creme	.32	$$
Estee Lauder Cheek Color	$$	
Flori Roberts Radiance Blush	.20	$$
Iman Luxury Blushing Powder	.15	$$
Lancôme Blush Subtil	.18	$$$
M.A.C. Powder Blush	.10	$$
Prescriptives Powder Cheek Color (refillable compact)	.20	$$
Shiseido Gradation Colors Blush & Eye Shadow	.24	$$$
Ultima II Wonderwear Cheek Color	.34	$$

DRUGSTORE PRODUCTS

PRODUCT	SIZE (OZ)	PRICE
L'Oréal Blushesse Endless Color Powder Blush	.16	$
Maybelline Shades of You 100% Oil Free Powder Blush	.25	$
Max Factor Lustrous Sponge-On Satin Blush	.20	$
Revlon Naturally Glamorous Blush-On	.21	$

SPECIALTY BRANDS

Astarte Blush	.12	$
The Body Shop Powder Blush (refillable)	.21	$
Matrix Colors Velvette Treatment Blush	.20	$$
Origins Blush-On Color Compact (refillable)	.14	$$

THE EYES HAVE IT

More than anywhere else, the eyes give away your age and make many women look older than they are. In addition to crow's-feet, crepey eyelids, and bagginess under the eyes, you may eventually have to deal with puffiness, unmanageable eyelashes, dark circles, recessed eyes, spider veins, and tiny whiteheads. Skin care and plastic surgery can correct many of these problems, but carefully applied makeup can hide all kinds of problems and enhance your best features all at once and for a fraction of the cost. Remember that when it comes to eye makeup, the adage that "less is more" has never been more applicable.

Eyebrows

Eyebrows should frame your eye, starting at the inner corner of your eye and extending to the outer corner. Never wax or tweeze away eyebrows and then pencil them back in, or tweeze them into a one-hair line.

The older I get, the more I think waxing eyebrows is a good option. As my eyesight gets a little poorer, it's easier for me to manage the shape of my eyebrows with a once-a-month waxing. I can handle the occasional stray with my tweezers. I like Revlon or Tweezerman tweezers because they are accurate and easy to work.

Eyebrow color should coordinate with your hair color, so if you are a bleached blond, have someone lighten your eyebrows, too. Like your hair, eyebrows can become gray and the color can fade, so I recommend the powder "brush-on brows" to accent the color. Eyebrow pencils work great if you can apply them in short feathery strokes, but too many women end up with visible lines that just look fake, so I think the brush-on brows work better. Again, choose a color that coordinates with your hair color. *Do not try to color your eyebrows with at-home hair color.*

EYEBROW PRODUCTS

Price Key: $ under $10; $$ $11–$20

PRODUCT	PRICE
Clinique Brow Shaper	$$
Elizabeth Arden Dual Perfection Brow Shaper and Eyeliner	$$
Lancôme Mode le Sourcils Brow Groomer	$$
L'Oréal Brow Elegance Browliner	$
Revlon Natural Brow Color & Style System	$

Eye Shadows

The very first rule of eye shadow for older eyes is to avoid any pearl or frosted eye shadows because the pearlescence will enhance wrinkles and crepiness. If you have some in your drawer, throw them out and don't buy any more. A semimatte shadow, or something labeled "age-defying" or "dewy" is better. Those products will give you just a little moistness without the aging frostiness. Use the same guidelines that directed your blush color choices in choosing eye shadows. If you have pink undertones in your skin, choose warm shadows. If your complexion is warm, and has yellow undertones, choose cool-colored shadows.

Elaine's Exclusive

EYE CARAMBA!

If your eye shadow seems to stop abruptly with a definable line, apply a dry sponge, ever so lightly to the edges to eliminate the harsh line.

For mature eyes, I recommend neutral shades such as cinnamon, honey, taupe, mocha, or reddish browns in a matte finish. Highlight the brow bone with soft pinks, beiges, or peach colors. Steer clear of trendy fashion colors, and remember, the more muted shades will camouflage crinkly eyelids.

To prevent eye shadow from creasing and to hide redness or darkness around the eyes, apply a little foundation or eye shadow primer to the eye area. If you plan to go without eye shadow, smooth your foundation over your lids to give yourself a more polished look and highlight your brow bone with just a touch of your blush. Makeup artists do this all the time, but because blushes very often contain coal tar dyes that irritate eyes, I usually caution against it unless you use a blush, like Shiseido's, that you are certain is free of coal tar dyes.

Deeply recessed eyes can benefit from a little highlight on the bottom lid, very close to the lashes, and a medium shade on the outer corner of the eye, followed by just a touch of highlight on the brow bone.

Eye shadows come in creams, cream powders, and pencils or crayons and the best one to use is mostly a matter of personal preference.

Powders offer the widest variety of colors and finishes, but some people find that the powders come off too easily. Applying loose powder over the lid, before the shadow, will help absorb any extra moisture and a quick brush of finishing powder will help set it when you're done. I particularly like powder shadows because they are very blendable and often sold packaged with complementary shades for highlighting.

Cream shadows may be too greasy for older, wrinkled eyelids, but the tubes make application easy.

Pencils and crayons deposit color right where you want them, but test them before buying to be sure that they glide on easily. Pressing too hard is no good for delicate skin.

EYE SHADOWS

Price Key: $ under $10; $$ $11–$21; $$$ $21–$30; $$$$ $31–$40; $$$$$ over $40

DEPARTMENT STORE BRANDS

PRODUCT	PRICE
Adrian Arpel Mix & Match Shadow Kit duo (refillable; includes one-time cost of compact)	$$$
Elizabeth Arden Eye Color Naturals single	$$

PRODUCT	PRICE
Elizabeth Arden Eye Color Naturals duo	$$
Estee Lauder Compact Disk Eye Shadow	$
Iman Luxury Eye Shadow	$
Lancôme Maquiriche Creme Powder Eye Colour Duo Personalized Selection (includes one-time cost of compact)	$$
M.A.C. Eye Shadow small	$
M.A.C. Eye Shadow large	$$
Philosophy Word of Mouth	$$
Prescriptives Eye Shadow Doubles Refillable (includes one-time cost of compact)	$$$
Prescriptives Eye & Cheek Compact Refillable (includes two shadows & blush and one-time cost of compact)	$$$$
Princess Marcella Borghese Shadow Milano single	$$
Princess Marcella Borghese Shadow Milano duo	$$$
Princess Marcella Borghese Shadow Milano trio	$$$$
Shiseido Gradation Colors blush & shadow	$$$
Shiseido Petit Shadow duo	$$$
Ultima II The Nakeds Eye Color	$$
Ultima II Wonderwear Eye Color Duets	$$

DRUGSTORE BRANDS

Almay Easy To Wear Long Lasting Eye Color	$
L'Oréal Soft Effects	$
Maybelline Natural Accents Eye Shadow	$
Revlon Age Defying Eye Color	$
L'Oréal Colour! Colour! Eye Shadow Trios	$

SPECIALTY BRANDS

Matrix Colors Eye Silks	$

Eyeliner

Eyeliner will give your eye definition and, unless your eyes are particularly recessed or there is a great deal of darkness above or below the eyes, no one should leave home without it.

Eyeliner comes in pencil or liquid. I recommend using pencils to line the eyelids, especially for older women whose hands may not be as steady and whose eyes may be a little too weak to apply liquid eye-liner straight. Also, liquid eyeliner can appear harsh. Choose any inexpensive pencil that is not so hard that it tugs at the eye, or so soft that it crumbles. There is no reason in the world to spend $12 for a department store brand eye pencil.

Apply the pencil to the outer three-quarters of the lower lid and all across the upper lid as close to the lash line as possible, smudging the color just a bit with a Q-tip.

When applying eyeliner, choose a color that coordinates with your eye shadow and work from the outside of the eye toward the middle. Dark black eyeliner should be reserved for the darkest complexions, everyone else should stick with soft blacks, gray, navy, or brown.

EYELINERS

Like lip liners, there's no need to spend lots of money on eyelining pencils, and as I've said before, liquid eyeliners are not the best for women with failing eyesight and shaky hands. The following pencils do a fine job for less than $10. Lancôme, Prescriptives, and Princess Marcella Borghese make particularly good pencils in a wide range of colors that you may wish to spend more for. The Borghese pencil even comes with a sharpener and a smudging tip.

PRODUCT
L'Oréal Le Grand Kohl Perfectly Soft Liner
Max Factor Eye Designer Shadow Liner with sponge tip
Max Factor Pensilks Glide-On Eye Pencil
Maybelline Smoked Kohl Eyeliner
Origins Eye Pencil
Revlon Colorstay Eye Liner
Revlon Soft Stroke Powder Liner
The Body Shop Eye Liner

Mascara

As we get older, mascara, the staple product of the makeup drawer, becomes more of a necessity because our eyelashes become thinner and more sparse. Applying mascara is as easy as passing the wand over the lashes from base to tip and choosing the right color—

black for women with dark hair, brown for everyone else, and never navy, green, or turquoise (leave them for the teenagers). Couldn't be simpler.

Unless you'll be swimming, crying a lot, or you have allergies, stick with nonwaterproof mascara. The waterproof variety is hard to remove without eye-makeup remover and many women pull out half of their lashes trying to get it off.

Elaine's Exclusives

A REAL EYE-OPENER

An eyelash curler will help open up your eyes, so use it every day, but always remember to curl first and apply mascara second to avoid breaking lashes. Maybelline makes the very best eyelash curler on the market.

LASHING OUT

For the longest lashes ever, press loose powder on top and bottom lashes. Apply mascara. Allow mascara to dry and apply a second coat. If you wear contacts, do this before putting in your lenses.

Most mascaras are created equally and since they should be replaced every three months to avoid the buildup of bacteria, I recommend choosing an inexpensive drugstore brand product. Within any given brand there will be several mascara products. Some contain fibers to lengthen lashes, others are thicker formulations that coat the lashes more heavily to make them look fuller. Choose the product that suits your particular needs. Women who wear contact lenses should avoid lash-lengthening mascaras. They contain rayon and nylon fibers, which can get underneath the lenses.

Whatever product you choose, when applying mascara, be sure to avoid overcoating lashes and ending up with clumps. Nothing ages the eyes more. If you get clumps, use an eyelash comb to detangle the mess.

MASCARA

Mascaras fall into the same category as lip- and eyeliners. There's no need to spend extra money for department store products when the $5 to $7.50 drug-store products are as good as they get. Also, to reduce the risk of eye infections, you'll want to buy new mascara every three months anyway. Many women love Lancôme mascaras, and I can't argue with their endorsement, but there's no need to spend twice as much for them. I've listed my favorite products below. Contact-lense wearers should be sure to avoid lash-lengthening products. Most packages labels will tell you if the products are appropriate for those who wear contacts. All of these mascaras sell for under $10.

PRODUCT

Almay One Coat Waterproof Mascara
Almay Amazing Lash Mascara
Avon Full Figured Mascara
The Body Shop Mascara
L'Oréal Voluminous Mascara
L'Oréal Sensitique Mascara
Max Factor 2000 Calorie Mascara
Max Factor Stretch Mascara
Maybelline Great Lash—Pro Vitamin
Revlon Colorstay Mascara
Revlon Lashful Mascara
Revlon Quick Thick Mascara

LIP COLOR: DON'T LEAVE HOME WITHOUT IT

Lipstick works with blush to add color to your face and, as such, lip color should always coordinate with your blush.

Always define your lips with a liner that coordinates with your lip color. Forget about trends like the one that showed dark lip liner and lighter lip color, says Janet Paolucci from Manhattan's Gerard Bollei Salon. Leave the trends to the kids. If your lips are too full, apply the liner just inside the natural line, and if they are too thin, which is more likely for older women, apply the liner just outside the natural line.

Matte lip colors leave something to be desired for older women who want the dewy look of youth, so choose a cream that has a little gloss in it. If you just love your matte color, smooth on a little gloss to give it shine. Frosted colors are best used sparingly because they can draw attention to lines around the lip area.

The biggest problem most older women have is bleeding lipstick. In the morning you look like a million dollars, but by lunchtime your lipstick has run halfway to your nose, traveling up those highways etched into your upper lip.

There are several tricks to stop that from happening and a few products, namely Estee Lauder's Lip Zone and Sorme, that really keep lipstick in place without burning or drying out the lips. In addition, try applying powder or foundation to your lips before putting on your lipstick. Lip liners made with silicone derivatives such as Revlon's Colorstay help keep lipstick in place, too.

Many women find that lipstick tends to darken after a while and cosmetics company chemists tell me that's because the lipstick is reacting to the woman's saliva. If this happens to you, just choose the next shade lighter, even if it looks too light when you test it. It will probably darken as you wear it.

Because there are so many great, inexpensive lipsticks that come in a wide variety of colors, I generally don't recommend spending $15 or $20 for a tube. But, because the right lipstick can really make or break your look and can greatly improve your own morale, if the color that's just perfect for you costs a little more, buy it. You're worth it.

Elaine's Exclusive

LIP SERVICE: THE FOOLPROOF WAY TO FIND THE PERFECT LIP COLOR

- Test lipstick on the palm of your hand.
- Draw a line in the V between your thumb and forefinger and hold it next to your mouth.
- Remember that yellow-based lipsticks will accentuate yellowing teeth. Blue-based reds will whiten teeth, but older women should avoid blood-reds because they are too harsh.

LIPSTICK

Lipstick selection is a very personal choice driven mostly by color and texture. Some women swear by Chanel products, while others, myself included, have found drugstore and private label products in a wide range of colors that feel nice and stay on for hours. Even though I don't recommend matte lipsticks for older women, if you have a favorite shade in a matte formulation, just brighten it up with a little lip gloss. The products recommended here were chosen because they are creamy-moist, wear well, and come in a broad range of shades.
Price Key: $ under $10; $$ $11–$20; $$$ over $20

DEPARTMENT STORE BRANDS

PRODUCT	PRICE
Clinique Long Last Soft Shine	$$
Christian Dior Rouge Aleures	$$
Estee Lauder True Lipstick	$$
Estee Lauder Perfect Lipstick (SPF 4)	$$
Iman Luxury Moisturizing Lipstick	$$
Lancôme Rouge Absolu Lipstick	$$
M.A.C. Lipstick	$$
Prescriptives Extraordinary Lipstick	$$
Princess Marcella Borghese Lip Treatment Moisture (SPF 15)	$$
Princess Marcella Borghese Lumina Lipstick	$$
Shiseido Staying Power Lipstick	$$
Shiseido Advanced Performance Lipstick	$$
Ultima II Super Luscious Lipstick	$$

DRUGSTORE BRANDS

Almay Color Basics Lipstick	$
L'Oréal Colour Endure Stay-On Lipcolour	$
Max Factor Lasting Color Lipstick	$
Maybelline Shades of You Cream Lipstick	$
Moon Drops Lipstick	$
Revlon Super Lustrous Lipstick	$

HOME SALES/SPECIALTY STORES

Astarte Lipstick	$
Avon Beyond Color Triple Benefit Lipstick (SPF 12)	$

PRODUCT	PRICE
Avon Perfect Wear Color	$
The Body Shop Colourings Lipstick	$
Origins Lipcolor	$

LIP LINERS

There are any number of private label and inexpensive lip liners that are priced starting at $1.99. Because lip liners all do the same job and come in a variety of colors, there's no real reason to spend more than $10 for a lip pencil, unless you buy a department store lipstick and want the exact pencil to match. Ordinarily, though, you'll be able to find an inexpensive pencil that matches closely. When shopping for a pencil, look for something that applies easily without a lot of pulling or pressing.

PRODUCT	PRICE
L'Oréal Lip Precision	$
Revlon Colorstay Lipliner	$
Revlon Time Liner for Lips	$
Nat Robbins Lip Liner	$
Maybelline Shades of You Lip Liner	$
The Body Shop Colourings Lip Liner	$
Origins Lip Pencil	$
M.A.C. Lip Pencil	$

KNOCK IT OFF

Companies like Russ Kalvin have been knocking off designer formulas of hair products and fragrances for years, but now a company in San Antonio known as DCA (Designer Classic Alternatives) is knocking off lipsticks. They sell Chanel, Lancôme, and Estee Lauder lipstick knockoff that are remarkably similar to the original for only $2.99. Usually an imitator's packaging leaves a lot to be desired, but DCA even does a good job of packaging their products. The one drawback is that they imitate only a few shades from each brand, so the selection is limited.

POWDER: PUFF UP YOUR COSMETIC CONFIDENCE

There's nothing like light, luxurious powder to set your makeup, and tone down any shine that breaks through, and today's ultrafine powders are the best ever. If you are an older woman who gave up powder years ago because it was getting caked into your wrinkles, I urge you to give it another try. Today's products are fabulous. Revlon's Julio Ross explained to me that tiny spherical materials, often called microbubbles by the marketing departments, make it possible for even the most wrinkled women to wear powder again.

I prefer loose powder, because it doesn't get stuck in the creases the way even the new compact powders sometimes can. When I'm away from home, I keep a small amount of loose powder in an old eye-shadow container and sponge it on for touch-ups. At home, I use a large, soft brush, tap off any excess powder, and then fluff on a very light coating to set my makeup for the day.

If you buy pressed powder, apply it lightly with a brush and throw away the puff. Pressed powder can deliver a nice, sheer finish, but not if you use the powder puff that comes with the compact.

POWDER

*Even though today's powders are all finely milled, if you don't want to look like you're wearing a mask, it's important to apply only a light dusting of powder with a wide, fluffy brush instead of the powder puff that comes with the product. I prefer loose powder, but have recommended a few pressed powders for those of you who prefer a compact. The following products are recommended because each is a silky, luxurious product that I am sure you will enjoy wearing. You may be interested to know that blindfolded samplers could not tell the difference between the L'Oréal loose powder and any of the department store brands.
Price Key: $ under $10; $$ $11–$21; $$$ $21–$30; $$$$ $31–$40; $$$$$ over $40*

DEPARTMENT STORE PRODUCTS

PRODUCT	SIZE (OZ)	PRICE
Christian Dior Loose Powder	.88	$$$$$
Clarins Face Powder	1.4	$$$
Clarins Powder Compact	.28	$$$
Estee Lauder Moisture Balance Translucent Face Powder	.2	$$$
Flori Roberts Gold Chromatic Loose Powder with Silk Oil-Free	1.2	$$

PRODUCT	SIZE (OZ)	PRICE
Iman Luxury Loose Powder	.7	$$
Lancôme Poudre Majeur Pressed Powder	.38	$$$
Lancôme Poudre Majeur Loose Powder with Microbubbles	.7	$$$
M.A.C. Face Powder	.87	$$
Prescriptives All Skins Powder	.8	$$
Princess Marcella Borghese Pressed Powder with sunscreen	.33	$$$
Shiseido Pressed Powder	.49	$$$
Ultima II The Nakeds Pressed Powder	.32	$$

DRUGSTORE PRODUCTS

PRODUCT	SIZE (OZ)	PRICE
L'Oréal Hydra Perfecte Loose Powder	.5	$

SPECIALTY PRODUCTS

PRODUCT	SIZE (OZ)	PRICE
Astarte Portable Finish Powder	.5	$$
Origins Loose Powder	1.4	$$

WISH LIST

The following items are truly fabulous products, although they cost much more than other products of their kind. Can you live without them? Absolutely. But if you're in the mood to spend money on yourself, you may want to consider splurging on one of these items.
Price Code: $ under $20; $$ $20–$50

PRODUCT	PRICE
The Body Shop Peppermint Foot Lotion	$
Chanel Maximum Moisture Lip Treatment (SPF 8)	$$
Christian Dior Eye Shadow Duo	$$
Christian Dior Face Powder	$$
Clarins Bio-Ecolia Perfecting Cream-Mask	$$
Donna Karan Cashmere Hand and Body Lotion	$$
Elizabeth Arden Smooth Lining Eye Pencil	$
Lancôme Mascaras	$
La Prairie Bronzer	$$
M.A.C. Shave Rasage	$

PRODUCT	PRICE
Prescriptives Softlining Eye Pencil dual-ended	$
Shiseido Absolute Lipstick Remover	$
Yves St. Laurent Radiant Touch Concealer	$$

HOT TIPS FROM THE PROS

Makeup artist Cheryl Stuart from David J. Witchell Salon in Newtown, Pennsylvania, offers the following tips for great makeup:

1. If your makeup gets cakey in certain areas, dampen a sponge with water or alcohol-free toner. Smile hard to accentuate the lines and press the sponge into the cakey area. The dampness will hydrate the area and the sponge will lift out the excess foundation.
2. To give eyes a lift, dot concealer on the top of the brow bone and under the eyes near the brow bone. Blend with a sponge.
    Or: Carry eyeliner across eye and lift top and bottom corners just a little. Apply lighter color shadow under eye and blend up toward corner.
3. Run away from anyone offering permanent makeup, which is essentially tattooing. The promise of never again applying eye makeup may be alluring, but with age, lips thin, cheeks lose their fat pads, eyes become recessed, and jowls sag. Eventually you'll end up with makeup where you don't want it.
4. Over time, foundation will oxidize and become one or two shades darker, so if your foundation doesn't seem right all of a sudden, it may be time for a new bottle.

Mari Aldin of Astarte makes these recommendations for Black women:

1. Choose alcohol-free, fragrance-free, and oil-free cosmetics with built-in sunscreen to prevent reactions from super-sensitive Black skin.
2. Select a foundation that matches the cheeks by applying three stripes on the cheek in line with the nostrils, in a vertical direction. Do not match foundation to the hairline, which tends to be darker than the rest of the face.

3. To prevent ashiness, use a gentle scrub product once or twice a week.
4. Black skin reflects light and therefore appears shiny, but don't just assume it is oily. Check your skin type to be sure.

Janet Paolucci, of the Gerard Bollei Salon, says:

1. To make creamy makeup a little more sheer, add a little bit of moisturizer to it.
2. Avoid clumpy mascara by applying two light coats and using an eyelash comb to separate lashes.

Elaine's Exclusive

NOTHING LASTS FOREVER

Despite all of the preservatives and advanced chemistry that's applied to cosmetics, no product will last a lifetime. To avoid using products that are past their prime, remember these simple rules.

1. Date your cosmetics at the time of purchase.
2. Buy from reliable retailers, never from a flea market.
3. Don't accept a dusty package or one that has two price stickers on it. The product may have been sitting for months.
4. If a product separates or has a foul odor, don't use it.
5. Clean out your makeup drawer every six months.
6. Discard products after the following time periods:

mascara	3 months
eye pencils	3 years, if there is no eye irritation
foundation	1 year
powder	3 years
eye shadow	3 years, if there is no flaking or eye irritation
lip color	2 years; keep away from heat and discontinue use if irritation develops.
fragrance	5 years; keep away from heat and light.

Laura Geller of Laura Geller Make Up Studios in New York offers these tips for selecting blush and eye makeup colors based upon hair color:

Blondes: Select muted, almost watercolor-like colors from muted mauves to coral pinks. Avoid strong, defined lines and colors.

Black or brunette: Use color to create contrast and pay attention to lips and eyes. Don't use oranges or corals and go easy on the blush to avoid looking like a Kewpie doll.

Redheads: Your hair brings color to your face anyway so use warm, muted colors on your cheeks, but not too much brown and certainly not strong orange. Play up your eyes.

Elaine's Exclusive

BACK TO M.A.C.

M.A.C. encourages customers to recycle their products' packages through an innovative program that is part recycling initiative, part frequent-buyer program. Every time a customer returns an empty M.A.C. plastic container, M.A.C. puts a Back to M.A.C. sticker on a special card. When the customer collects six stickers, she can select a free lipstick. M.A.C. takes responsibility for ensuring that the containers are properly recycled.

Helen Lee of the Helen Lee Day Spa, New York, offers these tips for Asian women.

1. Choose blush and lipstick that are rosy or soft pink and even reds that lean a little toward the blue spectrum. They will stand up nicely to yellow-toned skin without making it look monotone or flat.
2. Buy a yellow foundation toner to even out your skin color.
3. Use a medium or light color shadow over the entire eyelid, brushing upward and outward to give the eye lift, hide puffiness, and avoid a dark or dirty look.

KEEP IT SIMPLE

Everyday makeup needn't be an involved process. Once you've selected the right colors for your skin tones, you can get a great look every day in less than ten minutes and with fewer than ten steps. Just be sure to select your products ahead of time, so you don't waste time fumbling in your makeup drawer.

Step 1   apply concealer (30–45 seconds)

Step 2   apply foundation (1.5–2 minutes)

Step 3   apply cheek contour (optional; 15 seconds)

Step 4   fluff on cheek color (15 seconds)

Step 5   blend, using buff & puff technique (15 seconds)

Step 6   apply eyeliner, shadow, and mascara (2 minutes)

Step 7   accent brows if needed (15 seconds)

Step 8   apply lip fix, lip liner, and lipstick (30 seconds)

Step 9   admire yourself and add more color if needed (30 seconds)

Chapter 11

HAIR TODAY

"When I go to the beauty parlor, I always use the emergency entrance. Sometimes I just go for an estimate."
—PHYLLIS DILLER

Perhaps more than any other part of the body, our hair says a lot about us. It's the first thing many people notice, and one of the first characteristics used to describe us to others. She's a blond, redhead, brunette. Her hair is long, short, braided, teased, bobbed, cornrowed, bleached, frosted—you get it.

Some of us let our hair make political or social statements for us. Skinheads choose a certain hairstyle, or lack thereof, so that the world immediately knows something about their point of view. In the sixties, everyone who was young and questioning authority conveyed that message by growing their hair long. People in the armed forces wear short, no-nonsense haircuts. Corporate women tend to have stylish haircuts that reflect a minimum of fuss—very professional and to the point.

We use hair to communicate emotions, tossing it back when we're feeling free, exhilarated, and confident, twirling it when we're shy or unsure, running our hands through it when we're stressed, running them through someone else's when we're feeling sexy. How many of us go out for a new haircut, permanent, or color when we need an emotional lift?

We remember people for their hair. Farrah Fawcett's tresses made her famous and Barbara Bush's white mane made women everywhere feel more comfortable. Certainly boxing promoter Don King has a singular style and poor Hillary Clinton attracted an awful lot of unwanted attention as she tried on different hairstyles.

Hair has even made it into the vernacular. When everything seems to go uncontrollably wrong, we're having a bad hair day. When everything is going our way and we look great besides, it's a good hair day. Hair has even had its own Broadway musical.

Because of the important role hair plays in our lives, magazines are constantly filled with articles about the season's newest cuts and colors. Companies fill store shelves with shampoos, conditioners, at-home coloring products, and styling aids, and spend a bundle in advertising to convince us that "we're worth it." In fact, we spend more than $2.5 billion a year in shampoo and conditioner alone, according to Packaged Facts.

So many products and so much advice can make it difficult to keep our crowning glories looking and feeling glorious, but having shiny, healthy hair really isn't complicated at all.

THE ANATOMY OF HAIR

Like skin and nails, hair is made of protein, mostly keratin, and each strand is comprised of three layers. The cuticle, which is the outer layer, is formed by cells that overlap like roof shingles. Below the cuticle is the cortex, which makes up the hair's bulk and color, and at the center is the medulla, a thin core of cells and air space. Each strand springs forth from the hair follicle and each follicle has its own blood, nerve, and muscle supply.

Illness, injury, poor nutrition, poor circulation, lack of exercise, and any number of systemic problems manifest themselves in the way hair looks because hair cells reproduce faster than any other cells in the body, except bone marrow. As a result, even the slightest changes or upset to the status quo can impact the hair. This is why hair falls out during cancer treatment. Chemotherapy is essentially poison that is administered to the entire body to kill off cancer cells. The poison in the bloodstream finds its way to the hair follicles, too, killing off cells and causing hair loss.

There has been much written about hair being dead. Indeed, the hair shaft does not have a blood supply, nerves, or muscles, notes Philip Kingsley, an internationally known trichologist, salon-owner, and author of *Hair, An Owner's Handbook*. In that sense, it is dead. But it is remarkably resilient considering how we color it, cut it, apply chemicals to it, brush, curl, and comb it.

"Even though hair is dead, it can still be affected," says Muggs Lerberg, director of education for Redmond/Aussie hair products. "You still dye your clothes, bleach them, and put in fabric softener. Clothing is dead, too, but it can be affected and changed."

HAIR QUALITY

Once we simply described hair as dry, normal, or oily and chose products accordingly, but today, we know that those descriptions are incomplete at best. Hair also has other qualities that can be addressed with hair-care products, so it is best to know not only whether your hair is dry, normal, or oily, but also the following qualities:

Texture: Is your hair, fine, medium, or coarse?

Shape: Limp, straight, wavy, curly, or frizzy?

In general, thin hair tends to be limp; coarse, thick hair is more likely to be wavy and full of body. Choose products that claim to give your hair what you want. For example:

If your hair is frizzy, you want control, manageability, and moisture.

If your hair is limp, you want body or volume.

If your hair is curly, you may want something to soften the hair.

If your hair is straight, you may want extra body to hold a style.

If your hair is fine, you may want to add moisture and volume.

If you have coarse hair, you may want to smooth and soften it.

The message here is don't try to select products based on one descriptive. Take a good look at your hair and then choose products that will address all of your needs.

AGING HAIR

Just as your skin becomes thinner, drier, and less elastic with age, so too does your hair. And just as we tend to slow down physically, so does hair growth. The hair does everything the rest of your body does.

Hair is thinner in diameter and there is less of it by the time most people reach age forty. Unfortunately, the thinning and slow growth causes many people to do more with their hair in terms of permanents and regular colorings, which spawns a need for more careful and frequent hair care. Daily shampooing and conditioning are important to maintaining the health of chemically treated hair or hair that has simply become drier with age.

When you've reached a stage where you notice that you have less hair, be sure to be especially diligent about covering your head to protect your scalp from sunburn. In the winter, covering your head will protect your body from heat loss as well as sunburn.

Gray Hair

I know women who can point to their gray hairs and tell you the incident and child responsible. "I got my first gray hairs when my fifteen-year-old was two hours late coming home from her first car date," remembered one friend. Stress is probably the main factor most people blame for their gray hairs and according to Kingsley, stress really can cause gray hair, although probably not isolated incidents like dating daughters. Stress eats up the body's vitamin B reserves, which nourish the hair. People who are constantly under high stress can, indeed, turn gray ahead of schedule. He adds that patients have been known to reverse the graying process by taking high doses of vitamin B.

More than stress, gray hair is most commonly associated with old age, but the truth is, it can happen at almost any age—people in their twenties will start to turn gray if it's a family trait, and pregnant women have also been known to sprout gray hairs because of their hormonal fluctuations.

"Gray hair is simply a loss of pigment, like a pen running out of ink," says Manhattan salon-owner Beth Minardi. And it can be caused by anemia, thyroid problems, and diabetes as well as heredity. Contrary to popular opinion, gray hair is not necessarily coarse. In fact, it is usually thinner than the original hairs. What's different is that the hair tends to be drier because the oil glands are not functioning as well as they once did. The loss of pigment can make gray hair wiry, so you may need to begin using a styling gel to tame the wild hairs. Permanents also help control hairs that have a mind of their own.

Most women I know start out covering their few strands of gray with hair color, but there comes a time when the gray starts winning the race for dominance over your head. That's when some women decide to forsake their every six-week touch-up in favor of the "natural look." I'd like to be able to help you decide whether or not you should let your hair go, but the choice is really only a matter of personal preference. Gray or white hair can be stunning—just look at Barbara Bush, Kenny Rogers, or former Texas governor Ann Richards. Also it's certainly easier to care for than hair that requires regular coloring. While you're toying with the decision, go to a wig shop and try on a gray or white wig to see how you'd look, or seek out a fancy salon that has an imaging computer that can show you how you'd look with any color or style.

Once you decide to keep the gray, be sure to wash your hair daily, as gray hair shows dirt more readily. Also, if you still smoke or if you perm your hair, consider a blue rinse or blue shampoo to help keep the color from yellowing. (Try limiting your use of the blue shampoo or rinse to once or twice a week to avoid getting a blue cast to your hair.)

Gray hair also tends to absorb light, so you might want to use a small amount of shiner or glosser to add luster. Don't use too much, though, or your hair will look greasy.

ETHNIC HAIR

Black hair tends to be thin, which you would not normally want to condition much for fear of weighing it down. But because the tight curls often need additional moisturizing and conditioning for detangling purposes, it is important to use a conditioner so that you can comb and detangle the hair without breaking it. Pulling and combing without the benefit of a conditioner can result in broken hair and stress to the hair follicle.

Asian hair is just about perfect. It tends to be thick, straight, and full of body, requiring little special treatment except for styling purposes. What's more, Asian women tend to turn gray later in life than their Black or Caucasian counterparts, and they are least likely to experience hair loss.

HAIR LOSS

We all lose hair every day—that's natural. Thinning hair, however, is cumulative hair loss that suddenly becomes noticeable. Usually by the time it becomes noticeable, it's been happening for some time and women are thunderstruck.

There are any number of reasons why twenty million normal, healthy women, like men, begin losing their hair; so before you can decide to do anything about it, you first need to determine the cause.

Illness or Medication

Anemia, thyroid problems, hormonal changes, nutritional deficiencies, stress, and high fever are among the many ailments that can cause hair to fall out. In fact, hair loss can be one of the first indications of a medical problem. If you notice that you are suddenly losing your hair, see your doctor immediately for a complete physical or consult with an endocrinologist.

Certain medications, including thyroid drugs, birth control pills, cortisone, tranquilizers, amphetamines, antibiotics, blood thinners, aspirin, and even an excess of vitamin A can cause hair loss. If you're taking any of these drugs and experience hair loss, be sure to discuss it with your doctor, as he or she may be able to prescribe an alternate medication for you.

Heredity

Heredity plays a role in male- and female-pattern hair loss, which is primarily dictated by the presence of the male hormone, androgen, on the hair follicle. But everyone has androgen, and not everyone loses their hair. Therefore, the only people who will become sparse on top are those who are genetically susceptible. For unknown reasons, blondes tend to experience more hair loss than other Caucasian women. According to Kingsley, it is a myth that baldness is inherited only from your mother's side of the family.

Female baldness patterns tend to come in two types: diffuse hair loss when the hair thins out all over, and the female version of male-pattern baldness, a thinning on the top of the head only. Typically the first inch of the hair line, above the forehead, remains intact and the thinning happens on the top.

Chemotherapy

This form of cancer treatment is essentially cell-killing poison that is intended to wipe out cancer cells. Unfortunately, in doing so, it also weakens other body systems, making us more prone to infection and causing hair loss. The good news is that hair grows back, usually quickly, once the treatment is stopped.

Dermatologist Dr. Wilma Bergfeld recommends using minoxidil, commonly sold as Rogaine, as a prophylactic measure against hair loss. Other than that, there is not much you can do to prevent the loss from occurring. You can, however, keep your scalp healthy by treating it to gentle cleansing and moisturizing until the hair grows back—and it will. Often hair returns much different from its original state. Curly-headed people suddenly have straight hair and vice versa.

Friction

Frictional hair loss is especially common among Black women due to attempts to straighten the hair by pulling it with rollers or irons. Choosing chemical straightening techniques can help lessen this kind of traction hair loss. Women who wear severely pulled-back hairstyles and those who sleep on tight rollers can also develop this kind of hair loss.

REMEDIES FOR HAIR LOSS

Unless you are experiencing pattern hair loss that is due to changing hormones and heredity, chances are very good that your hair will eventually grow back.

If your condition is hereditary, and therefore likely to be permanent, you can seek out permanent solutions in the form of hair transplants. Those who suffer from the female-pattern-type baldness described earlier are the best candidates for transplant therapy, says Dr. Robert Leonard, a Cranston, Rhode Island, hair transplant specialist.

Hair Transplants

Today's transplants involve removing hair from the sides and back where it is abundant and transplanting it where hair has ceased to grow. Under local anesthesia, doctors remove hair follicles a few at a time and then reinsert them in the scalp using small incisions. The new techniques are vastly improved from the old plugs that gave the recipient a Barbie-hair look that was aesthetically unpleasing—but for some people preferable to baldness. These newer methods, moving a few follicles at a time, can give a much more natural look.

The transplanted hair brings with it its own genetic message so it will continue to grow as if it were on the sides of the head. Keep in mind, though, that pattern baldness is progressive, so repeat grafts may be necessary to avoid having an island effect on the top of your head. The cost for transplants starts at around $2,000 and goes up depending on how thick you want the hair. According to Dr. Leonard, 5 to 8 percent of his patients are women.

Minoxidil

Experts disagree on how well minoxidil, now sold over the counter and best known as Rogaine, actually works. It was originally sold as minoxidil lonitin, a blood-pressure medication, and patients who were taking the drug discovered that they began regrowing body hair, which caused Upjohn's researchers to develop a topical application for the product. Until 1996 it was available only by prescription.

Even the ads for Rogaine state that it doesn't work for everyone and doctors caution that patients must be dedicated to the twice-daily application of the product for at least four months in order for it to work. As with most things, there are no guarantees, but since Rogaine is the best thing going for stopping hair loss, it's certainly worth a try.

Massage

As we age, each hair naturally becomes thinner, eventually creating a noticeable loss of volume. Scalp massage can stimulate blood flow to the hair follicles and possibly help keep them from thinning.

> **HAIR AND HORMONES**
> **The male hormone androgen is part of the recipe for pattern hair loss. In addition, menopause's declining estrogen levels can leave hair thinner and drier as we age. But just as hormone replacement therapy is known to provide a youthful glow to skin, it can also restore hair's luster and bounce and, more importantly, keep you from losing your hair.**

SHAMPOOING AND CONDITIONING

As in skin care, there are so many products on the market claiming to provide truly amazing benefits, it's hard to know what you need and which products to buy. But just as skin care doesn't need to be complicated, neither does hair care. Remember this: Cleansing and conditioning are the only things we must do to our hair to keep it healthy.

SHAMPOOING

Just as you bathe and wash your face everyday, you should shampoo daily to remove pollutants, dirt, and styling products, to leave hair clean and ready for the next day's style. Some years ago, daily shampooing got a bad rap for supposedly causing hair to dry out and for overstimulating oil production. The fact is that shampoo won't dry out hair and if your scalp is oily, daily shampooing will help keep hair from becoming greasy.

I know many older women who make a weekly visit to their local beauty salon for a wash and style and they don't do anything to their hair in between visits except for spraying on more hairspray and fluffing up their 'do. If it works for you, who am I to argue, especially if holding your arms over your head to wash and style is a problem, as it is for many older women. However, if your hair feels dry or unhealthy, you may want to consider more frequent cleansing and conditioning.

The trick, according to Kingsley, is to shampoo properly. He advises thoroughly soaking the hair first. Next, pour a small amount of shampoo into the hands and then run hands over the hair, distributing the shampoo as you go. Massage shampoo into the hair and scalp gently for about three minutes. Never scratch the scalp or use a massage brush. Run your fingers through your hair to prevent tangling and then rinse thoroughly. Once you've finished rinsing, he says, rinse again. Too often, dull hair is caused by shampoo residue.

Shampoo is essentially soap, with other ingredients mixed in, says Matthew Gurrola, director of quality assurance for Sebastian. The other ingredients are intended to cling to the hair, making it stronger, fuller, shinier, or less dry, depending on the type of hair the product was formulated to serve.

Elaine's Exclusives

LET'S CLEAR THIS UP

Clarifying shampoos that are created to clean away weeks of built-up conditioners and styling agents will also dull your hair color or even strip it away. Stay away from clarifiers if you color your hair.

ENEMY HAIR DRYER

Don't overdry the hair. Squeeze the excess moisture out of your hair with a towel (aggressive rubbing will cause tangling and breakage), and then use a blow-dryer until almost completely dry. Finish drying with your dryer on a cooler setting and a lower speed to avoid damaging the hair.

Essentially shampoos all do the same thing, which is cleanse the hair. The price difference in shampoo, says Gurrola, reflects the difference in the price of raw ingredients. "It's like a car," he says. "A '65 Volkswagen and a '96 Mercedes will both get you where you want to go, but one gives a better ride and has more style."

Some shampoos bill themselves as serving color-treated hair, gray hair, a permed hair, which generally means that they are gentle formulations with conditioning agents targeted for the hair's particular needs. Gray hair, for example, can look dull in daylight because gray absorbs light, so a shampoo for gray hair may have more silicones to make it shinier. Gray hair also tends to be wiry, so a gray-hair formulation may have more conditioners to make hair more manageable.

Specialty Shampoos

MOISTURIZING SHAMPOO These products contain more botanicals and humectants and are good for dry, frizzy, and chemically treated (permed or colored) hair. Look for ingredients like plant extracts and oils, panthenol, and glycerin in the formulation.

VOLUMIZING SHAMPOO If your hair is thin and limp, a volumizing shampoo will coat it with proteins or vitamins like panthenol (vitamin B5), says Redken's Lerberg. But, just as collagen cannot penetrate the skin, protein and vitamins cannot penetrate the hair shaft or "nourish" the hair. As ingredients in shampoo, the only thing protein and vitamins can do is coat the hair and provide temporary protection.

CLARIFYING SHAMPOO If you use a lot of styling aids, gels, mousses, or sprays, you may want to buy a bottle of clarifying shampoo, which strips away all of the built-up chemicals, leaving behind just naked hair. (Look for chelating agents, ingredients that end with the initials EDTA, or sodium aspartate on the label.) If you use a lot of products and find your hair feeling weighed down, this is a good way to get back to basics. Then, if your hair is still limp or lifeless, you can begin using new products that target that particular problem.

SPORT SHAMPOO These products are growing in popularity for their advertised ability to wash away perspiration, salts, chlorine, and pool chemicals, but truly, any shampoo will wash away those things along with dirt, dust, and pollution. Some of them, however, serve as shampoo and conditioner in one bottle, or double as a body wash, too, which makes them handy for the locker room.

SHAMPOO AND CONDITIONER All-in-one products that clean and condition may be handy, but they don't work as well as the individual products. In a pinch, they sure won't hurt and if you tend to shower at the gym or tennis club, it's certainly easier to take along just one bottle.

HORSE SHAMPOO Just as horse groomers discovered that the creams they applied to the horse's hooves strengthened their own fingernails, groomers also started using the shampoo used on horse's manes and tails on themselves. Those who've used it say that it makes hair manageable and silky, but I don't think it's worth spending extra money just for something that seems exotic or unusual.

SHAMPOO BARS In an effort to reduce trash, some companies have boiled the water out of their shampoos and turned them into bars, just like body soap, wrapped in paper. The formulations are made for every type of hair, so if you're environmentally concerned, you may want to try one of these.

EXPENSIVE VERSUS INEXPENSIVE
Do you *need* to spend $10 for a bottle of shampoo? Certainly not. Just as facial cleansers don't need to be expensive to clean the skin, shampoos don't need to be expensive either. If you like the way your hair looks and feels using inexpensive products, by all means stick with them. There are many fine products on the market. On the other hand, if you're having a hard time finding something you like, ask your stylist for a recommendation. It may cost more, but, in my book, anything that prevents a bad hair day is worth the price.

CONDITIONING

The purpose of conditioner is to improve the condition of the hair. Conditioners are intended to coat the hair in order to smooth the outer cells of the hair shaft, preventing tangles, eliminating static, adding moisture, body, or whatever the hair needs.

Again, the key to getting the most from a product without weighing down the hair is proper application: smoothing the product over the hair, especially the ends, avoiding the scalp, and then rinsing thoroughly.

Limp, lifeless hair is the most common complaint about conditioner, and if you have fine, limp hair that can be a real problem. Try using a conditioner on the hair and then applying a styling aid that adds volume and body, to counteract any additional softness problems that the conditioner creates.

Conditioners usually do one of two things: they either add moisture or body. Body-building conditioners give your hair bounce by coating each hair with proteins. Moisturizing conditioners are good for dry, brittle hair and for chemically treated (permed, colored) hair. Deep, leave-in conditioners are particularly good for coarse or curly hair, while daily conditioners work just fine for everyone else. TRE-Semme makes a great hot-oil treatment that does an excellent job of deep conditioning the driest, most damaged hair. For less than $3, it is worth trying if your hair is in bad shape.

SHAMPOOS AND CONDITIONERS FOR DRY, DAMAGED, AND CHEMICALLY TREATED HAIR

Price Key: $ under $5; $$ $6–$10

SHAMPOO

PRODUCT	SIZE (OZ)	PRICE
Aussie Moist Shampoo	16	$
Logics COLOReserve System Balancing Shampoo (color treated)	12	$$
L'Oréal ColorVIVE Gentle Shampoo (color treated)	11	$
Matrix Essentials Nourishing Shampoo (dry, damaged)	16	$$
Pantene Pro-V Shampoo Plus Pro-Vitamin Conditioner in One Revitalizing Formula (color treated/permed)	16	$
Pantene Pro-V Shampoo Plus Pro-Vitamin Conditioner in One Moisturizing Formula (dry-damaged)	16	$
Paul Mitchell Moisture & Shine Shampoo (dry/chemically treated)	9	$$
Redken One 2 One Moisturizing Shampoo (dry)	10.1	$$
Revlon Outrageous Moisture-Rich Shampoo for Dry, Permed, Color-Treated Hair	15	$
Sebastian Cello Shampoo (dry, color-treated, permed)	10	$$
TRESemme European Color-Treated & Permed Shampoo	32	$

CONDITIONERS

Aussie 3 Minute Miracle (dry, damaged, color treated)	8	$

PRODUCT	SIZE (OZ)	PRICE
L'Oréal ColorVIVE Creme Conditioner	11	$
Matrix Essentials Nutrient-Rich Conditioner	4	$$
Paul Mitchell Super-Charged Conditioner	4	$$
Revlon Outrageous Moisture Rich Conditioner (dry, color treated)	15	$
TRESemme European Color Treated Conditioner	32	$

SHAMPOOS AND CONDITIONERS FOR FINE, THIN, FRAGILE HAIR

Price Key: $ under $5; $$ $6–$10

SHAMPOO

PRODUCT	SIZE (OZ)	PRICE
Aussie Real Volume Shampoo	16	$
Helene Curtis Salon Selectives Level 6 (extra body)	15	$
L'Oréal FortaVIVE Conditioning Shampoo	11	$
Pantene Pro-V Shampoo Plus Pro-Vitamin Conditioner in One Extra Body formula	13	$
Redken One 2 One Volumizing Shampoo	10.1	$$
Revlon Outrageous Volumizing Shampoo	15	$
Sebastian Performance Active Shampoo	8.5	$$
Vavoom Shampooing	16	$$
Vidal Sassoon Ultra Care All-in-One Shampoo, Conditioner & Protective Finishing Rinse, Extra Body (Fine or Thin Hair)	10	$

CONDITIONERS

Aussie Leave-In Volumizer	8	$$
Aussie Slip Detangler	12	$
Aveda Rosemary/Mint Equalizer	8.45	$$
L'Oréal FortaVIVE Clean Rinse Conditioner (fine/fragile)	11	$
Redken One 2 One Daily Recovery Conditioner	10.1	$$
Revlon Outrageous Volumizing Conditioner	15	$
Vavoom Conditioning	16	$$
Vidal Sassoon Ultra Care All-In-One Rinse Extra Body for Fine or Thin Hair	13	$

SHAMPOOS AND CONDITIONERS FOR NORMAL HAIR

Price Guide: $ under $5; $$ $6–$10

SHAMPOO

PRODUCT	SIZE (OZ)	PRICE
Aussie Mega Shampoo	16	$
Clairol Herbal Essence Shampoo (moisture-balancing)	8	$
Helene Curtis Salon Selectives Level 5 (regular)	15	$
L'Oréal HydraVIVE Gentle Shampoo	11	$
Matrix Essentials Systeme Biolage Normalizing Shampoo	16	$$
Paul Mitchell Awapuhi Shampoo	8	$
Revlon Outrageous Moisturizing Shampoo (normal)	15	$
Sebastian Sliplene Shampoo	10	$
Senscience Energy Shampoo	8.4	$$
Vidal Sassoon Ultra Care All-In-One Shampoo, Conditioner & Protective Finishing Rinse, Balanced for Normal Hair	13	$
Volumax Shampoo	15	$

CONDITIONER

PRODUCT	SIZE (OZ)	PRICE
Aussie Slip Detangler	12	$
L'Oréal HydraVIVE Creme Conditioner (normal/dry)	11	$
Matrix Essentials Conditioning Balm Conditioner	4	$$
Revlon Outrageous Daily Beautifying Conditioner (normal/dry)	15	$
Volumax Conditioner	20	$

SHAMPOOS AND CONDITIONERS FOR GRAY, WHITE, PLATINUM, AND SILVER HAIR

Price Key: $ under $5; $$ $6–$10

SHAMPOO

PRODUCT	SIZE (OZ)	PRICE
Aussie Moonlight Reflections Shampoo	10	$
Aveda Blue Malva Shampoo	8.4	$$
Clairol Shimmer Lights Shampoo	8	$
Matrix Essentials So Silver Shampoo	12	$$
Nexxus Simply Silver Toning Shampoo	8.4	$$

PRODUCT	SIZE (OZ)	PRICE
Paul Mitchell Creatives Color Infusing Shampoo-In-Violet	8	$$
Paul Mitchell Shampoo One	8	$
Schwartzkopf Igofleur Prescription Color Shampoo—Gray Hair	8.5	$$

CONDITIONER

Clairol Shimmer Lights Conditioner	8	$
Matrix Essentials Simply Silk Detangling Rinse	12	$$
Nexxus Ensure Acidifying Conditioner	8.4	$$
Paul Mitchell, The Detangler	6	$$

DANDRUFF SHAMPOOS AND CONDITIONERS

Price Key: $ under $5; $$ $6–$10

SHAMPOO

PRODUCT	SIZE (OZ)	PRICE
Head & Shoulders Dandruff Shampoo	15	$
Matrix Systeme Biolage Anti-Dandruff Shampoo	16	$$
Nexxus Dandarest Dandruff Shampoo	8.4	$$
Zotos Bain de Terre Alpine Mist Dandruff Shampoo	16.9	$$

CONDITIONER

Matrix Systeme Biolage Daily Leave-In Tonic	12	$$
Paul Mitchell Creatives Lite Detangler	8	$$

THE COLORING BOOK

Years ago, no one wanted to admit to coloring their hair, because having to color your hair was an admission that you were getting old. Fortunately that's changed and today we have entire supermarket, drugstore, and beauty-supply aisles dedicated to coloring products. You can frequently hear women telling a friend or coworker that they have a date with Clairol #103 when they get home.

Unlike a few years ago, today we have a huge variety of good products from the three major players, Clairol, Revlon, and L'Oréal, to choose from and new products from new companies are entering the market all of the time. The problem with having such a variety is that making a selection can be very confusing. Thankfully, companies are beginning to remedy that problem by providing hair swatches in the store. L'Oréal supplied me with the following guide to hair coloring terminology that will make your shopping easier.

TEMPORARY COLOR Also called a rinse, temporary color washes out with the next shampoo. A blue rinse will help keep gray hair from yellowing, but be careful to avoid using too much or you'll end up as a blue-haired lady.

SEMIPERMANENT The hair cuticle is coated with color, but the hair's natural pigment is not altered. Semipermanent colors contain no ammonia and they can only add color to the hair, not lighten it. Semipermanent color will cover up to 50 percent of the gray, and will wash out in six to twelve shampoos.

TONE-ON-TONE These products deposit color on the cuticle and cortex but do not alter the natural pigment. Tone-on-tone colors add a complimentary color to the hair's natural color to enhance and brighten. They contain no ammonia and because there is no lightening, only the addition of color, you will not develop roots. Tone-on-tone will blend away 25 percent of the gray and will wash out after twenty or more shampoos.

PERMANENT COLOR Permanent color works on the cortex, where the natural pigment is lightened and then the new color is added. The color will last until the hair is cut off, which is why touch-ups are necessary to color new growth. Permanent color will cover gray completely. Blonding, lightening, highlighting, and frosting are also permanent processes.

PROGRESSIVE HAIR COLOR Progressive color uses metallic dye on the cuticle of the hair, and can only darken the hair. If you have this kind of coloring done, be sure to read the label of any new coloring product you may wish to use at a later date as some coloring products are not compatible with metallic dyes.

VEGETABLE DYES Vegetable dyes are a good choice for women who are allergic to chemical dyes. The process is safe, yet time-consuming, and can only add color to the hair, not lighten it. Henna is a common vegetable dye.

CHOOSING A COLOR

Once you've decided how long you want your color to last, then you must decide how you want your hair to look. Are you looking for a dramatic change or do you simply want to recapture some of the territory lost to gray hairs? Do you want highlights and a little brightness and luster or would you like to try a shade lighter or darker? You can really achieve just about any look you like with today's over-the-counter hair colors, but keep these hints in mind.

1. Because gray is an absence of color, it takes more hair color to cover it, so choose a shade darker than your regular color.
2. Select colors based on your skin tones:

    If your complexion is *cool*—that is pink or ruddy-toned—and tends to burn easily, and you have blue, green, or gray eyes, choose cool hair colors with words like Ash, Champagne, or Beige in the name.

    If your complexion is *warm*—dark, golden, or olive skin that tans easily—and you have brown, black, or amber eyes, select a hair color with words like golden, copper, auburn, or red in the name.

    If your complexion is a *dark, rich brown*, choose black, dark, warm brown, or dark auburn shades.

    If your complexion is *tawny*, choose dark or light brown, light auburn, or dark blonde shades.

    Keep in mind that if you're turning gray, your skin tone may be changing, too. Take a good, honest look in the mirror before going to the store.
3. Using the color charts provided in the store, identify your own *natural* hair color and then select a shade that is no more than two tones lighter or darker than your own color.
4. If you are debating between two shades, go for the lighter of the two colors for more contrast between your hair color and complexion.

When to Spring for Salon Color

One in three women color their hair. Most women I know go to the salon occasionally and use at-home products in between visits because today they really do get good results. It's been years since I've heard an at-home hair-coloring disaster story. The products do a nice job of coloring and leave hair feeling soft and manageable. But sometimes, doing it yourself is not the best option.

If you're considering permanent color for the first time, I'd recommend doing temporary color first to see how you like the look and then letting a trained salon colorist do it for you. Once you've had the first successful coloring under your belt, then try doing the touch-up yourself.

If you're contemplating a look that requires coloring, then frosting, or some other multiple process, or if you're having color removed for some reason, I'd let the professionals handle it.

And finally, if you're planning a new look for a big night out—a company awards dinner, child's wedding, big anniversary party, fiftieth birthday bash—don't try something new yourself. Call in the pros.

Prices for salon coloring will vary geographically and depend on the salon you use and the reputation of the colorist. Talk over your options with your salon's colorist (who is just as important to your look as your stylist), and pay attention to other women leaving the salon before you decide to make the leap. Remember, permanent color is just that, so don't do something drastic on a whim that you might regret later and have to live with for several months.

If you find that your gray comes back quickly after going to the salon for permanent color, go back to the salon and ask to have it redone. At the very least, be sure to mention it to the colorist the next time you are in the shop. There may be something she or he can do to help the color last longer the next time.

HELPFUL HINTS FOR HAPPY HAIR

1. Follow package instructions carefully, performing any patch tests for allergies and strand tests that are recommended.
2. Do not color damaged, bleached hair or apply color when there is a scratch, scab, or other scalp condition.
3. Wait forty-eight hours after a permanent or relaxing process before applying permanent color. Tone-on-tone products can be applied the same day as a permanent or relaxing procedure.
4. If you are unhappy with the results of your hair coloring, wait twenty-four hours before trying again.

SENSATIONAL STYLES

Many mature women operate under the mistaken notion that women of "a certain age" should only wear short hair. What nonsense. Any style that flatters the face and frame of the woman wearing it should not be considered off limits.

Certainly, good taste should prevail. You don't want to look like you're trying to emulate your teenaged granddaughter, but by the same token, there's nothing wrong with a little length and curl. In fact, a shoulder-length style will go a long way to hide a sagging jawline or a crinkly neck.

Consider the following guidelines provided by Manhattan's Minardi and Minardi Salon for selecting a style:

Height: Anyone under 5'5" should keep hair above the shoulders. Anyone 5'5" and taller can carry off additional length as long as the hair is in good condition.

Frame: Small, slender women can get lost in "big" hair or cascades of hair. Tall, heavy women need more hair to soften features and counterbalance the extra weight.

Rosario Acquista, director of the Kim Lepin salon in New York, recommends a style that sweeps away from the face, and she cautions women to update their look every so often so as not to become stuck in another decade.

Bangs, which should always skim the eyebrows, camouflage a wrinkly forehead and can take years off your face.

Curls are always in style. For older women, they are especially helpful because they eliminate the need for a lot of styling or holding the arms over the head. But don't think of a permanent like the old-lady perms of yesterday. A permanent can give you soft, loose curls that frame the face with a minimum of fuss, or it can add body and volume to hair that is thinning. Unless you have sculpted features and perfectly smooth skin, a stark, straight look will not be as flattering as soft curls or waves.

A perm is a great option for many women, but this is a process I wouldn't trust to a home kit. Let a professional handle this one to avoid damaging your hair. And remember: If you've permed your hair, don't bleach it, or you'll end up with cotton candy on your head and trust me, it won't be sweet. You can color permed hair, but the stripping action of bleach is guaranteed to cause disaster.

STYLING AIDS

I remember a time when styling aids were limited to setting gels, like Dippity Do and Alberto VO5 (good products that are still on the market, by the way), and nasty-smelling aerosol hairspray. Today we have mousse, styling gel, gel spray, pump and aerosol hair spray, shiners, volumizers—you name it. Here's a quick reference to help you know which products do what.

SHINERS These products add a light oil or silicone coating to the hair to make it shiny. You can also find shining ingredients in shampoos, according to Dr. Ronald DiSalvo, director of research and product development for Paul Mitchell. Look for ingredients that end in "one" like dimethicone or cymethicone. Lanolin or lanolin derivatives increase shine, as do cetyl, ceteraryl, stearyl alcohol, chamomile, rosemary, jojoba, and safflower.

MOUSSE Feels like whipped cream and is a body enhancer and style holder best used on fine or frizzy hair because it does not weigh the hair down. Too much mousse can leave the hair feeling crispy, so remember, a dab will do.

SCULPTING GEL Tames thick hair for styling or will coerce hair into defying gravity, or its own nature, to meet your demands. Gels can leave hair stiff and wet-looking. Avoid gels if your hair is thin or frizzy because the gel can be too heavy for your hair. Sculpting gel can also come in a spray pump.

DETANGLER Coats the hair so that the "shingles" of the cuticle don't overlap and get stuck. It also keeps hair from ending up like steel wool.

DEFRIZZERS Provide a coating of silicone to keep the hair in place and prevent it from absorbing moisture from the air. If a product claims to eliminate frizz for long periods of time, steer clear. It may not wash out and will eventually dry out the hair simply by doing its job, which is to inhibit moisture absorption.

HAIRSPRAY Hairsprays now come in non-aerosol pumps (better for the environment) or aerosol cans (now using fewer fluorocarbons, and therefore not as bad for the atmosphere as they once were). I find that the pump bottles tend to be wetter and stickier than the aerosols, which tend to spray on drier. Either way, the trick is to hold the bottle eight to twelve inches from your hair so that the product sets the style without blasting a new one into place.

Elaine's Exclusives

DON'T GO UP IN FLAMES

Because of the high alcohol content of styling agents and hairsprays in particular, these products carry warning labels advising consumers that they are flammable. Be sure to heed the warnings about using the products around open flames. Many people have been burned when they sprayed their hair near a stove or while smoking a cigarette.

Because your hair is one of the first things people notice about you, and because it dictates to some extent how you feel about yourself, don't take your hair for granted. Give your cut, style, and color some extra thought and attention to ensure that your outward appearance matches the way you feel inside. And certainly, don't let your prim and proper inner voice talk you into an "appropriate style for your age" unless it is truly flattering and what you really want.

STYLING AIDS THAT VOLUMIZE
AND MAKE HAIR SHINE

Research and development employees say that alcohol is used as a carrier in styling aids and to help the product dry fast. They say that alcohol does not damage the hair because the products themselves contain conditioners to soften the hair. But, just to play it safe, the products recommended here are all alcohol-free.

Price Key: $ under $5; $$ $5–$10

PRODUCT	SIZE (OZ)	PRICE
Aussie Natural Gel	7	$
Bain de Terre Mint Balm Spray Stylizer	7	$$
Clairol Herbal Essence Styling Mousse	8	$

PRODUCT	SIZE (OZ)	PRICE
L'Oréal Invisi-Gel Mega Body	6.8	$
L'Oréal Invisi-Mousse	6	$
Nexxus Styling Gel Regular Hold	8.4	$$
Nexxus Mousse Plus Alcohol Free	3.3	$
Paul Mitchell Extra-Body Sculpting Foam	6	$$
Paul Mitchell Extra-Body Sculpting Gel	6	$$
Sebastian Hi-Contrast Gel	5.1	$$
Sebastian Shaper Slipline Clean Hair Gel	10.2	$$
Tres Gelee Styling Gel Fixative	9	$
Vidal Sassoon Alcohol-Free Styling Mousse	8	$
Vidal Sassoon Styling Gel Extra Hold	8	$

Elaine's Exclusives

BAKED-ON GREASE

Do not apply a curling iron or hot rollers to hair that has already been moussed or gelled. You'll literally cook the product into your hair and could cause it to become dried out or damaged.

Chapter 12

LIVING WELL IS THE BEST REVENGE

"To be 70 years young is sometimes far more cheerful and hopeful than to be 40 years old."
—OLIVER WENDELL HOLMES, SR.

SO THIS IS GROWING OLDER GRACEFULLY?

Dry skin, varicose veins, menopause, facial hair—isn't growing older grand? Yes, it's true that accumulated years cause us to spend more time than ever before tending to our own maintenance. My overnight bag once contained a toothbrush, shampoo, deodorant, cologne, and mascara. Now I've got an arsenal of skin care, makeup, beauty lifts, vitamins, hormones, and reading glasses. But that's okay. I'm in good company.

There's never been a better time to be a fifty-something-year-old woman and there are millions of others following right behind me. Everyday I see women my age making a mark on the world in their own way. Most of them aren't famous people either. They're hardworking, ordinary women who are getting the most from the second half of their lives.

A few years ago, my mother's best friend ran a marathon in Pittsburgh at age sixty-seven.

My friend Marilyn Miller lost her husband two years ago, but rather than curling up and fading away, she took up square dancing. Now she travels the country with a much younger partner, competing in square-dance competitions. I'm not surprised that she recovered so well from her loss. She was the first woman to win the Mrs. Kansas pageant and has always said, "If you're constantly active, you'll never have time to grow old. I will be a little old lady in size only."

In my mother's day, there wasn't much left for women to do once the children were reared and launched. Today, I see older women who retire from their jobs and can't imagine how they ever had time to work because they're so busy doing things they enjoy.

There's never been a better time to be growing older, but the truth is that even though we can identify plenty of positive aspects—more free time, more disposable income, grandchildren—most of us are not too pleased with what happens to our bodies.

Nobody, except hairdressers, likes going gray, and nobody, except gynecologists, truly likes menopause. We no sooner have extra time, energy, and confidence than nature starts reminding us that the clock is ticking.

Let's all stomp our feet over the unfairness of it all.

Now that you've read up on all of the latest potions and procedures to help you look and feel your very best, take a few minutes to pick up some advice on living a full and happy life from some of the most vivacious and wonderful women I know. They didn't start out savoring the sweet days of middle age, but once they stopped looking back at the half of their lives that had passed, they started working on making the second half even better.

Several years ago, when a friend's mother died, I met three elderly women who were making a mourning call on the family. They were all friends from the deceased's bridge club who volunteered together at the local hospital. Each of the women were perfectly dressed and neatly, but not elaborately, coifed and made up. They looked terrific and their vitality showed in the way they spoke and carried themselves. Despite their ninety-plus years, they all wore heels and stepped lively (no feet shuffling for them), and each demonstrated such grace and dignity that I thought to myself, "This is how I want to be when I grow up."

KEEPING BUSY

I didn't start my career until I was forty-one, when I was fired from the cosmetics counter for recommending what I felt were the best products for a particular customer. The problem was that the products weren't made by the company I worked for but they were the best products for this particular woman. So shoot me, I'm honest. After I dusted off my confidence, I took my cosmetics knowledge to the local adult schools and taught self-improvement classes. Then I began lecturing and writing for a local newspaper. That led to my first book, then a second book, and here I am today.

The point is that my children were grown, I had time on my hands, and I found a good outlet for my talents. Sure, when I was fired I felt like it was the end of the world. Nobody likes to be rejected. But it turned out to be the best thing that ever happened to me. I got up and got back to doing what I love—helping other women to look their best. I realize that I'm not going to win a Nobel Prize for what I do, but it's what I'm good at and it's something I can share with other people, so it's just fine with me.

I try to encourage other women to pursue their dreams, but you'd be amazed how many people think they have nothing to offer.

"I just cooked and cleaned and raised kids all my life," said one woman I met recently. "What can I contribute?" She was amazed by how many suggestions I came up with off the top of my head. How about taking dinner to someone who can't get out or cook for themselves? Or inviting someone who's lonely to your house for dinner? Could you go grocery shopping or run errands for a new mother who's home alone with her new baby? Could you do a load of wash for someone? Maybe you could teach a household budgeting class for newlyweds. If you ran a home and raised kids, I'll bet you're pretty organized. You could volunteer to run a benefit for your favorite charity. Maybe you could start a cleaning service and earn some money for what you've done for free all of these years.

You could also do things for yourself that you never had time to do. Take up bird-watching so that you'll be able to identify more than just a robin at first glance. Read the complete works of Charles Dickens, or Jackie Collins, if that's more your style. Learn to do needlepoint. Knit. Take piano lessons. Learn to golf. Check out the fifty out-of-the way places that are less than three hours from your home.

She stopped me after suggestion number 23, but I think she got the message. Everyone has something to contribute and it's important to seek out work or activities that will be satisfying to you.

But not everyone's an empty-nester looking to fill time.

Grace worked full time while raising two children and was a bank vice president when she finally retired. She wasn't looking for fulfillment in her golden years, she was looking for fun.

"Retire while you're young enough to enjoy it," she says. At seventy-eight, Grace has had close to twenty years of retired life with her husband, Bob, who is an active and enthusiastic eighty-five. "My granddaughter used to tease us that we had a better social life than she did—and she was right. When we first retired, we traveled, went dancing, belonged to clubs, and spent time learning about things we never had time for when we were working and raising our daughters. Now that time has slowed us down, we don't feel like we've missed anything, but if we had worked longer, we would have missed out on some of the best years of our lives."

Shelly, fifty-four, sees things a little differently. She earned her Ph.D. after her kids were grown and intends to make good use of her hard-earned skills and education. "As long as I can continue to help people and make a difference, I never want to retire," she says. As she recalls, Shelly was tongue-oiling her furniture when she realized she had to go to work and do something meaningful with her life. Now she is the happiest person in the world. "What I do is what I love."

What you do doesn't really matter. What's important is that you do something, preferably something that is satisfying—either monetarily, intellectually, spiritually, or even just socially.

STAYING POSITIVE

Keeping busy is probably the most important factor in living well as you grow older, but I think that staying positive runs a very close second. Unfortunately, it's not something that comes easily to a lot of people. For too many, it's much easier to focus on what's wrong with themselves and others than it is to point out what's right.

Just recently, I met a woman at the beauty parlor who was in her eighties or nineties. She was there for her weekly shampoo and blow-dry. Her nails were done, her clothes casual and neat. I struck up a conversation with her, admiring how great she looked. She couldn't have been any sweeter and her advice couldn't have been more relevant.

"Always say kind things," she told me. "Kindness is spread so sparingly these days that you would think it cost a fortune, but a few kind words don't cost anything and to the recipient they are priceless."

She's right. It's easy to be critical and to find fault. Anyone can do that. It's the rare and wonderful person who always has a good word for someone else, who is well remembered and welcome anywhere. What's more, if you practice being positive with others, it will bounce back on you and you'll start focusing on the good things in your own life, rather than what could be improved. And then, when you have constructive criticism to offer, you can be sure someone will be listening.

"It's your attitude, not your aptitude, that determines your altitude," says Carol, quoting Dr. Ernst G. Schmidt.

You can only go so far and accomplish so much with a poor attitude. If you expect things to turn out poorly, they probably will, but if you anticipate good things, that's what you'll get. Norman Vincent Peale was the first to talk about the power of positive thinking. As we grow older I think that a positive attitude can truly be our greatest source of power.

Gladys, eighty-one, adds that, "If you always do what you always did, you will always get what you always got." Never stop learning and never stop changing if you want life to be rich and meaningful. It is very easy to get into a rut, but you'll be much more interesting if you work at staying out of them. Gladys stays away from ruts by counseling abused women, taking classes, and belonging to a support group. "If you don't like the way things are, change them, or change the way you view them."

Positive thinking and constant activity will hold you in good stead, especially as you move beyond your sixties and seventies and you start to slow down.

In her book, *Gifts of Age—Portraits and Essays of 32 Remarkable Women,* Charlotte Painter quoted eighty-four-year-old Julia Child as saying: "If you pretend that old age is not going to happen, it will fall right on you. I think it is very selfish of people not to have planned ahead for the day they slip off the raft."

Despite the fact that Julia cooks with pounds of butter, she's still going strong teaching cooking and making television shows. Her point about recognizing and accepting age is important to maintaining a positive outlook. If the fact of your aging catches you by surprise, it can be a real emotional setback.

SPUNK/RISK TAKING

Everyone loves a spunky old lady. Feisty women are always on the move and always have plenty of company because they have such good stories to tell.

"I can die at home, or I can die at the mall. If something happens to me, they'll call you," said eighty-year-old Annie Fletcher as she heads out the door of her daughter's home to catch the bus to the mall.

Don't let anyone convince you that you are too old to take part in activities that you feel capable of enjoying. Annie would have loved my friend Muz, whose real name is Grace. "It's better to wear out than rust out" she says. Muz, who travels every year to far-off places like Norway or the Panama Canal with several eighty-something widows says that, "Every time we go somewhere we wonder how much longer can we climb these stupid mountains? I'll keep climbing them until I just can't do it anymore."

Queen Elizabeth has been quoted as saying that "One can't dance really wearing a tiara." And she's right. If you're busy being a princess, you can't really let loose and have a rollicking good time.

Many of us have spent our entire lives being "good girls" who do everything that's expected of us. But playing by the rules and living up to everyone else's expectations can be awfully dull, not to mention restricting. I think that by the time you've reached a certain age, you shouldn't have to worry about what other people will think of your behavior—unless it's dangerous, criminal, or hurtful to someone else. So if you want to go out and dance naked in the moonlight— why shouldn't you? I'm sure this isn't exactly what Queen Elizabeth had in mind when she uttered those words, but I'll bet after a lifetime of living up to very exacting standards she could use a little tiara-less dancing herself.

"The one advantage to being old is that you can speak your mind and be a little outrageous as long as it doesn't hurt anyone," adds Sylvia, sixty, who certainly isn't old yet, but is enjoying the freedom of gently speaking her mind just the same.

This reminds me of the poem that many of you have probably read called "Warning" by Jenny Joseph that was published in the book *When I Am an Old Woman, I Shall Wear Purple.* In it, the author talks about doing all kinds of "outrageous" things that we wouldn't normally do for fear of people talking about us, like wearing colors that don't suit us or learning to spit, or picking flowers from other people's gardens or wearing slippers in the rain. The message is that it's okay—heck, it's necessary—to let loose a little and not worry about what the neighbors will think.

Think about the older women you enjoy. Chances are good that they are kind, interesting, spunky women who have great stories to share and weren't afraid to take risks and do what suited them. Even if you haven't been especially adventurous until now, you still have plenty of time to tally up a few wild tales that you can recount with relish when you are an old woman wearing purple.

HANG LOOSE

In Hawaii, the locals have a kind of state motto that comes with it's own hand symbol. You make the *shaka* sign by making a fist and then extending your thumb and pinky—it means hang loose— don't worry—relax—have fun. It's this worry-free attitude that is part of what makes Hawaii paradise; it's easy to forget your troubles there.

But, you don't have to go to Hawaii to practice the hang-loose way of life. (I would strongly recommend it, though, if you haven't been there yet.) In fact, there's really no other way to live. Have you ever solved a problem by worrying about it? Is there very much, besides your own behavior, that you can really control anyway? Is any-one handing out trophies for the best brow knitter? No, no, and no.

Okay then—just hang loose.

"You should never worry about yesterday, because it is spent. Never worry about tomorrow, because it's a promissory note. There are 86,400 seconds in a day. Don't waste one of them. Spend them wisely and don't throw one of them away," advises Carol, who is fifty-six. Worrying never solved a single problem and I'm fairly certain that worrying causes wrinkles.

"Take a nap," says ninety-three-year-old Winnefred, who shovels snow, mows the lawn, and tends her garden in northern Michigan. Winnefred takes things in stride and believes that we should not take ourselves quite as seriously as we often do. Whenever she has a prob-lem to solve, Winnefred takes a nap, after which things always look better. "Either the problem goes away while you are sleeping, or you will have more energy to deal with it when you wake up."

"Women should not dwell on fine lines, because nature is kind to lovers, for when wrinkles and sagging begin to increase, our eyesight begins to diminish," says my friend Frieda, sixty-one. Despite all of the creams and surgical procedures, there's only so much most of us are willing to do to get rid of wrinkles and since you can't stop them alto-gether, there's no sense in worrying about them.

Worrying is a total waste of time.

TREAT YOURSELF

Most of us have worked hard all of our lives, raised children, kept a home, volunteered, you name it. We've taken care of others and now it's okay to take care of ourselves. When your teenagers had athlete's foot, you bought them some foot spray, right? Now it's your turn to be pampered a little.

I know that many of us were taught to take care of everyone else in our lives first and those habits die hard. To some women, the idea of having a pedicure seems selfish, fussy, or a waste of money and varicose veins are something you just live with. I disagree. Paying attention to the dry skin, brittle nails, and frightful feet will make you feel infinitely better and getting medical advice for aching swollen legs or your first signs of menopause will pay off in good health and long-term peace of mind.

"It's not about *need,*" Anne, fifty-two, used to tell her husband when he questioned purchases that seemed unnecessary to him. "When you get right down to it, we don't *need* most of the things we have; we can survive with much less. But if you can afford something you want and it makes you feel good, why not get it? A used Chevy will get me to the grocery store, but it's more fun to go there in a convertible."

"Women are under a lot of pressure to look great, but a man only has to be a little bit better looking than a monkey," said Gladys's grandmother Toba, who liked to treat herself to pretty things. "My looks may fade with age, but I can still have my hair done and dress stylishly."

You go, girls.

If you've spent most of your life neglecting yourself or only doing what's absolutely necessary to maintain your health and looks, now is the time to pay yourself back with a little extra Tender Loving Care. And, if it will make you feel less guilty, think of it this way: If you're looking and feeling better, you'll be more inclined to do for everyone else.

FAMILY

Years ago I heard a woman say that the best thing about motherhood was grandchildren. I've been five-times blessed and I understand her feelings perfectly. It's not that my own children were not a joy, but you really do enjoy grandchildren more.

These days, families are spread out all over the country and not everyone is able to spend much time with their families. I'm always encouraged to hear that Mother's Day is AT&T's busiest day and that Thanksgiving weekend is the most heavily traveled weekend of the year.

Dolores's husband and seven children decorated her hospital room and made a party to celebrate their thirtieth wedding anniversary, even though Dolores had just learned that her cancer had spread. "I know this is bad news, but I can't do anything about the cancer—that's up to God and the doctors. What I can do is enjoy my husband and my kids no matter where I am and no matter what the circumstances. Don't let anything keep you from enjoying your family," she said.

If you're not fortunate enough to have your family nearby, try to get to know another family in your neighborhood. Work, church, synagogue, and volunteer groups are other good places to find people who are separated from their own families. Remember that if you're on the East Coast and your daughter and her family are living in Colorado, there's probably a woman like you in Colorado, with a daughter and grandchildren living in the East. Go find them. Your family doesn't have to be limited to the people who are related to you.

FOCUS ON THE FUTURE

All of the women in this chapter have different thoughts to offer, but the common thread through each of their ideas is that they are all looking toward to the future. Whether it's learning something new, spreading kindness, buying a treat, spending time with family, or going somewhere, each woman's words focused on the future.

None of us knows what's around the corner. What I know is that people are much more interested in hearing someone talk about what they are doing next, rather than what they've already done, and that there are many things I want to do yet. Maybe I'll start a cosmetics company and become the "Dr. Ruth" of skin care, or maybe I'll teach cooking. What I won't do is spend the rest of my days living in the past.

I want to learn to play bridge, which is something Gladys recommended. She points out that bridge is a universal game. If you know bridge, you can play cards with someone, even if you speak different languages. No matter how old you become, if your mind still works, you can play bridge.

I also want to learn to Rollerblade, which I should probably work on soon.

I want to play with my grandchildren and hopefully see great grandchildren. I want to travel with my husband and grow old with him and my friends. The list is long and varied.

What's on my list isn't what's important. The important thing is to have one. Putting anything on a list gets your sights set on the future, rather than on the past. It doesn't even matter if you get to everything on your list. What matters is working on it.

"Keep yourself interested and interesting," says Cheryl, fifty. "Your chronological age may be determined by time, but your real age is determined by your attitude. You can be old at twenty-five or young at seventy, it all depends on whether you are open-minded and continue to grow."

"Compared to the alternative, growing old isn't bad," says fifty-something Annalee.

Dear Abby quoted an essay by Samuel Ullman that I think eloquently describes aging in the nineties:

> Youth is not entirely a time of life — it is a state of mind. It is not wholly a matter of ripe cheeks, red lips, or supple knees. It is a temper of will, a quality of the imagination, a vigor of the emotions. Nobody grows old by merely living a number of years. People grow old only by deserting their ideals. You are as young as your self-confidence, as old as your fears; as young as your hope, as old as your despair.

As we get older, we come to recognize the truism that outer beauty is, indeed, fleeting and that inner beauty is what really counts. (That may be a convenient shift in attitude that coincides with wrinkles and gray hair, but I don't think so.)

If you are a productive and positive person whose life is filled with activity, what difference do gray hair and wrinkles make? Friends, family, and strangers will be attracted to you for your inner beauty — your wisdom, sense of humor, ideas, and perspective. If you keep your mind and body active and consider every day a new adventure, you are sure to remain forever. . . Ageless.

Seven Tips for Enjoying the Second Half of Your Life

- It's all in your head. It doesn't matter how great you look if you are focused on the past instead of the future. If you need one, get a new attitude — and the sooner the better.

- Laugh it off. As serious, mature adults, we sometimes forget to laugh and enjoy life. Remember, you really can't control what other people do, you can only control your own reaction to it. So don't worry about what you can't control. Be happy. After all, your mother was right, your face will freeze that way if you keep frowning.
- Be good to yourself. Treat yourself to a massage, facial, day of beauty, or even a weekend at a spa. Local beauty salons offer all kinds of treatments and if you're in the market for a day, weekend, or week-long trip to a spa, you can call 1-800-ALL SPAS for a directory of more than two hundred spas nationwide. From California's famous Golden Door and the Canyon Ranch in Massachusetts to lesser-known retreats in the mountains of nowhere, this directory has them all.
- Take up yoga, or any other feel-good practice. Learn to meditate, delve into crystals or aromatherapy, or learn some self-relaxation techniques that really work. Do something that will make you feel great and relieve stress. Your local high school or community college probably offers inexpensive evening classes if you call for a directory.
- Keep a journal. Once you get in the habit, you'll look forward to the time you spend with yourself, and just think of the surprises your grandchildren will discover when they read your memoirs years from now.
- Find yourself a role model for growing older, or if you've gotten good at it, be a mentor to someone who is struggling with her first wrinkle and the realization of her own mortality.
- Go back to college and earn a degree, or just take a class in something you've always wanted to know more about.

GOOD READING

Getting Over Getting Older, Letty Cottin Pogrebin
Choice Years, Judith Paige and Pamela Gordon
When I Am an Old Woman, I Shall Wear Purple, Various authors
Is It Hot in Here, or Is It Me?, Gayle Sand
Forever Fifty, Judith Vorst
Silent Passages, Gail Sheehy
Rich with Years, Malcolm Boyd

BEAUTY BARGAINS

It's easy to save money on beauty items if you know where to look. In addition to these budget boosters, also watch your drugstore circulars for advertised specials and visit your neighborhood beauty supply store. A little comparison-shopping can save you a lot of money.

The following beauty chains offer the best products at tremendous savings. Use the 800 numbers listed to find a store near you.

SALLY BEAUTY SUPPLY (1,000 STORES NATIONWIDE)
800-284-SALLY

COSMETIC CENTER (76 STORES, MOSTLY IN THE EAST)
800-638-8700

CLUBS

The following members-only clubs offer substantial savings when you purchase giant-size products. Especially good for products that you use often like cotton swabs, baby powder, shampoo and conditioner, soap, body lotions, etc.

PRICE CLUB
800-774-2678

BJ'S WHOLESALE
800-BJS-CLUB

SAM'S CLUB
800-WALMART

Sam's Club also has a home page on the World Wide Web where you can enter your zip code to find a store near you. You can find them at *HTTP://www.samsclub.com*.

COSMETIQUE BEAUTY CLUB
800-621-8822

This club features eight exclusive lines of products and a monthly mailing of products suited to your skin type and coloring. There is no purchasing minimum and the prices are very good. An introductory kit of full-size products, including a blush, mascara, and tinted moisturizer in a small purse, is only $4.95 and subsequent mailings never exceed $20 for at least $30 worth of products.

Catalogs

YVES ROCHER
800-321-YVES

French, natural beauty products offered through mail order. Discounts vary with each catalog.

At-Home Sales

NUSKIN
800-487-2121

AVON
800-367-2866

Heavenly Savings from St. Ives

St. Ives makes many terrific products from shampoos and conditioners to AHA facial and body lotions, but the best thing about these products is their prices. I think they're a great value. The bad thing is they are not sold everywhere. To solve that problem, St. Ives will mail you any product you'd like for only $1 extra if you write to them at St. Ives Laboratories, Inc., Los Angeles, CA 91311.

AGELESS PHONE DIRECTORY

AARP
800-456-2277

ACCREDITATION ASSOC. FOR
AMBULATORY HEALTH CARE
708-676-9610

ADRIEN ARPEL
800-215-8333

ALBERTO CULVER, USA, INC.
708-450-3000

ALLERGAN SKIN CARE
800-253-9499

ALMAY
800-473-8566

ALPHA HYDROX
800-552-5742

AMERICAN ACADEMY OF
COSMETIC SURGEONS
800-A NEW YOU

AMERICAN ACADEMY OF
FACIAL PLASTIC AND
RECONSTRUCTIVE SURGERY
800-332-FACE

AMERICAN ASSOCIATION
FOR ACCREDITATION OF
AMBULATORY PLASTIC SURGERY
FACILITIES
708-949-6058

AMERICAN BOARD OF MEDICAL
SPECIALITIES
800-776-2378

AMERICAN PODIATRIC MEDICAL
ASSOCIATION
800-366-8227

AMERICAN RUNNING AND
FITNESS ASSOCIATION
800-776-2732

AMERICAN SOCIETY FOR
AESTHETIC PLASTIC SURGERY
888-ASAPS-11

AMERICAN SOCIETY OF
DERMATOLOGIC SURGERY
800-441-2737

AMERICAN SOCIETY OF
PLASTIC AND RECONSTRUC-
TIVE SURGEONS
800-635-0635

ASTARTE
212-206-8095

AQUA GLYCOLIC
800-253-9499

AQUANIL
800-423-2341

AUSSIE HAIR PRODUCTS
800-947-2656

AVEDA
800-AVEDA-24

AVON
800-445-2866

BAIN DE SOLEIL
800-743-5423

BAIN DE TERRE
800-242-9283

BANANA BOAT
800-869-2224

BASIS
800-926-4832

BIOMEDIC
800-736-5155

BJ'S WHOLESALE
800-BJS CLUB

BOBBI BROWN
212-980-7040

THE BODY SHOP
800-541-2535

CARESS (LEVER BROS.)
800-451-6679

CELLEX-C
800-423-5539

CETAPHIL LOTION
800-582-8225

CHANEL
212-688-5055

CHRISTIAN DIOR
212-418-0459

CLAIROL
800-223-5800

CLARINS
212-980-1800

CLINIQUE
212-572-4200

⏂PERTONE
⏂4090

⏂NTER

⏂AUTY CLUB

⏂-2219

⏂RMABLEND
800-631-2158

DONNA KARAN
212-789-1500

DOVE (LEVER BROTHERS)
800-451-6679

ELIZABETH ARDEN
212-261-1179

ESTEE LAUDER
212-572-4200

ETHOCYN
800-227-2085

EUCERIN
800-227-4703

EUROPEAN TOUCH EXUVIANCE
800-225-9911

FACIAL FLEX
800-469-FLEX

FLORI ROBERTS
800-631-2158

FREEMAN
310-286-0101

GLYDERM
800-321-4576

GUERLAIN
212-751-1870

HAWAIIAN TROPIC
904-677-9559

HEALTH MEDIA OF AMERICA
619-688-0377

HELENE CURTIS
312-661-0222

HELEN LEE
212-888-1233

HYMED/HYLUNIA
800-547-1232

IL MAKIAGE
212-371-0551

IMAN
800-631-2158

JAN MARINI PRODUCTS
800-347-2223

JERGENS
800-222-3553

JOHNSON PRODUCTS
800-631-2158

JOHNSON & JOHNSON
800-526-3967

JOINT COMMISSION ON
ACCREDITATION OF HEALTH-
CARE ORGANIZATIONS
708-916-5600

KERI LOTION
800-468-7746

KIEHLS
800-KIEHLS-1

LAC-HYDRIN
800-333-0950

LANCÔME
800-LANCÔME

LAURA GELLER
212-570-5477

LA PRAIRIE
800-821-5718

L'ORÉAL
800-322-2036

L'ORÉAL HAIR
800-631-7358

LUBRIDERM
800-223-0182

LUMINIQUE
212-535-9200

M.A.C.
800-387-6707

MARKRON NAIL PRODUCTS
503-635-7723

MARY KAY
800-627-9529

MATRIX
888-777-6396

MAX FACTOR
800-526-8787

MAYBELLINE
800-944-0730

MD FORMULATIONS
800-253-9499

MD FORTE
800-253-9499

MOISTUREL
800-333-0950

MONTEIL OF PARIS
212-850-2460

MURAD
800-242-1103

NAIL MAGIC
503-225-9303

NAILTEK
800-676-2457

NATIONAL CANCER INSTITUTE
800-4-CANCER

NATIONAL HEART, LUNG, AND
BLOOD INSTITUTE
301-251-1222

NEOSTRATA
800-628-9904

NEUTROGENA
800-217-1136

NEXXUS
805-968-6900

NIVEA
800-227-4703

NOVA SKIN
800-379-6682

NUSKIN
800-487-2121

OIL OF OLAY
800-285-5170

ORIGINS
212-572-4200

ORLANE
800-775-2541

OSMOTICS
303-293-2087

PANTENE
800-285-5170

PAUL MITCHELL
800-321-JPMS

PHYSICIAN'S FORMULA
800-227-0333

POND'S
800-243-5804

PRESCRIPTIVES
212-572-4200

PRINCESS MARCELLA
BORGHESE
212-572-3303

PROCTOR & GAMBLE
800-526-8787, 800-285-5170

PURPOSE
800-526-3967

REDKEN
800-545-8157

RENOVA
800-992-9689

REVLON
800-473-8566

SALLY BEAUTY SUPPLY
800-284-SALLY

SAM'S CLUB
800-WALMART

SCHWARTZKOPF
800-234-4672

SEBASTIAN
818-999-5112

SENSCIENCE HAIR CARE
800-242-9283

SHISEIDO
212-805-2300

SKIN CANCER FOUNDATION
212-725-5176

SMOKENDERS
800-828-4357

SORME
818-908-5335

ST. IVES
818-709-5500

SUDDEN CHANGE
201-330-1400

SUN PRECAUTION
800-882-7860

SUNSOR, INC.
800-492-9815

TOPIX PHARMACEUTICALS
800-445-2595

ULTIMA II
800-473-8566

UNIV. OF CALIFORNIA,
BERKELEY, WELLNESS LETTER
800-829-9170

VASELINE INTENSIVE CARE
800-243-5804

VAVOOM
800-282-2822

VIDAL SASSOON
800-285-5170

WARNER LAMBERT
800-223-0182

WESTWOOD SQUIBB
800-333-0950

YEARS AWAY BEAUTY LIFTS
800-207-4411

YVES ROCHER
800-321-YVES

YVES ST. LAURENT
908-417-0202 ext. 3900

RESOURCES

Karen Andes. *A Woman's Book of Strength.* Berkley Publishing Group, 1995.

Denise Austin. *Jump Start.* Simon & Schuster, 1996.

Howard C. Baron, M.D., F.A.C.S., and Barbara A. Ross. *Varicose Veins.* Facts On File, Inc., 1995.

The Boston Women's Health Book Collective. *The New Our Bodies, Ourselves.* Simon & Schuster, 1992.

Charles B. Clayman, M.D., Ed. *The AMA Home Medical Encyclopedia.* Random House, 1989.

Patricia Fisher, Ed. *Age Erasers for Women.* Rodale Press, 1994.

Thomas Goodman, M.D., and Stephanie Young. *Smart Face.* Prentice Hall Press, 1988.

Ronald P. Grelsamer, M.D., and Suzanne Loebl, Eds. *The Columbia Presbyterian Osteoarthritis Handbook.* Macmillan, 1996.

Robin Marantz Henig. *How a Woman Ages.* Esquire Press, 1985.

Diana Lewis Jewell and Rex Hilverdink. *Forever Beautiful with Rex.* Clarkson N. Potter, Inc., 1994.

Philip Kingsley. *Hair, An Owner's Handbook.* Aurum Press Ltd., 1995.

Earl Mindell, R.Ph., Ph.D. *Earl Mindell's Anti Aging Bible.* Simon & Schuster, 1996.

Judith Paige and Pamela Gordon. *Choice Years.* Villard Books, 1991.

PDR Family Guide to Nutrition and Health. Medical Economics Company (Montvale, NJ 07645), 1995.

Prevention Magazine, Eds. *The Complete Book of Cancer Prevention.* Rodale Press, 1988.

Letty Cottin Pogrebin. *Getting Over Getting Older, An Intimate Journey.* Little, Brown & Co., 1996.

D.S. Thompson, Consulting Ed. M.D. *Every Woman's Health: A Complete Guide to Body and Mind by Top Women Doctors.* Simon & Schuster, 1993.

Joyce Vedral. *Bottom's Up!* Warner Books, 1994.

Kathleen Walas. *Real Beauty — Real Women.* MasterMedia, Ltd., 1992.

Jon Winokur. *True Confessions.* Plume Books, 1992.

INDEX

One of the things I like best about being an author is the opportunity to hear from women all over the country. In the past, women have written to me asking about specific beauty problems and sharing tips and helpful hints of their own. I invite you again to write to me with your questions or ideas and I promise to answer your letters. Also, if there is enough interest for ongoing information, I may develop a newsletter sometime in the future. If you would be interested in such a periodical, please drop me a postcard with your name, address, and telephone number and I will contact you if and when that project is developed.

Elaine Brumberg
P.O. Box 301
Jenkintown, PA 19046